Principles of
Neuropsychological
Rehabilitation

PRINCIPLES OF NEUROPSYCHOLOGICAL REHABILITATION

George P. Prigatano, Ph.D.

Barrow Neurological Institute
St. Joseph's Hospital and Medical Center
Phoenix, Arizona

New York   Oxford
OXFORD UNIVERSITY PRESS
1999

Oxford University Press

Oxford   New York
Athens   Auckland   Bangkok   Bogotá   Buenos Aires   Calcutta
Cape Town   Chennai   Dar es Salaam   Delhi   Florence   Hong Kong   Istanbul
Karachi   Kuala Lumpur   Madrid   Melbourne   Mexico City   Mumbai
Nairobi   Paris   São Paulo   Singapore   Taipei   Tokyo   Toronto   Warsaw

and associated companies in
Berlin   Ibadan

Copyright © 1999 by Oxford University Press, Inc.

Published by Oxford University Press, Inc.
198 Madison Avenue, New York, New York 10016
http://www.oup-usa.org

Library of Congress Cataloging-in-Publication Data
Prigatano, George P.
Principles of neuropsychological rehabilitation /
George P. Prigatano.
p.   cm.
Includes bibliographical references and index.
ISBN 0-19-508143-9
1. Brain damage—Patients—Rehabilitation.
2. Clinical neuropsychology.
I. Title.
[DNLM: 1. Brain Injuries—rehabilitation.   WL 354 P951p 1999]
RC387.5.P754   1999   616.8'043—dc21   DNLM/DLC   for Library of Congress   98-50681

1 2 3 4 5 6 7 8 9

Printed in the United States of America
on acid-free paper

This book is dedicated to R. Barton Carl, M.D., neurosurgeon, friend, and mentor, and to Robert F. Spetzler, M.D., neurosurgeon and Director of the Barrow Neurological Institute, who has continued to support clinical neuropsychology during the most difficult of times.

Preface

The principles described in this book are my own interpretations derived from a variety of experiences in examining and later in attempting to rehabilitate young and middle-aged adults who sustained sudden and unexpected brain damage. Initially, most of the patients were victims of severe traumatic brain injuries. In the ensuing years, I have also had the opportunity to work with patients who have suffered from ruptured aneurysms, arteriovenous malformations, cerebral anoxia, brain tumors, and radiation treatment after the surgical removal of malignant tumors. Although patients inevitably bring different patterns of cognitive, linguistic, sensory, motor, and personality characteristics to their rehabilitation, the process of helping these patients to recover and adapt to permanent neurological and neuropsychological disturbances has convinced me that certain "principles" could guide the rehabilitation process.

Without guiding principles, clinicians can easily get lost in the maze of problems that brain-injured patients (and their families) can present. Furthermore, fiscal pressures, whether self-imposed or mandated by an administrative group, can engender inadequate or inappropriate treatment. Although fiscal realities may dictate the amount of time a therapist spends with a patient, they should not dictate a rushed attitude toward the patient or ineffective treatment during the patient's sessions. Clearly, clinicians must continually strive to clarify the types of problems that they can help patients with and the types they cannot. Consequently, establishing guidelines greatly strengthens the clinician and provides both a moral and scientific basis for the practice of neuropsychological rehabilitation and assessment. It is my hope that the principles of neuropsychological rehabilitation outlined here will help in that process.

In these introductory remarks, I would also like to acknowledge several sources of support and inspiration. My initial efforts to develop a neuropsychological rehabilitation program in Oklahoma City in 1980 would have been impossible without the active support of Dr. Barton Carl, neurosurgeon. I continue to be indebted to him in many ways. This book is dedicated to him because of the professional standards that he fosters. He continues to be a true mentor of professional behavior. The early work with my colleagues in Oklahoma City, especially with David Fordyce, Ph.D., Mary Pepping, Ph.D., and Robert Wienecke, M.D., also provided many useful discussions and considerable emotional support. Without each of their contributions, our early work would not have been possible.

In 1985, the efforts of Joseph C. White III, M.D., who was then Chairman of the Department of Neurology at the Barrow Neurological Institute (BNI), St. Joseph's Hospital and Medical Center, in Phoenix, Arizona, made it possible to develop a neuropsychologically oriented rehabilitation program in a major neurological and neurosurgical setting. After Dr. White's death, the administrative and fiscal support of the Institute continued under the gracious auspices of Dr. Robert Spetzler, Director of the BNI. Sister Nancy Perlick, RSM, former Vice President of Neurosciences, was also instrumental in supporting the neuropsychological clinical and research programs.

An invitation to take a brief sabbatical in 1991 at Massey University in New Zealand, which was orchestrated by Janet Leathem, Ph.D., provided the opportunity to start collecting my thoughts for this book. Also during that time, grant support from the National Institute of Disability for Handicapped Research and the World Rehabilitation Fund in the form of an International Exchange of Experts in Rehabilitation Fellowship allowed me to conduct a small cross-cultural study on altered awareness in patients with traumatic brain injuries. That experience further stimulated my ideas concerning the role of social and cultural factors in the rehabilitation of brain dysfunctional individuals. During my sabbatical, I also received an invitation from the Rehabilitation Institute of Chicago to present the James C. Hemphill Lectureship. This opportunity stimulated my strong desire to communicate about the role of "science and symbolism" in the process that we call neuropsychological rehabilitation. The requests to give several other lectures also helped me to commit to paper the ideas, impressions, and convictions that have evolved from the past 25 years of clinical work. Finally, an invitation to provide a series of lectures on neuropsychological rehabilitation at the University of Granada in Spain during February 1997 helped consolidate what I thought was the final effort in organizing and preparing this text.

An anonymous reviewer of this text obtained by Oxford University Press proved exceptionally helpful. All the reviewers' comments helped me recognize where the text lacked clarity and how different points of view needed to be incorporated in certain sections. Finally, an invitation to speak at a Consensus Development Conference on the Rehabilitation of Persons with Traumatic Brain Injury sponsored by the National Institute of Child Health and Human Development (NICHD) and the Office of Medical Application of Research (OMAR) of the NIH forced me to write an abstract on the efficacy of the impairment-oriented approach to cognitive rehabilitation. Sometimes the experience of saying things concisely further clarifies what is known and what needs to be studied in the future. Writing that abstract resulted in a major revision of Chapter 11, on outcome.

Finally, I would like to acknowledge many of my colleagues at the BNI who have directly and indirectly assisted me. I would like to acknowledge particularly those colleagues involved in the Adult Hospital for Neurological Rehabilitation for their dedicated clinical efforts and challenging questions concerning the management of patients with formidable cognitive and personality disturbances. The patient and skilled secretarial support of Barbara Todd, Judy Wilson, Eve DeShazer, Carol Carper, and Blanca Palencia and the editorial assistance of Shelley A. Kick, Ph.D., are greatly appreciated. Without the continued administrative support of Dr. Spetzler, our section of clinical neuropsychology would not have survived the ravages of managed care, and this book would never have been possible. I am greatly indebted to him.

Writing this text has been at times a slow and difficult process. The effort, however, has helped clarify my own thinking, and my hope is that it will serve the same role for other clinicians and researchers in the field.

August 1998   G. P. P.
Phoenix, Arizona

Contents

III   Theoretical and Empirical Issues

I

HISTORICAL AND CLINICAL
PERSPECTIVES

1

Introduction to the Principles in the Context of a Brief Historical Perspective

> There cannot be a philosophy, there cannot even be a decent science, without humanity.
>
> J. Bronowski, *The Ascent of Man*, 1973, p. 15

Throughout the United States and Europe, economic support for various health-related services is diminishing. As part of this economic tidal wave, rehabilitation services for persons with an acquired brain injury have likewise been reduced. The failure to clarify which types of rehabilitation services are efficacious for specific patient groups has further compounded this problem. Too often, no scientific database is available to counter decisions based more on economic concerns than on the needs of patients (Prigatano, 1996).

The field of neuropsychological rehabilitation needs such guidelines and underlying principles to orchestrate the work of clinicians. This book presents 13 principles of neuropsychological rehabilitation. They have evolved from clinical and scientific observations of persons who have attempted to regain a productive lifestyle and to reestablish meaning in their lives after sustaining significant disturbances of their higher cerebral functioning. The 13 principles are as follows:

Principle 1: The clinician must begin with patient's subjective or phenomenological experience to reduce their frustrations and confusion in order to engage them in the rehabilitation process.

Principle 2: The patient's symptom picture is a mixture of premorbid cognitive and personality characteristics as well as neuropsychological changes directly associated with brain pathology.

Principle 3: Neuropsychological rehabilitation focuses on both the remediation of higher cerebral disturbances and their management in interpersonal situations.

Principle 4: Neuropsychological rehabilitation helps patients observe their behavior and thereby teaches them about the direct and indirect effects of brain injury.

This may help patients avoid destructive choices and better manage their catastrophic reactions.

Principles 5: Failure to study the intimate interaction of cognition and personality leads to an inadequate understanding of many issues in cognitive (neuro)sciences and neuropsychological rehabilitation.

Principle 6: Little is known about how to retrain a brain dysfunctional patient cognitively, because the nature of higher cerebral functions is not fully understood.

General guidelines for cognitive remediation, however, can be specified.

Principle 7: Psychotherapeutic interventions are often an important part of neuropsychological rehabilitation because they help patients (and families) deal with their personal losses.

The process, however, is highly individualized.

Principle 8: Working with brain dysfunctional patients produces affective reactions in both the patient's family and the rehabilitation staff. Appropriate management of these reactions facilitates the rehabilitative and adaptive process.

Principle 9: Each neuropsychological rehabilitation program is a dynamic entity. It is either in a state of development or decline.

Ongoing scientific investigation helps the rehabilitation team learn from their successes and failures and is needed to maintain a dynamic, creative rehabilitation effort.

Principle 10: Failure to identify which patients can and cannot be helped by different (neuropsychological) rehabilitation approaches creates a lack of credibility for the field.

Principle 11: Disturbances in self-awareness after brain injury are often poorly understood and mismanaged.

Principle 12: Competent patient management and planning innovative rehabilitation programs depend on understanding mechanisms of recovery and deterioration of direct and indirect symptoms after brain injury.

Principle 13: The rehabilitation of patients with higher cerebral deficits requires both scientific and phenomenological approaches. Both are necessary to maximize recovery and adaptation to the effects of brain injury.

Chapters 2 through 14 will consider these principles and their implications in more detail. Before proceeding, however, a discussion of what the word "principle" means and how the term is used in this text is needed.

The Word *Principle*

The word *principle* has many definitions (Webster's, 1983, p. 1431), including the concept of "beginning." It also can refer to the *essential ele-*

ment of something or to *rules of conduct*. This text draws heavily from some of Goldstein's (1942) and Luria's (1948/1963) early or beginning observations about the rehabilitation of patients with disturbances of higher cerebral or cortical functions. Those observations are combined with my experiences in establishing two neuropsychological rehabilitation programs for adults and a beginning program for children. As such, it reflects an effort to highlight key or essential elements of such work and to suggest broadly defined rules of conduct for engaging in this clinical effort.

The word *principal* derives from the Latin word *principalis*, which in turn derives from the word *princeps*, meaning chief. The word principal also has several definitions (Webster's, 1983, pp. 1430–31). It can refer to the most important topics of debate or points of law. In finance, it means the amount of debt to which interest must be paid. In art, it refers to the chief feature to which the "rest are subordinate."

It would be presumptuous to imply that these principles of neuropsychological rehabilitation are the principal principles. They do, however, reflect the chief features of my own approach to the rehabilitation of persons with acquired brain injury. That approach has been influenced by several people.

Historical and Contemporary Influences on these Principles of Neuropsychological Rehabilitation

In his book *The Ascent of Man*, Jacob Bronowski (1973) discussed Paracelsus as a medieval example of a man who "steps out of the shadowland of secret and anonymous knowledge into a new system of open and personal discovery" (p. 140). He used Paracelsus to symbolize that progress in science assumes many forms, but in each form the observer or the scientist must have a passion for what he or she observes. Thus, Bronowski (1973) states: ". . . scientific discovery flows from a *personality* [italics added], and that discovery comes alive as we watch it being made by a person" (p. 141). Directly or indirectly, several "key" individuals have influenced current efforts at neuropsychological rehabilitation.

John Hughlings Jackson

J. Hughlings Jackson's (Fig. 1-1) influence in neurology, particularly in the study of epilepsy, is well known. He is credited with the observation that "localization of a deficit" after brain injury is not the same as localization of higher cerebral functions in an intact brain. His interest in diagnosis and the treatment of brain diseases also emphasized two important facts. First, studying the process of recovery after a brain insult is as important as analyzing the initial symptom profile. Second, an evolutionary conceptualization of the organization of the human brain of-

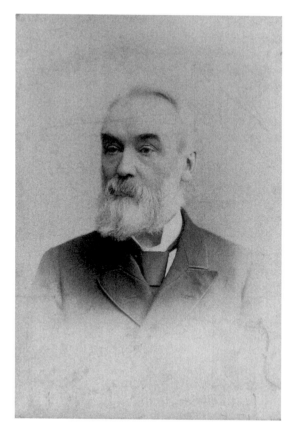

Figure 1-1. John Hughlings Jackson. *Courtesy of Wellcome Trustees.*

fers interesting insights for the field of neurorehabilitation. Consider Jackson's (1888) thoughts about recovery.

> The process of recovery is obviously of vast importance for our consideration in regard to rational treatment of some cases of very serious brain disease; for if recovery be spontaneous, we may err in attributing it to the effects of our remedies, and thus our opinions on therapeutics become untrustworthy (p. 114).

He continues:

> Why do patients recover from hemiplegia when the loss of nerve tissue is permanent? The reply is hypothetical. There are according to degrees of gravity of the destructive lesion, degrees of recovery. I should put down paralysis at the onset to the destruction effected, and attribute degrees of recovery to degrees of *compensation* [italics added]; nervous arrangements near to those destroyed, having closely similar duties,

come to serve, not as well, but, according to the degree of gravity of the lesion, next and next as well as those destroyed (p. 114; Jackson, 1888).

Jackson's first point about recovery is that the effectiveness of therapeutic or rehabilitation efforts cannot be assessed until the natural process of recovery after various brain disorders is understood. A major problem in the field of neuropsychological rehabilitation is the lack of scientific studies on the recovery process of language, motor and cognitive processes—not to mention the patient's emotional and motivational disturbances. The few studies that have considered the long-term consequences of traumatic brain injury (TBI) provide a rough yardstick for measuring the overall effectiveness of neuropsychologically oriented rehabilitation programs today. Specific information about recovery of various higher cerebral functions is often lacking.

A second point that Jackson makes is that recovery of (motor) function (the example he uses is hemiplegia) occurs by compensatory rather than restorative mechanisms. This is an important theoretical point that we will return to several times. Note that Jackson states that his opinion is theoretical—based not on fact, but theory. Later, we will consider the relevance of contemporary findings to this issue.

Besides Jackson's insights about the importance of recovery phenomena, his perspective on the nature of higher cerebral functions is also interesting. Apparently influenced by Darwin's theory of evolution, Jackson (1898) was among the first to apply evolutionary concepts to brain organization and function. In delivering the first Hughlings Jackson lecture to the British Neurological Society on December 8, 1897, Jackson (1898) stated the following:

It is necessary here to remark that such an expression as 'high organization' is not, when used with regard to the nervous system, synonymous with most complex . . . ; indeed, the most complex, nervous arrangements, centers and levels, are the least organized; the most simple are the most organized. Thus the centers of the lowest level are much more strongly organized than those of the highest level are. It is very important to bear this in mind. A man deeply comatose from sucking raw spirits out of a cask and whose highest level, or presumably most of it, is rendered quite functionless by much alcohol rapidly taken, recovers because the 'vital' centers of his lowest level are very strongly organized and go on working, although imperfectly, when the comparatively weakly organized centers of his highest level have 'given out.' If the 'vital' centers of the lowest level were not strongly organized at birth life would not be possible; if the centers of the highest level ('mental centers') were not little organized and therefore very modifiable we could only with difficulty and imperfectly adjust ourselves to new circumstances and should make few new acquirements (pp. 84–85).

When referring to the higher brain centers that govern "mental function," Jackson suggested that they are most complex but "less organized." That is, the arrangement of the neuronal networks that perform such complex processes as learning, attention, memory, perception, or language functions may have "broad" rather than "specific" representation in the brain. Current neuroscientific research has elucidated this issue, which is discussed later in the text. Jackson's observations, however, fueled the hope that the rehabilitation of higher cerebral functions might be possible because they are less organized compared to the lower brain functions (e.g., motor functions), which are more highly (i.e., specifically) organized. A. R. Luria, who recognized Jackson's contributions to his thinking, developed this idea further.

Working 100 years ago, Jackson was perhaps one of the first to apply Darwinian principles of evolution to explain the organization of brain function and structure. Edelman (1987), however, returned to this type of thinking in his text *Neural Darwinism: The Theory of Neuronal Group Selection.*

Shepherd Ivory Franz

Early in the twentieth century, Shepherd Ivory Franz (Fig. 1-2) was an American spokesman for the importance of studying recovery phenomena and rehabilitation interventions. In 1924, Franz criticized von Monakow's excellent work for its inadequate discussion of recovery of function and "re-education" after brain damage:

> It is generally conceded that a disease or a diseased condition can be adequately known only if it is thoroughly studied from its beginning until its end, from the time of the origin of an infection, let us say, until the patient has completely recovered or has died, and, in the latter instance, until he has been examined post mortem. If this view is acceptable, it certainly follows that the aphasias are not understood . . . because they have not been thoroughly studied throughout their courses. *The phenomena of recovery are just as important to note as the primary phenomena of defect* [italics added] (pp. 349–350).

Franz (1924) was a pioneer in developing quantitative methods for the evaluation of reeducation or retraining programs for aphasic patients. He observed that new learning often was acquired slowly and that the amount of time needed to reeducate brain dysfunctional individuals varied considerably. His observation that patients were slow to demonstrate new learning led him to test whether generalization effects were associated with retraining experiences.

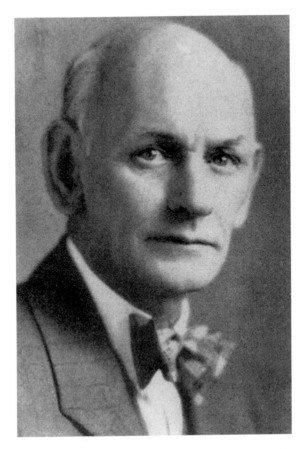

Figure 1-2. Shepherd Ivory Franz. *Courtesy of the University of Akron, Archives of Psychology.*

Although Franz's work has been cited in historical accounts of neuropsychological or cognitive rehabilitation (Boake, 1991), his contributions have rarely been recognized except perhaps in the work of Karl S. Lashley—a man whose own work has profoundly influenced theories of learning and brain organization.

Karl S. Lashley

In his 1929 book entitled *Brain Mechanisms and Intelligence*, Karl S. Lashley (Fig. 1-3) quantitatively analyzed behavioral disturbances associated with surgically induced brain lesions in rats. He summarized previous collaborative work with Franz (Franz and Lashley, 1917; Lashley and Franz, 1917) and attempted to systematize how the location and size of a lesion affected the performance of various learned habits.

For certain types of learning, Lashley (1929) demonstrated that the degree of "retardation" of a previous learned habit was proportional to

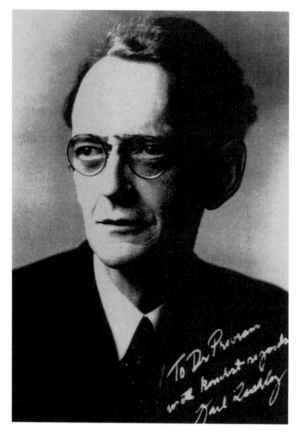

Figure 1-3. Karl S. Lashley, M.D. *Courtesy of Karl Pribram, M.D.*

the magnitude of the lesions (i.e., the Law of Mass Action). The average correlation between these two variables was 0.58, which would account for about a third of the variance. For the formation of new habits after a brain injury, the correlation was even higher and therefore the proportional relationship was significantly larger. On some tests, for example, the correlation was as high as 0.75, thus accounting for about half of the variance. Lashley also emphasized the rats' individual differences and the role of premorbid learning histories in understanding behavioral characteristics after brain injury.

In this early work, Lashley (1929) wrote that "the whole implication of the data is that the 'high level' integrations are not dependent upon localized structural differentiations but are a function of some more general, dynamic organization of the entire cerebral system" (p. 157). He continued as follows: "... the essential element of the stimulus is not the excitation of a pattern of specific sensory endings but the excitation of any endings in a particular spacial (sic) or temporal pattern" (p. 158).

This revolutionary assertion spurred further thinking on spatial and temporal representation within the brain, and the issue is still in the forefront of modern neuropsychological thinking (Pribram, 1991).

Although Lashley's early work emphasized important dimensions for understanding brain organization, his work also seriously challenged the reflex arc theory. That theory was the basis of Luria's concept of higher cerebral functioning, which is discussed below. Lashley also articulated important issues related to understanding the recovery of higher cerebral functions after brain damage.

In 1937, while serving as a professor at Harvard University, Lashley presented the second John Hughlings Jackson lecture at the Montreal Neurological Institute. The title of his talk was *Factors Limiting Recovery After Central Nervous Lesions*. He noted that after every injury to the central nervous system, function is recovered to some degree. Like contemporary observers (Poppel and Steinbuchel, 1992), Lashley (1938) asserted that multiple principles or mechanisms could underlie the recovery of function:

> We cannot understand the processes of recovery fully until we know the nature of the defects and know more than we do now of physiological integration within the cortex and lower centers. Functional loss may be due to destruction of essential structures, to temporary pathological changes in the cells, to shock or diaschisis, to metabolic disturbances, or to lowered tonic activity. In each case the mechanism of recovery will be different, and we rarely know, in any instance, to what extent these various factors have contributed to the symptoms (p. 735).

In emphasizing this point, Lashley clarified an important issue for neuropsychologically oriented rehabilitationists. The loss of a given higher cerebral function or its partial impairment may reflect several mechanisms. A corollary to this point is that brain dysfunctional patients may need different rehabilitation efforts depending on the nature of their symptoms and the related underlying mechanisms. Until the neurological basis of recovery of function is better understood, methods of neuropsychological rehabilitation can offer limited help to brain-impaired patients.

In his 1937 address, Lashley also stressed a point that others have since echoed—the problem of motivation:

> There are two aspects to the question of motivation. Many patients and, I believe, our experimental animals also, after long hospitalization develop functional disorders superimposed upon the organic. They are likely to have a passive attitude and to make little effort to utilize the capacities which they retain. This lack of motivation may lead us to an overestimation of the severity of the organic defect and to ascribe to

vicarious function a recovery which is really only an overcoming of a functional inhibition by the increased motivation of our retraining procedures.

On the other hand, there is some evidence that intense motivation is really effective in compensating for organic defects. . . . it is certainly true that the effort to learn, or the necessity of use, plays an important part in the recovery of functions.

. . . The experiments on motivation deal with the acquisition of specific reactions, not with the recovery of abilities and do not touch upon the fundamental problem of restoring motivation itself where it has been reduced by cerebral lesion. In no experiments have we evidence for any improvement in the general level of motivation (p. 752).

These observations are still germane. First, patients (or animals) can have reactionary problems that interfere with their motivation to learn a specific activity. Second, lesions to the brain can affect motivation negatively. And, as Lashley noted, there is no indication that "motivation itself" can be restored after it has been reduced by a cerebral lesion.

One other point concerning motivation is worth mentioning in relation to Lashley's contributions. As many theorists have noted (Hebb, 1949; Malmo, 1959; Simon, 1967), motivation and arousal are related. If an organism's arousal level is altered, its level of motivation also changes as well. Lashley (1938) cited Franz's (1916) work, which documented the "fluctuation of function in aphasic patients, indicating "that associative organization necessary for speech may still be present, but ordinarily at a low level of excitability" (p. 749).

In summary, Lashley's major contribution to the field of neuropsychological rehabilitation perhaps derives from his understanding that the size of a brain injury can play a crucial role in an individual's ultimate level of recovery. Second, he understood that because many mechanisms could underlie recovery of function, attempts to retrain partially impaired function must consider the multiplicity of mechanisms. Finally, Lashley, as well as later theorists, emphasized the role of motivation in teaching patients to learn new skills after brain injury even though motivation itself might be impaired. The tone of these observations is modern and easily appreciated by experienced clinicians.

Kurt Goldstein

The contribution of Kurt Goldstein (Fig. 1-4) to both personality (Hall and Lindzey, 1978) and neuropsychological theory (Luria, 1966) is well recognized. Trained in both neurology and psychiatry, Goldstein was in a unique position to describe the adjustment problems of brain dysfunctional patients and also to appreciate the importance of the underlying neurological factors that contributed to their symptom profile. Influenced by Hughlings Jackson (1898), Goldstein (1942) emphasized the impor-

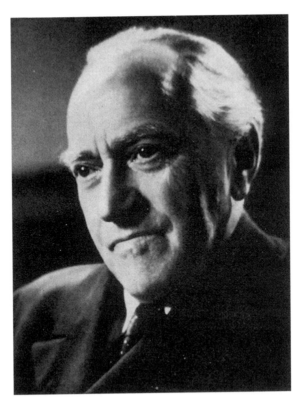

Figure 1-4. Kurt Goldstein, M.D. From *The Reach of the Mind* by M. L. Simmel, 1968. Springer, New York. *Courtesy of The Reach of the Mind by M. L. Simmel.*

tance of carefully observing the patient's symptoms and relating them to constructs about brain function and dysfunction. He devised a classification system for symptoms that is still extremely relevant today (see Chapter 3).

Goldstein suggested that some symptoms emanate directly from a specific lesion in the brain. For example, hemiparesis may reflect a direct injury of the sensorimotor cortex. He also described symptoms that reflected disturbances of what he called the "abstract attitude." Patients might behave inappropriately in certain social situations simply because cognitively they cannot grasp the complexity of the situation. Finally, he described symptoms that were in reaction to failures to cope with the environment. These reactions had compensatory and protective components (Goldstein, 1952). Patients overwhelmed by an environmental situation may exhibit what Goldstein described as a *catastrophic reaction* (see Chapters 2 and 3).

Goldstein's background was unique and one of his mentors was Karl Wernicke. Thus, his professional background emphasized the importance of focal lesions and their impact on specific neuropsychological syndromes. Yet, he reacted against this tradition and emphasized the importance of the entire organism struggling to cope with any type of adversity. His theories and concepts are summarized by Hall and Lindzey (1978) in a chapter dealing with the organismic theory of human personality.

Goldstein's (1942) approach to the rehabilitation of brain dysfunctional patients was extremely practical as well as humane. He recognized the need to document and evaluate systematically disturbances of higher cerebral functions via psychological tests. He discussed the importance of protected work trials for his patients and gave them rehabilitative experiences that increased their sense of personal competency. He understood their personality reactions and described them in exquisite detail (Goldstein, 1952). He reinstated words such as "joy" and "pleasure" into the scientific discussion of what these men may or may not have experienced.

Concerned about the entire person (in contrast to just knowing the objective effects of a brain lesion on behavior), Goldstein provided a humane approach to rehabilitation that later emerged in the work of Luria (1948/1963) and the more recent contributions of Diller and Ben-Yishay (Diller and Gordon, 1981; Ben-Yishay and Diller, 1983). Goldstein's concept of the catastrophic reaction and its important role in neuropsychological rehabilitation are considered throughout this text.

A. R. Luria

After World War II, Oliver Zangwill (1947), a noted British psychologist, raised a number of important theoretical points about recovery of function and retraining procedures for impaired higher cerebral functions (Prigatano et al., 1986). These issues were the very ones that Alexander Romanovich Luria (Fig. 1-5) had been working on in Russia during the same period. Luria's classic text, *Restoration of Function After Brain Injury*, translated by O. L. Zangwill, then Professor of Experimental Psychology at the University of Cambridge, was published in English in 1963.

Luria's work now is well known, and his contributions are not detailed in this text. In this brief introduction to the principles of neuropsychological rehabilitation, however, a few points about Luria's work need to be mentioned. First, Luria insisted on the importance of performing a careful, detailed neuropsychological examination of brain-injured patients to determine the underlying nature of higher cerebral dysfunctions. Establishing the core underlying disturbances for a given neuropsychological syndrome was the primary purpose of Luria's neuropsychological examination. Second, he emphasized the need for extensive practice during the retraining process after brain injury. Rebuilding new habits (complex reflex processes according to Luria) was necessary

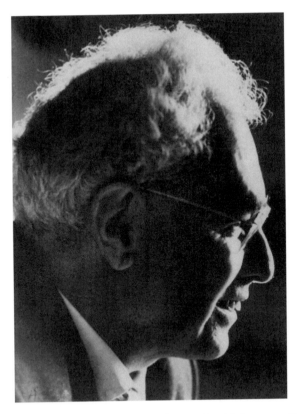

Figure 1-5. A. R. Luria. *Courtesy of Anne-Lisa Christensen, Ph.D.*

after brain injury, and this activity was always individually tailored (see Luria et al., 1969; Christensen et al., 1992). Third, like Lashley, Luria was impressed with the problem of motivation in the rehabilitation process. In fact, chapter 7 of his 1948 text was entitled *"Restoration of Functions After Brain Injuries: The Problem of Motivation."* Within this chapter, a sub-section was entitled *"The Principal Factors Determining the Success of Restoration of Function"* (p. 223).

Consider his words carefully:

We have studied the complicated path of restoration of disturbed brain functions through their reorganization. It remains for us now to analyze the last essential problem, which is one of equally great theoretical and practical importance.

Restoration of deranged brain functions is not equally successful in all cases. Sometimes the disturbed brain function is restored very quickly, and after a short time the physician can only detect a residual functional defect with great difficulty. In other cases the restoration of the deranged brain function drags on for a very long time. Finally, sometimes the disturbed function may not be restored at all, and the defect is irreversible.

How can we account for the variations in rate and success of restoration of deranged brain functions?

Classical neurology fails to supply a fully satisfactory answer to this question. As a rule in clinical practice there are two main factors determining inequality in restoration of functions in different cases: differences in the nature of the wound, and the pre-morbid features of the personality.

Other things being equal, we know that the severity of the brain wound, the volume of brain tissue affected, and the presence of complications of the brain injury are factors on which depends the success of restoration of deranged brain functions. For reasons which are perfectly well understood, the defect will be much more permanent in cases of large, severe wounds complicated by suppuration or inflammation than in wounds similarly located but following an aseptic course and not causing great destruction. . . .

The second factor influencing the rate and completeness of restitution of a defect is the state of the brain before injury. Other things being equal, we know that the brain of a young person possesses greater powers of compensation of a defect and of restoration of disturbed functions than the brain of an old person with an impaired cerebral circulation and having lost some of its original plasticity. . . .

These two clinical factors, however justified, do not tell the whole story. The present level of our knowledge demands much more concrete evidence and further development of these influences in accordance with our ideas of the type of restoration of function with which we have to deal, and of the psychological evaluation of the disturbance of function caused by wounds in a given situation. With differences in the type of compensation of a defect, and differences in the character of disturbance of the functional systems of the brain, there can be many different factors influencing the success of restoration of disturbed functions (pp. 223–224).

Luria devoted a considerable portion of his book to discussing many of these potential factors. Like Lashley before him, he emphasized the importance of the size of the lesion as a major determinant of outcome. He also stressed an individual's premorbid characteristics as an important determinant of the course of recovery. Although these two factors are extremely important, he further noted other influences on the manifestation of symptoms. These influences focus on the types of compensations that patients use to cope with a deficit (Chapter 3). This idea, also suggested by Lashley and Goldstein, is echoed in the writings of many other individuals in the field. Thus, a clear understanding of the important underlying dimensions of a symptom profile is the core of whatever principles of neuropsychological rehabilitation can be expli-cated. And understanding these potential factors requires knowledge of recovery mechanisms, the damaged areas of the brain, how higher cere-bral functions are most likely organized in the brain, and patients' in-dividual premorbid personality and cognitive characteristics as well as their manner of coping with their deficits. As discussed later, these and other issues must be synthesized to develop a true clinical neuropsy-chological approach to brain dysfunctional patients.

Leonard Diller and Yehuda Ben-Yishay

Any account of contemporary neuropsychological rehabilitation would be remiss if it failed to recognize the substantial contributions of Leonard Diller (Fig. 1-6) and Yehuda Ben-Yishay (Fig. 1-7) at New York Univer-

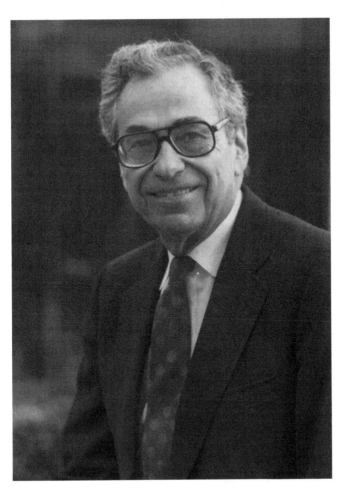

Figure 1-6. Leonard Diller, Ph.D. *Courtesy of Leonard Diller, Ph.D.*

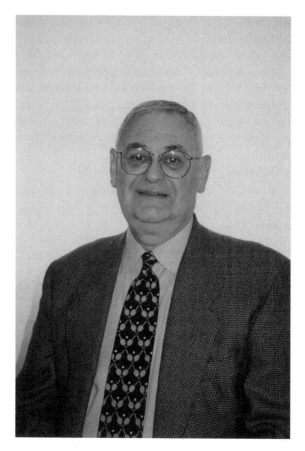

Figure 1-7. Yehuda Ben-Yishay, Ph.D. *Courtesy of Yehuda Ben-Yishay, Ph.D.*

sity and the Rusk Institute of Rehabilitation Medicine. They pioneered
the application of concepts from neuropsychology and clinical psychology to the rehabilitation of a variety of brain dysfunctional patients. They
attempted to apply the modern armamentarium of experimental psychology to the behavioral problems of people who had suffered strokes
or TBIs. They and their many colleagues have provided the models by
which neuropsychological rehabilitation has developed in the United
States and elsewhere.

Although Diller has made substantial contributions to the field of neuropsychological rehabilitation (Ben-Yishay et al., 1970; Ben-Yishay and
Diller, 1983; Diller, 1992; Diller and Gordon, 1981; Diller and Weinberg,
1972), one of his most outstanding contributions has been his ability to
conceptualize how a clinical problem should be approached in a scientific manner. He has also developed practical strategies to help persons
to compensate for a variety of disabilities.

Conversely, Diller's colleague, Yehuda Ben-Yishay, has infused neuropsychological rehabilitation with a considerable degree of personal energy, and he has successfully engaged patients in the rehabilitation process, in part, by virtue of the force of his personality. He instills a realistic sense of hope in patients: If they work systematically to ameliorate their higher cerebral deficits, they can, in fact, live more productive lives. Ben-Yishay's emphasis on small-group interaction and on teaching patients rules by which to interact is an extremely important contribution, particularly for patients with frontal lobe disturbances.

The most recent work of Diller, Ben-Yishay, and their colleagues has assessed both the general and specific effects of different combinations of therapies for certain forms of cognitive remediation (Rattok et al., 1992). Their approach has emphasized the systematic assessment of the efficacy of various rehabilitation activities. Clinical neuropsychologists involved in rehabilitation have gained tremendously from this legacy.

Edwin A. Weinstein

In 1955, Weinstein and Kahn published a text on the problem of altered awareness after brain injury. Their book, entitled *Denial of Illness: Symbolic and Physiological Aspects*, attempted to establish scientifically the biological and psychological determinants underlying the lack of insight that patients often display about their disabilities after brain injury. Weinstein (Fig. 1-8), who is both a neurologist and psychiatrist, was es-

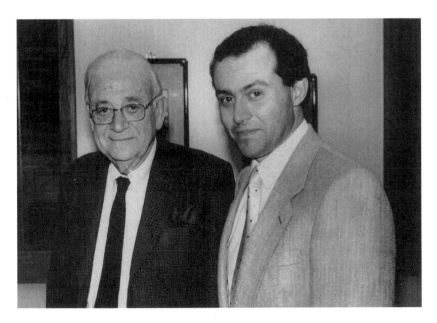

Figure 1-8. Edwin A. Weinstein, M.D. *(left)*, and George P. Prigatano, Ph.D. *(right). Courtesy of George P. Prigatano, Ph.D.*

pecially attuned to the role of neurological factors in producing this symptom. However, he was aware that how patients describe their symptoms potentially also conveys important personal or symbolic meaning. His research highlighted this problem as it relates to aphasia and amnesia (Weinstein and Kahn, 1952; Weinstein et al., 1962; Weinstein et al., 1966). His work is notable as a contemporary attempt to combine a phenomenological perspective with a scientific approach to understanding brain dysfunctional patients. This integrated approach is the foundation of this text, and I am personally indebted for the inspiration that Weinstein has provided. His contributions to neuropsychological rehabilitation have recently been reviewed (Prigatano and Weinstein, 1996).

Karl Pribram

Karl Pribram (Fig. 1-9) was trained as a neurosurgeon but quickly became interested in the questions of physiological psychology. He was

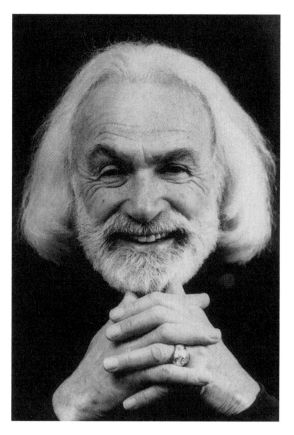

Figure 1-9. Karl Pribram, M.D. *Courtesy of Karl Pribram, M.D.*

greatly influenced by his mentor, Karl Lashley. Pribram's career is still active and cannot be easily summarized in a few words. His holographic theory of brain function attempts to deal with the problem of how learning and memory (including recognition memory or perception) are distributed over wide regions of the brain. His writings are not always easily understood (e.g., *Languages of the Brain: Experimental Paradoxes and Principles of Neuropsychology*, 1971), but his concepts and ideas are always challenging and are well worth the effort to understand them.

Pribram has attempted to integrate ideas from quite disparate areas of inquiry, and he is perhaps one of the true Renaissance men in the neurosciences. His collaborative work with Merton Gill (Pribram and Gill, 1976) attempted to revisit some of Freud's earlier ideas and to compare them to a number of concepts found in information theory as well as to the laws of thermodynamics. The later discussion of personality disturbances related to brain injury summarizes some of those ideas and illustrates Pribram's influence on my own thinking about how cognitive deficits and affective disturbances are interconnected.

Pribram has also worked extensively with other neuroscientists (Pribram et al., 1952) as he has attempted to understand the interconnection of the limbic system and basal ganglia with cortical centers. He has also collaborated with A. R. Luria (Pribram and Luria, 1973) in an attempt to integrate contemporary ideas concerning the neuropsychology and pathophysiology of the frontal lobes. His contributions are progressively becoming appreciated by other theorists in the field (Stuss, 1995). His concepts of "intention" as well as "attention" have clarified the relative roles of frontal and parietal systems on learning and, possibly, human consciousness (Pribram, 1987). He has appreciated the relative role of activation and "effort" in influencing cognitive systems and has been ahead of his time in this regard (Pribram and McGuinness, 1975).

On a personal note, Pribram exerted considerable influence on my own perceptions of the relative strengths and limitations of the scientific method. He has observed that within the scientific enterprise, we frequently collect facts. On numerous occasions, he has commented to me that when science resolves paradox, true knowledge emerges. This spirit of inquiry coupled to the need to resolve the paradoxical behavior of brain dysfunctional patients forms the pneuma of this text.

Freud and Jung

Perhaps the works of Sigmund Freud and Carl Gustav Jung are better known to psychiatrists than to neuropsychologists and neurologists. However, even during the training of the most experimentally oriented scientists, Freud is recognized for his iconoclastic attempt to understand the development of mental processes. Freud (1924) first proposed that nonconscious or unconscious processes are important determinants of complex behaviors and that biological urges during infancy play a role in the emergence of higher cerebral functions. The reemergence of interest in consciousness and the scientific examination of what is now called the nonconscious (see Kihlstrom, 1987) reflect Freud's continued impact on our thinking. Despite the subsequent criticisms of his theory, Freud's courage in reporting his observations about his patients and in an attempting to construct a comprehensive theoretical model to explain the observations was unique at the time.

This process parallels the task of contemporary clinical neuropsychologists confronted with the assessment and rehabilitation of brain dysfunctional patients. Clinicians must observe the events of the clinical arena carefully and then develop models to account for their observations, irrespective of how those models might be viewed by contemporary scientists or peers. Jung is an outstanding example of such intellectual resolve, and his break with Freud was the consequence of his disagreement about the theory of the libido. His text on the unconscious and symbols of libido (Jung, 1912/1952) irreversibly ruptured his relationship with Freud.

Nonetheless, these two theorists formulated practical ideas that are still important in the psychotherapy of brain dysfunctional patients. As discussed later, they emphasized the importance of personal productivity, sustaining interpersonal relationships that have a component of love, and individuals' capacity to delve into fantasy and to realize their potential in order to maximize their psychological health. Thus, any account of the principles of neuropsychological rehabilitation must acknowledge its indebtedness to these two archetypal figures of psychiatry and the study of human behavior.

Roger Sperry

Roger Sperry is usually recognized for his work with split-brain patients; yet his neuropsychological investigations opened new vistas for understanding consciousness and the role of the cerebral hemispheres in various higher cerebral functions. Sperry (1974) summarized his observations of patients who had undergone surgical resection of the corpus callosum to control seizures. Not only did he demonstrate the unique role of the left cerebral hemisphere in language functioning, he also demonstrated the importance of the right cerebral hemisphere in self-recognition tasks and in social judgment. Perhaps even more startling, he demonstrated that the right hemisphere actually stores information that it cannot report verbally via the left hemisphere when the corpus callosum is transected. His concept of a dissociated consciousness set the stage for later work on how altered awareness of brain injury manifests itself in different forms given the locus and the extent of the cerebral lesion (Prigatano and Schacter, 1991). Certainly the problem of altered awareness has become a major issue in the neuropsychological rehabilitation of brain dysfunctional patients, and Sperry's work was instrumental in highlighting this important issue from a scientific perspective.

B. F. Skinner

The work of B. F. Skinner (1938) is well known to American psychologists. One can hardly attend an amusement park, such as *Seaworld* in San Diego, California, without being struck by how powerfully the behavior of animals and man can be controlled according to the principles of learning as defined in the tradition of behaviorism. Wood (1987) and, more recently, Jacobs (1992) have documented how the principles of behavioral analysis can be used systematically to facilitate the rehabilitation of certain patients with brain dysfunction. Clinicians working with a variety of patients, including those with brain dysfunction, must be aware of Skinner's observation that behavior is a function of its environmental consequences.

Although useful, the behavioral model, in and of itself, is inadequate as an approach to neuropsychological rehabilitation as well as to other therapeutic endeavors. It is insufficient because it fails to consider how higher mental processes and feelings influence behavior. Rogers (1961), the well-known proponent of phenomenology, debated this issue with Skinner, but neither scored a decisive victory. Both approaches, the scientific as well as the phenomenological, are needed when dealing with human beings and their problems. Like Jung (1912, 1952) before him, Rogers (1961) emphasized this point.

Donald O. Hebb

Surprisingly, Donald Hebb (Fig. 1-10), the noted Canadian neuropsychologist, made an observation that supports this holistic perspective in his 1974 article, *"What Psychology is About."* Hebb is best recognized for his theoretical work on brain organization and his innovative concept of the cell assembly, which Edelman (1987) has further elaborated. Hebb's 1974 observation, however, most influenced me as a clinical neuropsychologist involved in the rehabilitation of brain dysfunctional patients. Hebb stated that psychology, as a science, was dedicated to an objective understanding of how the mind works. He defined mind as the capacity for thought and thought as the integrated activity of the brain. He remarked, however, that psychology (and for that matter psychiatry) has a poor track record in teaching people to live well or wisely after any major change or tragedy. Hebb asserted that other sources of information were needed to help people with personal and existential issues. Information that flows, for example, from the humanities such as art, literature, and history is crucial in this latter endeavor.

Hebb's observation is important to the practice of neuropsychological rehabilitation. The scientific method is indispensable for the success of a

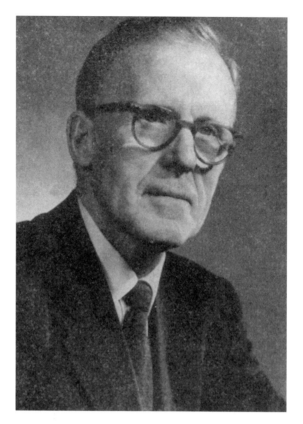

Figure 1-10. Donald O. Hebb, Ph.D. *Courtesy of McGill University.*

neuropsychologically oriented rehabilitation program. However, the patients' subjective (personal) perception of their rehabilitation experience can be an equally powerful influence on how they actually behave or cope with the residuals of neuropsychological impairment (Prigatano, 1991).

Summary and Conclusions

The field of neuropsychological rehabilitation needs guiding principles on which to base scientific inquiry and clinical practice. Thirteen principles of neuropsychological rehabilitation have been introduced. Historical and contemporary influences, which helped form these principles, have been briefly identified.

The historical concept in medicine that physicians should first do no harm and second, attempt to aid their fellow man to reduce suffering (i.e., the Hippocratic Oath) is as relevant today as it was thousands of years ago.

This text will attempt to emphasize, via its 13 principles, that both the scientific and phenomenological approach are needed for maximal effectiveness in patient care. The application of knowledge from human neuropsychology and related disciplines requires that practitioners sense what patients experience in order to plan treatment and to engage them in rehabilitation.

The remaining chapters will discuss each of the 13 principles and how they might guide the field of neuropsychological rehabilitation.

References

Ben-Yishay, Y., and Diller, L. (1983). Cognitive remediation. In M. Rosenthal (ed), *Rehabilitation of the Head Injured Adult*. F. A. Davis, Philadelphia.

Ben-Yishay, Y., Diller, L., Gerstman, L., and Gordon, W. (1970). Relationship between initial competence and ability to profit from cues in brain-damaged individuals. *J. Abnorm. Psychol*. 75: 248–259.

Boake, C. (1991). The history of cognitive rehabilitation following head injury. In J. S. Kreutzer and P. H. Wehman (eds), *Cognitive Rehabilitation for Persons with Traumatic Brain Injury: A Functional Approach* (pp. 3–12). Paul H. Brookes, Baltimore.

Bronowski, J. (1973). *The Ascent of Man*. Little, Brown, Boston.

Christensen, A. L, Pinner, E. M., Moller Pedersen, P., Teasdale, T. W., and Trexler, L. E. (1992). Psychosocial outcome following individualized neuropsychological rehabilitation of brain damage. *Acta Neurol. Scand*. 85: 32–38.

Diller, L. (1992). Introduction to the special section on neuropsychology and rehabilitation—the view from New York University. *Neuropsychology*6(4): 357–359.

Diller, L. and Gordon, W. A. (1981). Interventions for cognitive deficits in brain-injured adults. *J. Consult. Clin. Psychol*. 49: 822–834.

Diller, L., and Weinberg, J. (1972). Differential aspects of attention in brain-damaged persons. *Percept. Mot. Skills* 35: 71–81.

Edelman, G. M. (1987). *Neural Darwinism: The Theory of Neuronal Group Selection*. Basic Books, New York.

Franz, S. I. (1916). The re-education of an aphasic. *Journal of Experimental Psychology* 1: 355–364.

Franz, S. I. (1924). Studies in re-education: The aphasias. *Comparative Psychology* 4(4): 349–429.

Franz, S. I., and Lashley, K. S. (1917). The retention of habits by the rat after destruction of the frontal portion of the cerebrum. *Psychobiology* 1: 3–18.

Freud, S. (1924). *A General Introduction to Psychoanalysis*, (24th ed). Simon and Schuster, New York.

Goldstein, K. (1942). *Aftereffects of Brain Injury in War*. Grune and Stratton, New York.

Goldstein, K. (1952). The effect of brain damage on the personality. *Psychiatry* 15: 245–260.

Hall, C. S., and Lindzey, G. (1978). *Theories of Personality* (3rd ed). John Wiley & Sons, New York.

Hebb, D. (1974). What psychology is about. *Am. Psychol.* 29: 71–79.

Hebb, D. O. (1949). *The Organization of Behavior.* Wiley, New York.

Jackson, J. H. (1888). Remarks on the diagnosis and treatment of diseases of the brain. *British Medical Journal* July 21: 111–117.

Jackson, J. H. (1898). Relations of different divisions of the central nervous system to one another and to parts of the body. *Lancet* 1: 79–87.

Jacobs, H. (1992). *Behavioral Analysis Guidelines and Brain Rehabilitation: People, Principles and Programs.* Aspen Publishers, Gaithersburg, MD.

Jung, C. G. (1912/1952). *Collected Works (Vol. 5, Symbols of Transformation).* Princeton University, Princeton, NJ.

Kihlstrom, J. F. (1987). The cognitive unconscious. *Science* 237, 1445–1452.

Lashley, K. S. (1929/1964). *Brain Mechanisms and Intelligence: A Quantitative Study of Injuries to the Brain.* Hafner, New York. Originally published (1929) by University of Chicago Press.

Lashley, K. S. (1938). Factors limiting recovery after central nervous lesions. *J. Nerv. Ment. Dis.* 88(6): 733–755.

Lashley, K. S., and Franz, S. I. (1917). The effects of cerebral destruction upon habit formation and retention in the albino rat. *Psychobiology* 1, 71–139.

Luria, A. R. (1966). Kurt Goldstein and neuropsychology. *Neuropsychologia* 4: 311–313.

Luria, A. R. (1948/1963). *Restoration of Function After Brain Trauma* (in Russian). Moscow: Academy of Medical Science (Pergamon, London, 1963).

Luria, A. R., Naydin, V. L., Tsvetkova, L. S., and Vinarskaya, E. N. (1969). Restoration of higher cortical function following local brain damage. In P. J. Vinken and G. W. Bruyn (eds), *Handbook of Clinical Neurology* (Vol. 3, pp. 368–433). North-Holland, Amsterdam.

Malmo, R. B. (1959). Activation: A neuropsychological dimension. *Psychol. Rev.* 66: 367–386.

Poppel, E., and Steinbuchel, N. v. (1992). Neuropsychological rehabilitation. In N. v. Steinbuchel, D. Y. von Cramon, and E. Poppel (eds), *Neuropsychological Rehabilitation* (pp. 3–19). Springer-Verlag, Berlin.

Pribram, K. H. (1991). *Brain and Perception: Holonomy and Structure in Figural Processing.* Lawrence Erlbaum Associates, Hillsdale, NJ.

Pribram, K. H. (1971). *Languages of the Brain: Experimental Paradoxes and Principles in Neuropsychology.* Prentice-Hall, Englewood Cliffs, NJ.

Pribram, K. H. (1987). Subdivisions of the frontal cortex revisited. In E. Brown and E. Perecman (eds), *The Frontal Lobes Revisited* (pp. 11–39). IRBN Press, New York.

Pribram, K. H. and Gill, M. M. (1976). *Freud's 'Project' Reassessed.* Basic Books, New York.

Pribram, K. H., and Luria, A. R. (1973). *Psychophysiology of the Frontal Lobes.* Academic Press, New York.

Pribram, K. H., and McGuinness, D. (1975). Arousal, activation and effort in the control of attention. *Psychol. Rev.* 82(2): 116–149.

Pribram, K. H., Mishkin, M., Rosvold, H. E., and Kaplan, S. J. (1952). Effects on delayed-response performance of lesions of dorsolateral and ventro-medial frontal cortex of baboons. *Journal of Comparative Physiology and Psychology* 45: 565–575.

Prigatano, G. P. (1991). Science and symbolism in neuropsychological reha-bilitation after brain injury. *The Tenth Annual James C. Hemphill Lecture.* Rehabilitation Institute of Chicago, Chicago.

Prigatano, G. P. (1996). Neuropsychological rehabilitation after brain injury: scientific and professional issues. *Journal of Clinical Psychology in Medical Settings* 3(1): 1–10.

Prigatano, G. P., Fordyce, D. J., Zeiner, H. K., Roueche, J. R., Pepping, M., and Wood, B. C. (1986). *Neuropsychological Rehabilitation after Brain Injury.* The Johns Hopkins University Press, Baltimore.

Prigatano, G. P., and Schacter, D. L. (1991). *Awareness of Deficit After Brain Injury: Clinical and Theoretical Issues.* Oxford University Press, New York.

Prigatano, G. P., and Weinstein, E. A. (1996). Edwin A. Weinstein's contri-butions to neuropsychological rehabilitation. *Neuropsychological Rehabili-tation,* 6(4): 305–326.

Rattok, J., Ben-Yishay, D., Lakin, P., Piasetsky, E., Ross, B., Silver, S., Vakil, E., Zide, E., and Diller, L. (1992). Outcome of different treatment mixes in a multidimensional neuropsychological rehabilitation program. *Neu-ropsychology* 6(4): 3395–3415.

Rogers, C. R. (1961). *On Becoming a Person.* Houghton Mifflin, Boston.

Simon, H. A. (1967). Motivation and emotional controls of cognition. *Psychol. Rev.* 74: 29–39.

Skinner, B. F. (1938). *The Behavior of Organisms.* Appleton-Century-Crofts, New York.

Sperry, R. W. (1974). Lateral specialization in the surgically separated hem-ispheres. In F. O. Schmitt and F. G. Worden (eds), *The Neurosciences* (pp. 5–19). MIT Press, Cambridge, MA.

Stuss, D. T. (1995). Measurements of frontal lobe dysfunction for the clinician. *Conference on Neuropsychological Assessment and Rehabilitation after Brain Injury: Empirical and Theoretical Foundations,* Barrow Neurological Insti-tute, Phoenix, Ariz., May 1995.

Webster's New Universal Unabridged Dictionary (1983). New World Dictionar-ies/Simon & Schuster, Cleveland.

Weinstein, E. A., and Kahn, R. L. (1955). *Denial of Illness: Symbolic and Phys-iological Aspects.* Charles C Thomas, Springfield, Ill.

Weinstein, E. A., and Kahn, R. L. (1952). Nonaphasic misnaming (paraphasia) in organic brain disease. *Archives of Neurology and Psychiatry* 67, 72–79.

Weinstein, E. A., Lyerly, O. G., Cole, M., and Ozer, M. N. (1966). Meaning in jargon aphasia. *Cortex* 2: 165–187.

Weinstein, E. A., Marvin, S. K., and Keller, N. J. A. (1962). Amnesia as a lan-guage pattern. *Arch. Gen. Psychiatry* 6: 17–28.

Wood, R. L. (1987). *Brain Injury Rehabilitation: A Neurobehavioural Approach.* Croom-Helm, London.

Zangwill, O. L. (1947). Psychological aspects of rehabilitation in cases of brain injury. *Br. J. Psychol.* 37: 60–69.

2

The Patient's Experience and the Nature of Higher Cerebral Functions

As soon as I regained consciousness . . . I began to insist that I was soon to go home from the hospital . . . My visitors were apparently the living proof of my disability; I forgot their visits immediately upon their leaving, and disavowed that they had ever been there when asked . . . I became quite concerned about the groaning of some patients who shared the intensive care unit with me, attempting to care for them in the role of nonimpaired physician.

W. L. LaBaw, "Denial inside out: subjective experience with anosognosia in closed head injury," 1969, pp. 176–177

From the point of view of modern psychology, the higher human mental functions are complex reflex processes, social in origin, mediate in structure, and conscious and voluntary in mode of function.

A. R., Luria, *Higher Cerebral Functions in Man*, 1966, p. 32

The process of neuropsychological rehabilitation begins with understanding what the patient experiences regarding his or her higher cerebral functions (or dysfunction). What the patient experiences guides the neuropsychological interview and later examination. It is also crucial for planning rehabilitation strategies. If the patient does not experience, at some level, the usefulness of the examination or the rehabilitation program, he or she will resist treatment or only passively engage in it. Thus, the first principle of neuropsychological rehabilitation is that the clinician must enter the patient's phenomenological field in order to sense what he or she experiences. Frequently clinicians will encounter that the patient is frustrated and confused over what is happening. Therapy aimed at reducing this frustration and confusion will be eagerly met by the

A portion of this chapter is based on an invited lecture presented at the American Psychological Association (APA) Convention, Washington, D.C., on August 16, 1992, entitled: "What does the brain-injured person experience? Implications for rehabilitation."

patient, irrespective of whether such rehabilitation activities actually improve higher cerebral functions. The reality of helping patients not be alone with their disturbances and helping them deal with their disordered experience is of maximum value.

Let us begin, then, with the patients' experience of brain damage.

The Experience of Brain Damage

What is it like to suffer brain injury? What are the subjective or phenomenological experiences associated with brain dysfunction? Surely, certain experiences must be common to all brain dysfunctional patients, and others may be related to specific variables such as type of lesion, location, and acuteness of onset (Satz, 1966). The experience can also be colored by patients' premorbid history and how they attempt to make sense of their altered world.

In the case of a traumatic brain injury (TBI) associated with a significant disruption of consciousness and a resultant period of posttraumatic amnesia (Russell, 1971), patients may regain consciousness and demonstrate an ability to communicate with others—yet they may be totally unaware of their residual neuropsychological impairments. The first quote introducing this chapter is from an article written by LaBaw (1969), a psychiatrist who sustained a closed head injury. His article—entitled *Denial Inside Out: A Subjective Experience with Anosognosia in Closed Head Injury*—documented a common experience associated with TBI. After regaining sufficient consciousness to communicate, he engaged in various conversations that he later could not recall. During this time, he was disoriented and oblivious to his loss of insight about his neuropsychological disturbances, which, however, was obvious to observers.

Clinicians often assume that as posttraumatic amnesia resolves, patients not only become oriented to time and place but can remember daily events. During this initial period of recovery, patients' insight into their impaired higher cerebral functions seems to approach acceptable levels. Some patients may even perform reasonably well on many standardized neuropsychological tests (see, for example, the case M.L. referenced in Prigatano, 1991b). Clinicians therefore may be surprised to discover that some TBI patients appear to lack insight into their impairments and the resultant psychosocial consequences several months and even years after their injury (Prigatano et al., 1986; Prigatano, 1991a).

LaBaw (1969), for example, describes how he attempted to resume his hospital practice (apparently with a release from his attending physicians) only to be irritated when the nurses complained about his inefficient and ineffective professional work. He states that "At thirty months after my accident, I suddenly realized that surviving the wreck was one thing and that surviving the subsequent denial was another" (p. 184).

An essential thesis of this book is that disturbances in higher cerebral function often are associated with some disruption of self-conscious perception or experience of those disturbances. This fact not only has theoretical implications regarding the nature of the brain-mind relationship (Prigatano and Schacter, 1991) but also has important implications for rehabilitation (Prigatano et al., 1986). Consider a few clinical examples that support that contention.

The Clinical Evidence

A 35-year-old, right-handed nurse suffered a hemorrhage in the left parietal temporal area. A large arteriovenous malformation (AVM) was discovered and removed surgically. Postoperatively, the patient exhibited classic fluent aphasia (Benson, 1993). She made several paraphasic errors in her free speech. She could not repeat sentences. She could not execute complex two-step commands. Yet, the look of frustration on her face when attempting to speak suggested that she was aware of her language impairments. She improved progressively and the obvious signs of aphasia disappeared.

On neuropsychological testing, however, her performance on the auditory comprehension tests and the recall of short stories was impaired. She also had notable difficulty repeating sentences. Psychometric assessment of both verbal and nonverbal memory functions revealed scores one to two standard deviations below normal limits. She was willing to pursue speech and language therapy for these difficulties and did so religiously. One year after the onset of her neurological problems, neuropsychological deficits persisted in the form of impaired auditory comprehension and significant verbal memory difficulties.

The patient, however, insisted that she could return to her work as a nurse. When advised otherwise, she became suspicious of others and with time developed frank paranoid ideation that resulted in inpatient psychiatric treatment. Five years after her hemorrhage and surgery, she still had residual verbal memory deficits, auditory comprehension difficulties, and persistent paranoid ideation with auditory hallucinations. She continues to insist that she can return to nursing despite several academic failures in taking "refresher" nursing courses as well as a failure in successfully completing a course of neuropsychologically oriented rehabilitation of the type described by Prigatano and colleagues (1986).

In another example, a 27-year-old, left-handed woman with a high school education suffered a hemorrhage in the right frontal parietal region. A large middle cerebral artery aneurysm was detected and clipped surgically (see Fig. 1A and 1B in Prigatano and Henderson, 1997). She showed no gross neurological deficits on examination. She appeared, however, somewhat hyperverbal and hypermanic in her interview with the neurosurgeon. He also noted subtle euphoria. Six weeks after her surgery, she was referred for a neuropsychological examination because she insisted that she was ready to return to work, to drive a car, and to take care of her 3-year-old child.

On neuropsychological examination, she was grossly intact, but she showed subtle signs of right hemisphere dysfunction, including difficulties in spontaneously generating affect in her voice. More comprehensive testing revealed substantial visuospatial and visual memory difficulties. She also had difficulties with abstract reasoning and made a number of perseverative errors on the Wisconsin Card Sorting Test. Her higher cerebral functioning was clearly impaired, and she was in no position to resume her domestic or work responsibilities. Furthermore, in some instances, she obviously behaved in a socially inappropriate manner that could put her at risk for both physical and sexual abuse. The patient, however, insisted that she was completely normal, and she wanted to return to her previous job without undergoing any rehabilitation.

A 26-year-old, right-handed man suffered a spontaneous hemorrhage of undetermined etiology in the left basal ganglia. After his stroke, he was immediately aware of his residual left hemiparesis and subtle language difficulties. He agreed to physical and occupational therapy for his hand and leg. He was also willing to work at therapeutic tasks aimed at helping him improve verbal fluency, articulation, and reading. He recognized "some memory problems" but perceived them as relatively insignificant. He frequently, however, forgot assignments and responsibilities during the course of a rehabilitation day. When these lapses were brought to his attention and he was encouraged to use a "memory notebook" to help compensate for his memory problems, he became irritated and, at times, quite angry. He felt that others were exaggerating his difficulties, which he interpreted as part of his premorbid disposition.

A 21-year-old, right-handed man who suffered a severe TBI had an admitting Glasgow Coma Scale (GCS) score of 8. He demonstrated many of the predictable neuropsychological problems associated with this patient group, including notable memory difficulties and reduced speed of information processing (Levin et al., 1982; Levin et al., 1990). His affect was described as flat, but he was cooperative. He participated in a day-treatment rehabilitation program for almost 12 months. After a year of such rehabilitation activities, he was still perplexed about why he could not resume previous work responsibilities. Although his neuropsychological test scores documented improvement, he still demonstrated severe difficulties with memory and speed of information processing. He did not fully appreciate the presence or the extent of his impairments and later was seen for follow-up care. (This patient will be discussed further in Chapter 13.)

Each of these four case vignettes reflects different neuropathological, neurological, and neuropsychological findings. Each case, however, demonstrates some form of impaired self-awareness as it relates to the presence and degree of neuropsychological disturbance and associated psychosocial consequences. Each patient either actively or passively resisted certain rehabilitation activities that were considered potentially helpful. Not all patients show this phenomenon, but many do (see Ben-Yishay and Prigatano, 1990).

Historically, these patients might be described as "denying" their neuropsychological deficits. There is a growing appreciation, however, that these disturbances may be a direct as well as an indirect consequence of brain dysfunction (Prigatano and Schacter, 1991; Prigatano and Weinstein, 1996). Disorders of self-awareness are discussed in Chapter 12, and the question of "denial" is considered. For now, it is important to note that many brain dysfunctional patients undergoing neuropsychological rehabilitation seem to have only partial or implicit knowledge of their disturbances. This impaired awareness affects their behavior in interpersonal situations as well as in rehabilitation.

To work effectively with these individuals, clinicians must enter the patients' phenomenological field and try to obtain some sense of what they are experiencing (Principle 1). Appreciation of the patients' subjective experience can help clinicians to develop a rehabilitation program that at least partially reflects the patients' self-perceived needs. Otherwise, patients are prone to resist rehabilitative interventions or even to leave rehabilitation altogether.

Entering the Patient's Phenomenological Field and Encountering the Problems of Frustration and Confusion

Patients undoubtedly experience a wide variety of subjective states after a brain injury. They may have trouble talking, concentrating, and remembering important information. They may have difficulties in articulating speech sounds or in retrieving words. They may experience subtle difficulties with disorientation and, in some instances, show signs of reduplicative paramnesia. They may experience various degrees of "mental fatigue" or be euphoric and manic. They may "know" that their cognitive functioning has changed yet be unaware of the exact nature of the change or its impact on others. They may or may not have obvious motor difficulties, such as a hemiparesis. They may be complacent or angry. They may be depressed or display sadness appropriately. Whatever the patient's subjective state, clinicians must consider it when attempting to examine patients and to engage them in a rehabilitation program.

Once patients leave the hospital and attempt to resume activities that they are unable to do, predictable affective reactions can be observed. In the course of group psychotherapy with patients with various brain injuries, I specifically ask about these experiences. One question that frequently arises is "What is it like to be brain injured?" The responses from a recent group of rehabilitation patients captured two common reactions.

The most common reaction and the one typically mentioned first was the term "frustration." Despite variations in lesion location and in the age of the individuals, patients most often described themselves as "frustrated." Second, they spontaneously used the word "confusion" when describing their experiences after brain injury. Some expressed confusion about why they had certain physical or sensory symptoms. Others reported frustration and associated confusion in terms of their ability to understand therapists' and families' behavior. Some were particularly vocal about their feeling that therapists and family members restricted them needlessly. Often, they viewed the therapist's comments about their behavior as needless and unwanted interpretations or criticisms.

Although the terms frustration and confusion are used clinically when describing brain dysfunctional patients, these terms seldom appear in the titles of scientific papers devoted to understanding brain dysfunctional individuals. In a computer search of the literature published between 1985 and 1995, the words frustration and confusion were searched for in conjunction with the terms brain injury, head injury, stroke, cerebrovascular accident, cerebral aneurysms, or cerebral AVMs. Interestingly, more than 19,000 articles appeared with the terms stroke, AVM, or aneurysm in the title. An additional 7,600 articles appeared with the terms head injury and brain injury in the title. Together, more than 25,000 articles concerning some type of insult to the brain were published in this 10-year period.

During the same time, 321 articles appeared with the terms memory disorder or memory as well as one of the various terms mentioned above. In contrast, only 14 articles included the term confusion in the title with other terminology reflecting brain dysfunction. Furthermore, not one article included the term frustration in the title with terms such as stroke, head injury, brain injury, cerebral aneurysm, or cerebral AVMs. Four articles, however, included the term frustration in the abstract and three of these four abstracts discuss the frustration of family members or the therapists when dealing with TBI patients. Thus, despite the large number of scientific articles discussing these various nosological groups, the patients' problems of frustration and/or confusion were overlooked. Yet, patients affirm that these are two of their most common problems. Scientific investigation has failed to attend to patients' subjective experiences and to conduct research relevant to their perceived needs.

The Catastrophic Reaction in Response to Frustration and Confusion

In a seminal article, entitled *The Effect of Brain Damage on Personality*, Kurt Goldstein (1952) discussed disturbances in personality after acquired brain injury in adults. This work was based on the organismic theory of personality, which argues that the "organism is determined by one trend, the trend to actualize itself" (p. 246).

Goldstein repeatedly emphasized that brain dysfunctional patients attempt to impose order on the environment. When they are unable to cope effectively with an environmental demand, they are plunged into a state of disorder, or "a catastrophe." The form of the catastrophic reaction varies. It frequently, however, reflects a state in which patients are emotionally overwhelmed, upset, and withdrawn from environmental demands. The problem of the catastrophic reaction is observed repeatedly during the course of rehabilitation of brain dysfunctional patients. Unfortunately, this characteristic response is often poorly understood.

Goldstein emphasized that an impairment in abstract reasoning was frequently the basis of the catastrophic reaction. Patients who cannot grasp how to deal with a situation effectively may unexpectedly become emotionally overwhelmed. He (Goldstein, 1952) observed the following:

> They [the patients] are often afraid that they may not be able to react correctly, and that they will be in a catastrophic condition. Therefore, when they believe they have the right answer, they answer as quickly as possible. Because of impairment of abstraction, they are not able to deliberate: they try to do what they can do as quickly as possible because every retardation increases the tension which they experience when they are not able to answer. The quick response is an effect of their *strong necessity to release tension*; they are forced to release tension because they cannot handle it any other way. They cannot bear anything that presupposes deliberation, considering the future, and so on, all of which are related to abstraction" (p. 250).

Because these patients release their tension inappropriately, Goldstein believed that they are deprived of the feeling of joy produced by releasing tension. Goldstein was one of the few scientists and clinicians who incorporated such human terms when describing the plight of brain dysfunctional patients. We can now reconsider the importance of the phenomenological component in terms of Goldstein's scientific insights.

How can Goldstein's concept of the catastrophic reaction be related to what patients express about their frustrations and confusion? The term frustration has been used to describe the feeling states associated with the nonreward (or nonreinforcement) of behaviors that previously resulted in reward (Amsel, 1958). Although the concept of frustration has been criticized as prescientific (Lawsen, 1965), it is a useful phenomenological term. Frustration refers to a subjective state of discomfort associated with a real or anticipated blocking of attempts to achieve a goal or a state of comfort.

Many brain dysfunctional patients feel "blocked" in getting what they want. They are frustrated that they cannot drive a car or return to work. They are frustrated because they cannot remember something that is important to them. They get frustrated because they are told what to do rather than being able to do what they want. They are frustrated because they often feel dumb.

When brain dysfunctional patients fail to achieve a goal or to maintain a state of comfort, their frustrations can easily develop into a catastrophic reaction. Their judgment about the real significance of the failure may be poor, or they simply may be overwhelmed because they do not know how to handle the situation. If they do not identify their frustrations and work with therapists to eliminate or reduce them, a catastrophic reaction often occurs.

Therapists are wise to first list the patient's frustrations and to identify the ones most readily amenable to therapeutic assistance. As simple as this task may sound, many therapists fail to ask their patients to identify their most frustrating experiences and how they could work together to reduce at least some of those frustrations.

Dollard and Miller (1950) recognized that frustration often leads to some form of aggression and incorporated this concept into their psychotherapeutic approach to non-brain-injured individuals. Irritability, which might be considered a precursor to aggression, is common among TBI patients (Prigatano, 1992). Yet attempts to relate measures of irritability directly to the location, size, or severity of brain lesions have repeatedly failed. Still, irritability, at least partially, must be a reaction to frustration. And if frustration can be reduced in brain dysfunctional patients, irritability often declines, too (Prigatano et al., 1986). To avert a catastrophic reaction in brain-injured patients, therapists must attend to the patients' actual frustrations and work diligently to help them. Patients are also directly taught how to recognize catastrophic reactions in themselves and others (Principle 4).

Therapists must also attend carefully to what patients mean when they say that they are confused. For these patients, confusion does not simply refer to an impairment in abstract attitude or difficulty in thinking clearly. Rather, they state that their minds go blank when they attempt to solve problems and their problem-solving strategies fail. A major component to their sense of confusion is the experience that although their answers are wrong, they do not know how to reapproach the problem to obtain the correct solution. Not only does patients' capacity to think break down, but they have an associated sense of having a mental block or of going blank and not knowing how to reapproach the problem from another perspective. This feeling is a hallmark of confusion in brain dysfunctional persons, and therapists must understand it before they can enter the phenomenological fields of their patients.

For example, a patient suffered a large infarction of the right temporal-occipital lobes (Fig. 2-1). When asked to perform the subtraction "42 − 28 = what?" he began the task by stating, "Normally, I would subtract 30 from 42 and the answer is 14. Then I would subtract 2 from this in order to get the correct answer since 28 was two points less than 30." He said the answer must be "12" but seemed uncomfortable with his response. After pausing and thinking, he said it appeared that his answer was wrong. He sensed that something was wrong and was unsure of his answer. At that point, he said that his mind went blank, and he did not know how to try to reapproach the problem. He was obviously upset. Thus, confusion refers to more than the failure to solve a problem intellectually. By its nature, it takes the person out of a problem-solving loop. The patient becomes disorganized about how to proceed. This feature is a hallmark of a dysfunctional brain (see Chapman and Wolff, 1959, and Chapters 3, 4, and 5).

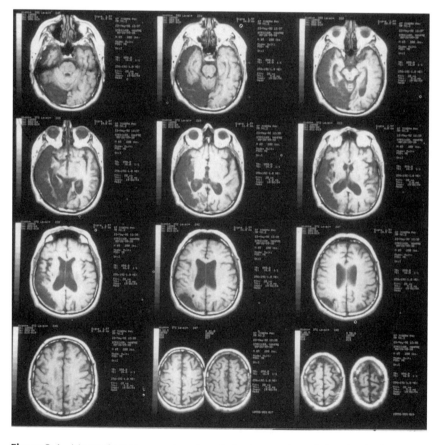

Figure 2-1. Magnetic resonance imaging study shows a large infarction in the region of the right temporal-occipital cortex in a patient whose thought processes were disorganized after failing to solve a simple arithmetic problem.

In addition to this disorganization, confusion connotes mental fatigue. The patient described himself as tired and as lacking the "will" to proceed. He was quick to add that this had *not* been his method of functioning before his injury. He viewed himself (and rightfully so) as previously capable of a considerable level of problem solving. His history documented that his level of intelligence and adaptive competency had been above average.

Obviously, further research is needed to clarify what patients experience when they become confused. Perhaps the clinical application of cognitive psychology can help elucidate this important issue. At present, however, clinicians must strive to understand their patients better when they say that they are frustrated and confused.

Mental Fatigue and Brain Dysfunction

Careful listening to patients' descriptions of their altered mental functioning after various brain lesions can produce extremely important clues for neurorehabilitation. In 1973, Professor A. Brodal published an extraordinary paper on what he experienced after "an infarction of part of the right internal capsule and its surroundings" (p. 676). He described the tremendous energy needed to "force" a paretic muscle to contract and how exhausting it was to exert "mental energy" during rehabilitation. He observed "clear cut changes in his handwriting" and how difficult it was for him to do almost any type of "mental work." Even though his verbal IQ was 142 and his performance IQ was 122 *after* his stroke, he found it difficult to follow arguments in scientific papers and to remember abstract concepts or symbols. He poignantly noted that although lesions of the left (dominant) hemisphere are often associated with frank aphasic disturbances, "the right (nondominant) hemisphere is not without influence on verbal functions" (p. 686). It was, for example, difficult to organize his thoughts and to convey his ideas clearly.

Brodal's (1973) description clarifies how easily patients can fatigue mentally even when they have only small subcortical lesions. What must it be like to have a larger lesion, particularly lesions that involve one or both cerebral hemispheres? Therapists who themselves are frustrated by patients who are slow to respond or who show difficulties in initiation should read Brodal's paper to gain greater insights into the subjective experience of patients with brain injuries. Patients undergo inevitable changes not only in their memory and motor functions but also in the actual energy that they must exert to perform a variety of cognitive and motor tasks. As discussed in Chapter 12, even disturbances of the motor system can affect conscious awareness of certain responses, the importance of which for rehabilitation cannot be overemphasized.

The more we listen to patients' comments about the nature of their higher cerebral dysfunctions, the more insight we will have about how to conduct their neurorehabilitation. Although psychometric tests can be useful, Brodal's test scores were misleading compared to how he was actually affected. If we rely solely on psychometric tests scores, we will often underestimate the true impact of brain dysfunction on a person's daily functioning and may attribute their behavior to emotional rather than neurological factors.

Barriers to Entering the Patient's Phenomenological Field

As important as entering the phenomenological field of the patient is, rehabilitation therapists (including competent clinical neuropsychologists) may have a difficult time achieving this goal for several reasons. First, the therapist, as well as the family members and physicians, can be confused about the nature of the higher cerebral dysfunctions that they observe in patients. Patients may appear unmotivated when they are in a hypoaroused state or have impaired initiation and planning skills (Stuss and Benson, 1986). They may appear to elect not to follow instructions when, in fact, they cannot remember the instructions. They may resist using certain compensatory techniques such as a memory notebook because they do not comprehend how the notebook will help them rather than just refusing to admit to difficulties. Entering the patient's phenomenological field means having the psychological capacity to sense life as the patient does. Both formal knowledge about brain-behavior relationships and a clinical psychological attitude toward the patient (Rogers, 1951; Kalff, 1980) are needed to succeed.

Second, therapists may draw conclusions about patients' resistance to treatment too quickly. Therapists may assume that patients are dishonest, uninterested, or unmotivated about working at their therapies. It is important to remember that therapists can easily misinterpret the causes underlying a given behavior. For example, a 30-year-old woman suffered a severe TBI and had an admitting GCS score of 4. Initially, she passively engaged in various rehabilitation efforts. With time, she resisted any form of cognitive remediation. She anticipated that the rehabilitation therapists and the program director would insist that she remain in the rehabilitation program contrary to her desires. Consequently, she was surprised when the director agreed to let her leave the rehabilitation program and to participate only in the physically oriented therapies that she had requested. Her "resistance" to cognitive rehabilitation may have been viewed as a lack of insight about or denial of her need for such therapies.

Several months later during a psychotherapy session, this woman's motivations become clear. Historically, she had resisted any opinion from an authority figure. Before her brain injury, her lifestyle centered around the theme that authority should be distrusted. When a perceived authority figure (the program director) agreed with her decision (i.e., to attend physical but not cognitive therapies), she was eventually able to discuss how other factors contributed to her initial "resistance." Once these factors were handled, she easily engaged with the neuropsychological rehabilitation program.

A third barrier to entering the patient's phenomenological field is the constant drain on the rehabilitation therapists' psychological resources and energy. Working with brain dysfunctional patients is confusing and emotionally draining. Animals studies have found that nonlesioned animals avoid brain-lesioned animals and show signs of emotional distress when exposed to the latter for prolonged periods (Franzen and Myers, 1973). This finding is extremely relevant and its importance should not be underestimated.

The rehabilitation day should be structured to allow therapists to deal with their own emotional reactions to patients and to provide an avenue through which they can improve their understanding of their patients' symptoms (Prigatano, 1989). If therapists structure their day to conserve energy and to improve their understanding of the complexity of their patients' problems, their interpersonal interactions with brain dysfunctional persons improve.

A fourth barrier is many therapists' growing sense that they lack sufficient time to listen to patients. With the tremendous push to meet productivity standards within hospitals and corporations, therapists are pressured to see as many patients as they can each day. In addition to individual sessions with patients, therapists write hospital notes, review records, and engage in numerous verbal and written communications about patients, among other duties. These tasks are necessary but are not directly reimbursable. Although the health care situation may dictate the number of hours patients can be seen, it should not dictate a rushed attitude during interactions with patients. Only when therapists can assume an attitude of quiet and calm is there a likelihood that they can enter the patient's phenomenological field.

A fifth common barrier is the problem of anger and suspiciousness (Gans, 1983). Patients often become angry with therapists, as do their families. There is increasing concern about litigation. The therapists must often document the rationale for their therapeutic choices (Bennett et al., 1990). These situations create an atmosphere in which therapists feel that they must protect themselves in the context of working with patients. Consequently, the empathic attitude that is so crucial to working with brain dysfunctional patients is eroded.

Portions of this text describe methods that can be used to overcome these barriers in an effort to increase the likelihood of therapists entering the patients' phenomenological field and thereby enhancing the efficacy of the neurorehabilitation effort. As Schafer (1967) indicated, psychologists need not only clinical sensitivity but clinical sensibility when working with their clients. This statement is as true for brain dysfunctional patients as it is for psychiatric patients.

Art and the Patient's Phenomenological Experience

Patients' artistic expressions can help clarify their personal experience. Over the years, I have collected many pictures from patients and have listened to their favorite music or fairy tales. The two pictures reproduced in this chapter illustrate how art can help therapists to enter patients' phenomenological fields. The first drawing is by a psychologist who had hemorrhagic contusions in the frontal and parietal areas after a severe TBI. The patient was a scholar as well as an artist. When asked during an art class to draw himself as a room in a house, he portrayed himself as a closet (Fig. 2-2). In our society, the phrase "coming out of the closet" refers to identifying one's self as having a special problem that is difficult to admit publicly. Admitting to having suffered a severe brain injury would be difficult for anyone, but perhaps especially so for scholars. This patient's picture is also rich with symbolism regarding the problem of impaired self-awareness and its positive and negative manifestations.

The second picture (Fig. 2-3) reveals a multitude of feelings and reactions a person experienced but could not easily discuss after brain injury. The artist, a young woman with a gunshot wound to the left hemisphere, had an intense negative reaction at one point in her neuropsychological rehabilitation. She literally was unable to talk about the issue. Within the context of a therapeutic relationship, however, she drew a picture that depicted her sense of anger as well as her feelings of sadness, depression and confusion—all common reactions after brain injury. This particular drawing is discussed in Chapter 9 and its importance in establishing a therapeutic alliance clarified. The drawing, however, helped the psychotherapist understand, for the first time, what this woman was actually experiencing.

A third picture (not presented in this text) revealed another side of brain injury. A person who suffered an apparently mild (but still significant) brain injury painted a picture for me after I gave a lecture on the problem of "lost normality" after brain injury. The surrealistic painting had a box in the upper left-hand corner that read "Y B N₀rmal."

The picture revealed a sense of depression, and it raises the provocative question of why patients should even consider psychotherapy after

Figure 2-2. Drawing made by a psychologist who represented himself as a closet in a house after he suffered a severe traumatic brain injury.

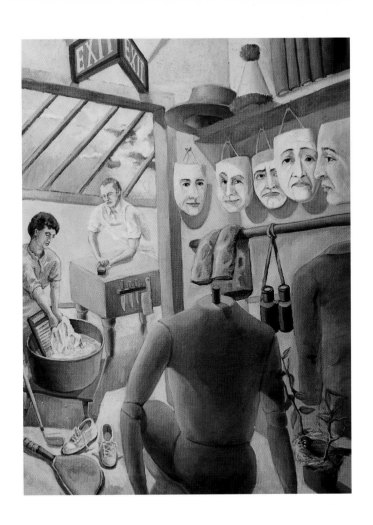

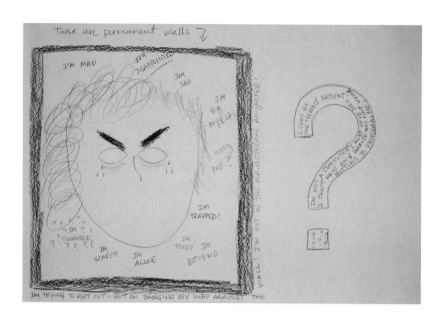

brain injury. When people ask "why be normal," they are often asking, "why should I follow the rules of society or attempt to behave in a manner that makes others happy with me?" This, of course, is not the goal of psychotherapy. Psychotherapy attempts to help individuals adjust interpersonally but not at the price of their individuality (see Chapter 9). Certainly, altered or lost normality (when defining normality as the premorbid state) is a problem of considerable importance after brain injury (Prigatano, 1995), and it must be approached through a variety of avenues. Drawings can convey a unique sense of the patient's phenomenological field.

The Nature of Higher Cerebral Functions in the Light of Human Experience

Does the experience of brain damage have anything to teach us about the nature of higher cerebral functions? A traditionally held view is that the higher cerebral functions are all "mental" and that the "lower" cerebral functions tend to be seen as "emotional" or reflexive (Mandler, 1984). These lower functions can affect higher cerebral functions, but should be separated from them. Also, higher cerebral functions are considered to make use of information processes in nonconscious systems (Kihlstrom, 1987; Posner, 1990), but that does not mean that the higher cerebral functions themselves are nonconscious. This traditionally held view is biased. It is biased because of our preoccupation with the view that "reason" and "intelligence" are the "true" higher cerebral functions. Observing brain dysfunctional patients, as well as gifted scientists and artists, teaches us something different.

More than one accomplished scientist has described his or her accomplishments in noncognitive terms. They may report having an intuition that the answer to a complicated mathematical problem was different from what the known rules of mathematics would have predicted. Artists will often describe themselves as simply a medium by which a poem, painting, or statue is created. They experience, in essence, something that leads to creative problem solving that is not purely rational. Why do theorists of higher brain function neglect this phenomenon?

Also, as just illustrated, brain dysfunctional patients often experience an integrated mixture of cognitive and affective disturbances. These observations should be considered when evaluating what is meant by the terms "higher brain function" or "higher cerebral functions."

Figure 2-3. Drawing made by a young woman after she sustained a gunshot wound to the left hemisphere: it depicts the anger, sadness, depression, and confusion associated with her altered state.

Higher Cerebral Functions—A Beginning Perspective

As noted in Chapter 1, J. Hughlings Jackson observed that higher mental functions are the "most complex, but least organized." That is, mental functions seem to emerge from a potentially wide array of possibilities. Undoubtedly, they follow some principles of organization, but these organizing principles seem to have considerable degrees of freedom (to use a statistical analogy) as they develop and function. These higher mental functions also seem to be distributed over wide areas of the brain and are not limited to the cortex. Brain activation studies have clearly documented this fact (Roland, 1993).

Luria (1966) constructed a useful definition of higher cortical functions. In his 1966 book, he states the following: "From the point of view of modern psychology, the higher human mental functions are complex reflex processes, social in origin, mediate in structure, and conscious and voluntary in mode of function" (p. 32). He continues to say: "Speech plays a decisive role in the mediation of mental processes" (p. 33).

The notion that higher cerebral functions are basically reflex processes has been challenged (Pribram, 1971) and has given way to broader information-processing models (Mesulum, 1990). Few would challenge, however, the notion that the higher cerebral functions are highly contingent on environmental inputs and may well be social in origin. The development of language is the classic example of this phenomenon. Whether we speak English or Japanese seems to depend on the speech sounds we hear as we grow and develop our abilities to communicate with our early significant others.

The question arises, however, are functions such as speech and language purely cortical in nature or do they involve subcortical regions as well? The use of positron emission tomography (PET) studies argues that various aspects of language require multiple brain regions, not simply the cortex (Wise et al., 1991).

Weinstein (Prigatano and Weinstein, 1996) reminds us of Sapir's interesting observation that "Language was not only a device for reporting experience, but also, to a considerable degree, defined experience for its speakers . . ." (p. 2). Thus, in its written and spoken forms, language allows us to define what we think, feel, and experience. Our choice of words clarifies for ourselves and others what we actually experience. This integrated activity suggests that the higher brain functions are not purely "cortical" in nature.

The most interesting and perplexing aspect of Luria's (1966) definition, however, is his statement that higher cerebral functions are "mediate in structure." What does this phrase mean? Luria appears to mean that an essential feature of these higher cerebral functions is that information is coded in such a manner that the structure of information is mediated by something that in and of itself has no information. His classical example was tying a knot in a handkerchief to remind oneself to do something. If, for example, I tie a knot in my handkerchief to remember to call a friend at night, there is no "information in the knot." Yet, when I return home, empty my pockets, and see the knotted handkerchief, I instantly remember there is something I must do and often immediately recall that I must call my friend. How the brain actually accomplishes this "mediate" function remains an essential mystery of the neurosciences.

Finally, Luria (1966) suggests that higher mental or "cortical" functions are conscious and voluntary in their mode of function. Despite our failure to define consciousness precisely (see Prigatano and Schacter, 1991), there is agreement about this issue. Otherwise, we all function within the context of our own personal psychotic fantasies. The higher cerebral functions, by definition, seem to be conscious, but are other aspects of higher brain functions beyond consciousness? Freud (1924) believed that this was indeed the case, as we will consider shortly.

What about the voluntary component of higher cerebral functions? When I *want* (that is, will or have a volition) to talk, I begin to say words. If I cannot do this, my higher cerebral functioning is impaired. An inability to perform when an individual desires to do so often indicates a disturbance in higher cerebral functioning. Thus, the voluntary mode of higher brain functions seems self-evident. Do higher brain functions, however, also have an involuntary component? Do they have a nonconscious component as some artists and scientists suggest?

Higher Brain Functions:
The Perspective of a Practicing Clinical Neuropsychologist

Observations from patients who have suffered brain injury as well as observations from normal childhood development suggest that a modification of Luria's (1966) definition may be useful.

Higher cerebral brain functions appear to be both convergent (meaning integrated) and emergent (meaning relational) information-processing systems that have both feedback and feedforward features that permit problem solving. Although social in origin, higher cerebral functions are not limited to conscious and voluntary modes of action but may be unconscious (or nonconscious) and "reflexive." They are constantly in a state of change because speech and language as well as memory and feeling states modify their structure and expression.

Starting with clinical observations, disturbances in self-awareness after brain injury seem to reflect more than a disturbance of perception or a failure of information to be matched or mismatched (Miller et al., 1960). Disturbances in self-awareness appear to be disturbances in experience. By definition, consciousness, an emergent brain function (Sperry, 1974), is more than a purely cognitive act. It is the act of human experience that, by definition, seems to include thinking and feeling.

Second, the act of spoken communication (speech), which is formed in a social milieu, is composed of specific vowel-consonant sounds and, ultimately, of words or phrases that are associated with more than a cognitive component (i.e., the denotation of the words). An affective component (i.e., the connotation of the word or message) is also present and can be purposely and simultaneously used.

It is also evident that the capacity for problem solving is inherent in what we mean by higher cerebral brain functions. Problem solving depends on information processing, but information processing, in and of itself, does not equal the type of problem solving that is meant by the term higher cerebral function. Often, solutions to problems arise when various sources of information converge so that they can be compared and contrasted—this is an integrated function. When this convergent activity occurs, something *new* for the problem solver (the person) seems to emerge. We often call this "insight," and the experience is frequently associated with a simultaneous affective sense of satisfaction. This feeling state associated with achieving the right answer should not be excluded from the definition of higher cerebral functions.

Are higher cerebral functions limited to conscious and voluntary modes of expression? It is highly doubtful that they are. Consider first the automatic or "reflexive" aspect of higher cerebral functioning. Listen to certain music (e.g., the American National Anthem) or certain speeches (e.g., Lincoln's Gettysburg Address or Martin Luther King's "I Have a Dream") and note the automatic and autonomic experience it invokes in people from that culture. Look at certain forms of art (e.g., the Mona Lisa or the Night Watch) and experience a reaction that seems uncontrolled or nonvoluntary. Our ability to respond to symbols, by definition, is possible through the higher cerebral functions. Symbols, by their nature, invoke not only a thinking component but a feeling component that is not immediately under subjective control. Jung (1964) recognized this aspect of symbols, which he tried to portray in his very important book, *Man and His Symbols*. We should not forget this component of higher cerebral functioning when attempting to define it.

What about the nonconscious aspects of higher cerebral functioning? This issue can be hotly debated, but any practicing psychotherapist who has stumbled on a repressed memory knows the reality that higher cerebral functions are not purely conscious. Patients may demonstrate in their behavior and in their subjective feeling states an intense anger that is disproportional to a specific incident. Patients experience this affect as uncontrollable and can recognize the illogical aspects of their behavior. Nevertheless, they still experience intense, uncontrollable anger with the slightest provocation. In the course of psychotherapy, they may suddenly remember an event that seems to be attached to the angry feelings they experience. Yet, previously they had no recollection of the event despite its tremendous impact upon them. Such was the case of a woman who suddenly remembered being raped by her brother but which she had not thought of for years. Suddenly she was aware of a feeling-memory that helped explain why she was so angry in her daily life. Collectively, these phenomena constitute what is meant by higher brain functions.

Summary and Conclusions

The first step in neuropsychological assessment and rehabilitation is to approach a patient's disturbance of higher brain functioning in a manner that reveals what the patient is experiencing. By entering the patient's phenomenological field, the therapist can identify a sense of what frustrates and confuses the patient. A beginning working relationship (or therapeutic alliance) can be established by taking initial steps to reduce this frustration and confusion. It is the first step in neuropsychological rehabilitation (Principle 1).

This chapter emphasizes the importance of the phenomenological method as an adjunct to the traditional scientific approach in the evaluation and care of brain dysfunctional patients. The strength of contemporary neuropsychology lies in its use of the scientific method. That method insists on careful controlled observations and reliable checks on information as it relates to brain-behavior disturbances. The phenomenological method is being invoked to supplement, not to supplant, the scientific approach.

This chapter also briefly considers the nature of higher cerebral or brain functions in light of human experience. While the nature of these functions can only be broadly defined, they provide a starting point for understanding the complicated symptoms caused by brain damage. Successful neuropsychological rehabilitation is built on understanding those symptoms and helping the patient and family cope with them. Often, the patient's symptoms reflect a complicated interaction of numerous factors, including the patient's premorbid state and the changes produced by altered brain physiology and structure (Principle 2). Chapter 3 thus considers Principle 2 in more detail.

References

Amsel, A. (1958). The role of frustrative nonreward in noncontinuous reward situations. *Psychol. Bull.* 55: 102–119.

Bennett, B. E., Bryant, B. K., VandenBos, G. R., and Greenwood, A. (1990). *Professional Liability and Risk Management*. American Psychological Association, Washington, D.C.

Benson, D. F. (1993). Aphasia. In K. M. Heilman and E. Valenstein (eds), *Clinical Neuropsychology* (3rd ed, pp. 17–36). Oxford University Press, New York.

Ben-Yishay, Y., and Prigatano, G. P. (1990). Cognitive remediation. In E. Griffith, M. Rosenthal, M. R. Bond, and J. D. Miller (eds), *Rehabilitation of the Adult and Child with Traumatic Brain Injury* (pp. 393–409). F. A. Davis, Philadelphia.

Brodal, A. (1973). Self-observations and neuro-anatomical considerations after a stroke. *Brain* 96: 675–694.

Chapman, L. F., and Wolff, H. G. (1959). The cerebral hemispheres and the highest integrative functions of man. *Arch. Neurol.* 1, 357–424.

Dollard, J., and Miller, N. E. (1950). *Personality and Psychotherapy.* Hill, New York.

Franzen, E. A., and Myers, R. E. (1973). Neural control of social behavior: Prefrontal and anterior temporal cortex. *Neuropsychologia* 11: 141–157.

Freud, S. (1924). *A General Introduction to Psychoanalysis* (24th ed). Simon and Schuster, New York.

Gans, J. S. (1983). Hate in the rehabilitation setting. *Arch. Phys. Med. Rehabil.* 64: 176–179.

Goldstein, K. (1952). The effect of brain damage on the personality. *Psychiatry* 15, 245–260.

Jung, C. G. (1964). *Man and His Symbols.* Doubleday Windfall, Garden City, NY.

Kalff, D. M. (1980). *Sandplay.* Sigo Press, Boston.

Kihlstrom, J. F. (1987). The cognitive unconscious. *Science* 237: 1445–1452.

LaBaw, W. L. (1969). Denial inside out: Subjective experience with anosognosia in closed head injury. *Psychiatry* 32(1): 174–191.

Lawsen, R. (1965). *Frustration: The Development of a Scientific Concept.* Macmillan, New York.

Levin, H. S., Benton, A. L., and Grossman, R. G. (1982). *Neurobehavioral Consequences of Closed Head Injury.* Oxford University Press, New York.

Levin, H. S., Gary, H. E., Eisenberg, H. M., Ruff, R. M., Barth, J. T., Kreutzer, J., High, W. M., Portman, S., Foulkes, M. A., Jane, J. A., Marmarou, A., and Marshall, L. F. (1990). Neurobehavioral outcome 1 year after severe head injury: experience of the Traumatic Coma Data Bank. *J. Neurosurg.* 73: 699–709.

Luria, A. R. (1966). *Higher Cerebral Functions in Man.* Basic Books, New York.

Mandler, G. (1984). *Mind and Body. Psychology of Emotion and Stress.* W. W. Norton, New York.

Mesulam, M-M. (1990). Large-scale neurocognitive networks and distributed processing of attention, language, and memory. *Ann. Neurol.* 28(5): 597–613.

Miller, G. A., Galanter, E. G., and Pribram K. H. (1960). *Plans and the Structure of Behavior.* Rinehart and Weinstein, New York.

Posner, M. I. (1990). *Foundations of Cognitive Science.* Massachusetts Institute of Technology, Cambridge, Massachusetts.

Pribram, K. H. (1971). *Languages of the Brain: Experimental Paradoxes and Principles in Neuropsychology.* Prentice-Hall, Englewood Cliffs, NJ.

Prigatano, G. P. (1989). Bring it up in milieu: toward effective traumatic brain injury rehabilitation interaction. *Rehabilitation Psychology* 34(2): 135–144.

ction`

Prigatano, G. P. (1991a). The relationship of frontal lobe damage to diminished awareness: Studies in rehabilitation. In H. S. Levin, H. M. Eisenberg, and A. L. Benton (eds), *Frontal Lobe Function and Dysfunction* (pp. 381–397). Oxford University Press, New York.

Prigatano, G. P. (1991b). Disordered mind, wounded soul: the emerging role of psychotherapy in rehabilitation after brain injury. *Journal of Head Trauma Rehabilitation* 6(4): 1–10.

Prigatano, G. P. (1992). Personality disturbances associated with traumatic brain injury. *J. Consult. Clin. Psychol.* 60(3): 360–368.

Prigatano, G. P. (1995). 1994 Sheldon Berrol, MD, Senior Lectureship: The problem of lost normality after brain injury. *Journal of Head Trauma Rehabilitation* 10(3): 87–95.

Prigatano, G. P., and Henderson, S. (1997). Cognitive outcome after subarachnoid hemorrhage. In J. B. Bederson (ed), *Subarachnoid Hemorrhage: Pathophysiology and Management* (pp. 27–40). American Association of Neurological Surgeons, Park Ridge, Ill.

Prigatano, G. P., Fordyce, D. J., Zeiner, H. K. Roueche, J. R., Pepping, M., and Wood, B. C. (1986). *Neuropsychological Rehabilitation After Brain Injury.* Johns Hopkins University Press, Baltimore.

Prigatano, G. P., and Schacter, D. L. (1991). *Awareness of Deficit After Brain Injury: Clinical and Theoretical Issues.* Oxford University Press, New York.

Prigatano, G. P., and Weinstein, E. A. (1996). Edwin A. Weinstein's contributions to neuropsychological rehabilitation. *Neuropsychological Rehabilitation* 6(4): 305–326.

Rogers, C. R. (1951). *Client-Centered Therapy: Its Current Practice, Implications, and Theory.* Houghton Mifflin, Boston.

Roland, P. E. (1993). *Brain Activation.* Wiley-Liss, New York.

Russell, W. R. (1971). *The Traumatic Amnesias.* Oxford University Press, London.

Satz, P. (1966). Specific and nonspecific effects of brain lesions in man. *J. Abnorm. Psychol.* 71: 56–70.

Schafer, R. (1967). *Projective Testing and Psychoanalysis.* International Universities, New York.

Sperry, R. (1974). Lateral specialization in the surgically separated hemispheres. In F. O. Schmitt and F. G. Worden (eds), *The Neurosciences* (pp. 5–19). Massachusetts Institute of Technology, Cambridge, Mass.

Stuss, D. T., and Benson, D. F. (1986). *The Frontal Lobes.* Raven, New York.

Wise, R. J., Hadar, U., Howard, D., and Patterson, K. (1991). Language activation studies with positron emission tomography. *Exploring Brain Functional Anatomy with Positron Tomography* (pp. 218–228). John Wiley & Sons, Chichester, England.

3

The Symptom Picture and the Neglected Problem of Premorbid Cognitive and Personality Factors

> The findings of the current study indicate that the personality alterations noted in DAT [dementia of the Alzheimer's type] are an integral part of the clinical syndrome. Like the intellectual deterioration, they reflect the structural and functional alterations produced by the disease process.
>
> S. Petry, J. L. Cummings, M. A. Hill, and J. Shapira, "Personality alterations in dementia of the Alzheimer's type," 1988, p. 1190

> ... irrational actions after the brain injury are not simply a manifestation of overall loss of judgment but can be selective and have a particular significance for the person.
>
> E. A. Weinstein, "Why do some patients confabulate after brain injury," 1995

Given that a clinical neuropsychologist has some understanding of what patients experience after brain injury and given that a psychologist can conceptualize, at least in broad terms, the nature of the patients' higher cerebral functioning, the next step is to reveal the patients' higher cerebral disturbances via a neuropsychological examination *without* overwhelming them.*

The examination must be conducted in a respectful manner. Consequently, the examining clinical neuropsychologist must have some sense of what patients were like before the brain damage was sustained and how they may be reacting to the disturbances that the brain damage has caused. The examining clinical neuropsychologist must also know how to put patients at ease and how to examine them in a way that allows both patients and the neuropsychologist to experience "what is wrong."

---

*For discussions of dimensions involved in a neuropsychological examination, see Prigatano, 1996, and Prigatano and Henderson, 1997.

This expertise is the "art" of a successful neuropsychological examination.

The importance of this approach for neuropsychological rehabilitation is that the ultimate goal of such rehabilitation is to teach patients in a humane fashion how to understand their disturbances, and, in so doing, better manage the effects of brain damage. It therefore becomes exceedingly important for the clinical neuropsychologist to understand what the predictable neuropsychological disturbances associated with various brain injuries are and how the patients' symptom picture may reflect both the direct and indirect effects of brain disturbance, to use Goldstein's (1942) terminology.

The Traditional Neurobiological Approach

It is well established that brain lesions produce predictable neuropsychological disturbances and syndromes (e.g., Bisiach and Vallar, 1988; Benson, 1988; Frederiks, 1985). If it were otherwise, neurologists and neuropsychologists would have no body of scientific knowledge on which to base the practice of behavioral neurology and clinical neuropsychology. When a patient shows a pattern of behavioral characteristics that has been studied in other patients with similar pathological processes in a particular region of the brain, the brain disturbance is attributed as the *cause* of the behavioral or psychological abnormality.

If important differences are noted among patients with common symptoms or syndromes, the differences are typically explained by two anatomical facts. First, no two lesions of the brain are exactly the same. Second, no two brains have exactly the same structure, physiology, or chemical features. Biological variation may therefore account for differences in symptom pictures. Another possibility, however, is that patients' cognitive, emotional, and motivational characteristics that predate the onset of their neuropsychological impairments interact with lesion location, size, and type in a very complicated way to produce variability in the symptom picture.

In other words, the observed symptom may reflect not only a disruptive process within the brain (i.e., the neurobiological approach) but also individuals' adaptive efforts to cope with the effects of brain damage (i.e., the psychosocial approach). Goldstein (1942, 1952) emphasized that an organism *always* attempts to adapt to its environment while it concomitantly attempts to actualize its potential. In some sense, the process is paradoxical: The goal of a given complex psychological process is simultaneously adaptation to external conditions and the expression of internal processes that reflect the individuals' desire to actualize their capacities and potentials. Goldstein (1942, 1952) emphasized this theory as organismic or holistic. In his theory of individuation, Jung (1957) emphasized this same concept from an analytic perspective.

If this premise is accepted, then the patient's preinjury or premorbid status always interacts with neuropsychologically based disturbances to produce the symptom profile (i.e., Principle 2). Although this problem has been recognized, it has not been studied sufficiently, presumably because many important premorbid factors are difficult to measure.

What Behaviors Are Directly Caused by Brain Dysfunction?

Cummings and his colleagues (Petry et al., 1988; Dian et al., 1990) have argued that patients with dementia show definitive personality changes that are a direct consequence of the disease state and are not a "release" of premorbid personality characteristics. From their perspective, the type and the location of the brain disturbance in demented patients greatly influence the symptom profile. Therefore, clinicians may erroneously attribute behavioral problems to premorbid states.

Weinstein (see Prigatano and Weinstein, 1996) notes, however, that patient behavior is related to several factors: (1) the type, severity, rate of onset, location, and extent of brain pathology; (2) the nature of the disability; (3) the *meaning* of the incapacity as determined by the patient's premorbid experience and values; and (4) the milieu in which the behavior is elicited and observed.

A recent clinical example* illustrates the heuristic value of this integrative approach. At his wife's request, a successful but aging Norwegian businessman resigned from his prosperous business, which he had established and which had made him independently wealthy. Apparently, his memory and judgment were declining slowly. Soon thereafter, his wife scheduled him for a neurological consultation. He was diagnosed with probable Alzheimer's disease. The medical authorities suggested that she contact various social agencies to help care for her husband. Dedicated and competent, she declined, preferring to manage her husband in their home.

The wife was successful until she herself became ill. One evening she had ominous chest pains and contacted her physician, who came to their home. Recognizing that she was gravely ill and that her husband could not be left home alone, the doctor hospitalized both of them. That evening, the patient's wife died of a heart attack. The nursing staff informed the husband (the Alzheimer's patient) that his wife had passed away and that he now needed to go to a rest home with a special unit that would care for his needs.

Before his wife's death, this patient had been cooperative and easy to manage. He never showed angry outbursts although he was easily con-

---

*The author thanks Hallgrim Kløve, Ph.D., for bringing this example to his attention on February 13, 1995.

fused about time and place. Under his wife's care and in familiar surroundings, he presented no behavioral problems whatsoever. After the abrupt change in his circumstances and the unexplained absence of his wife (he could not remember what he was told), he became belligerent and angry. He pounded on the walls and screamed, asking where his wife was. The absence of personal possessions, such as the family's silverware, also distressed him. His behavior deteriorated to such an extent that he was placed on Haldol®. This medication produced the predictable motor tremors but effected no change in his behavior.

An astute geropsychologist recognized that the patient had only fragmented memories of what had happened to him and decided to help him reconstruct his past. She took him to his wife's grave and videotaped him placing flowers on her tombstone. She took him to his home, which had been sold without his knowledge, and also videotaped him there. She repetitively told him that he had had a business, a loving and devoted wife, and a good life. After this repetitive reconstruction of his life via the videotapes and verbal rehearsals of significant events, his behavioral symptoms disappeared.

Without the efforts of a dedicated clinician, this patient's behavioral outbursts could easily have been attributed to the direct effects of brain dysfunction caused by his dementia. Only by attempting to understand the patient's feelings could the clinician determine the factors that contributed to the expression of his particular symptom profile. Retrospectively, it is easy to understand how the changes in the patient's life, coupled with his cognitive impairments, interacted to produce his belligerence. All too often, however, clinicians fail to consider the contributions of patients' subjective experiences to the expression of their symptoms, particularly if a higher cerebral dysfunction is present. Consequently, it is important to examine the meaning of the term, symptom, in relation to higher cerebral dysfunction.

What Is a Symptom?

Webster's (1983) states that a symptom is a sign that "indicates the existence or occurrence of something else" (p. 1849). In medicine (and related health care disciplines), a symptom refers to "... any condition accompanying or resulting from a disease and serving as an aid in diagnosis" (p. 1849). Webster's also describes it as a "perceptible change in the body or its function which indicates disease" (p. 1849). Many neuropsychological *symptoms* indicate or suggest brain dysfunction. Satz (1966) has classified such symptoms as both nonspecific and specific to different brain regions.

Memory impairment is perhaps the most recognized symptom. Depending on their severity and association with other symptoms, memory disturbances can reflect generalized brain dysfunction or specific syndromes. Thus, the term *amnestic syndrome* is used to describe memory impairment associated with normal problem-solving skills or general intelligence level. The term typically applies to specific subcortical dysfunctions (Squire, 1991). In other instances, memory impairment is associated with a generalized cognitive decline and may be associated with slowed information processing, impaired judgment, impaired intellectual ability, and language impairment. In these cases, memory disturbance is a part of a broader clinical syndrome that is sometimes termed *dementia* (see DSM-IV classification schema, American Psychiatric Association, 1994). *Syndrome* therefore refers to the blending or running together of specific signs (or symptoms) that characterize a specific disease state or condition (Webster's, 1983).

Given this definition, what is a neuropsychological symptom and how might it relate to premorbid factors? Frederiks (1985) comments about neuropsychological symptoms as follows: "A neuropsychological symptom is not quite the same as a classic neurological symptom. The neurological symptom is characterized by its predictable localizability" (p. 3).

Neuropsychological symptoms, however, are less easily predicted on the basis of anatomy and physiology. Many factors influence the manifestation of symptoms: the patient's age and sex; the site, lateralization, and size of the lesion; its nature and behavior (growth rate and recovery); the number of lesions and their stage; the presence of congenital anomalies; and, finally, the patient's "personality, education, skills, culture status, linguistic region, state of consciousness, motivation, etc." (Frederiks, 1985, p. 8). Lumping the latter higher-order factors into one category leaves much to be desired from a scientific perspective. Each of these factors is exceedingly important in understanding a patient's symptom profile, particularly in rehabilitation.

Positive and Negative Symptoms After Brain Damage

John Hughlings Jackson (as cited in Taylor, 1931–1932) distinguished between positive and negative symptoms associated with lesions of the central nervous system. Negative symptoms reflected a loss of function; positive symptoms reflected efforts to cope with the loss of function. Building on this distinction, Goldstein (1942) referred to negative and positive symptoms as *direct* versus *indirect* consequences of brain injury. This distinction is crucial when attempting to understand how premorbid factors influence the patient's symptom profile and how environmental factors may influence behavior after brain injury.

A direct neuropsychological symptom is a loss of some behavioral or psychological capacity as a direct consequence of disruption of a function or functional subsystem of the brain (Luria, 1966). It is, in the truest sense, a failure of production or accomplishment. It means a loss of the capacity to store, represent, or act upon information within the brain. For example, lesions affecting the pyramidal tract may lead to various losses indicative of motor dysfunction. Hand and arm movements are restricted. There can be a loss of finger dexterity, flexibility, and, at times "motor programming" (Angevine and Cotman, 1981).

Other examples of direct symptoms are language and memory disturbances. Left hemisphere lesions, posterior to the Rolandic fissure and involving the superior portion of the temporal lobe and the arcuate fasciculus, respectively (Benson, 1993), can lead to specific problems with auditory comprehension or sentence repetition. Lesions anywhere in the brain, however, can interfere with the ability to name objects rapidly (Geschwind, 1967). A substantial decrease in simple verbal fluency when asked to generate words that begin with certain letters is particularly associated with frontal lesions (Benson, 1993). As noted, changes in memory can be specific or can reflect diffuse damage within the brain (Squire, 1991). Premorbid factors likely have less impact (but not an absence of impact) on these negative or direct symptoms of brain injury.

In contrast, indirect or positive symptoms are the ones most likely to be influenced by premorbid factors and the social milieu. A positive neuropsychological symptom after brain injury is the brain's (mind's) attempt to satisfy an environmental demand or an internal biological need with existing or residual information processing systems. Positive symptoms are indirectly caused by brain injury insofar as they reflect the brain's residual capacity and struggle to adapt to the negative effects of brain injury or to avoid or escape that struggle (Goldstein, 1942, p. 69). In this case, premorbid factors or factors that exist in the brain (and emerge in terms of mental activity) that were not damaged directly exert a powerful influence on the individual's behavior and psychological functioning after injury.

At present, neuropsychological rehabilitation has more to offer patients in terms of their indirect neuropsychological symptoms than their direct symptoms. This fact explains why a healthy respect for how premorbid factors can and do influence the patient's symptom profile is badly needed and is useful in neuropsychological rehabilitation.

Premorbid Factors That Contribute to the Symptom Picture

When considering how individuals attempt to cope or avoid the struggles associated with brain dysfunction, clinicians must understand how preexisting characteristics naturally influence patients' behavior and functioning. Previous methods of coping seem to be highly influenced by the individual's age, stage of psychosocial development, educational background, level of intellectual functioning before the onset of brain injury, and the socio-cultural setting in which patients find themselves after brain injury (compared to before the brain injury).

Age and Psychosocial Stage of Development

Numerous studies have documented that an individual's age correlates with certain neuropsychological characteristics (Prigatano and Parsons, 1976; Prigatano et al., 1995). It is well known that in adulthood the speed of information processing declines as a function of age (Schaiel and Zelinski, 1978). Short-term memory also often declines (Gilbert and Levee, 1971; Storandt, 1991). For example, after the age of 70 years, normal individuals typically recall only two of four words after a brief distraction (Jenkyn et al., 1985) compared to young adults who can easily recall all four words.

In a recent normative study for a new screening test of higher cerebral function (Prigatano et al., 1991, 1993), only 70% of normal persons older than 60 years could recall three of three words after being distracted for 5 to 10 minutes. In contrast, 97.8% of the subjects between the ages of 15 to 39 years could perform this task. Age therefore clearly relates to memory and speed-of-information processing skills. In an older population, brain damage may exacerbate these already developing disturbances.

Studying the neurobehavioral consequences of closed head injury in patients 50 years of age or older, Goldstein and colleagues (1994) report significant sequela even when the judged severity of the brain injury was considered mild to moderate. They noted ". . . the classification of 'mild' head injury in a young person may represent a moderate injury in an older one" (p. 964).

At the other end of the age continuum, Levin and colleagues (1994) noted that the performance of children with traumatic brain injury (TBI) on the *Tower of London Test*, a test of abstract reasoning and the ability to follow rules, differed as a function of their age at injury. Compared to older children with TBIs (between 11 and 16 years old), younger children (between 6 and 10 years old) broke more rules in solving this task, particularly when the task became more complex. There was a three-way interaction among severity of injury, the child's age at testing, and the complexity of the task presented. Clearly, age affects the so-called direct effects of brain injury. Yet it has been difficult to differentiate the effects of these individual factors, and further research is needed.

What is, perhaps, better appreciated is that age, particularly once young adulthood is reached, influences how the indirect consequences of the brain injury are manifested. In the course of neuropsychologically oriented rehabilitation, how patients approach the rehabilitation experience differs predictably with their age. Older adolescents or young adults who have never faced a tragedy or major change in their life may find it particularly difficult to cope with the effects of brain injury. They display considerable resistance to various forms of rehabilitation and insist that they can return to school or work or drive a car before their therapists judge it wise.

In contrast, middle-aged and older individuals who have experienced a significant loss in their life often put their brain injury into a more realistic perspective because they have already made reasonable adjustments to the vicissitudes of life before their brain injury (Prigatano, 1991a). Older individuals, close to retirement, may even readily accept some of the changes as long as they do not impinge on their ability to enjoy their retirement years. Many of these patients, for example, are not eager to return to gainful employment but want the freedom to drive a car or to manage their money independently. Thus, an individual's age seems to influence which disturbances will likely provoke the most anxiety and which disturbances will be accepted as a part of everyday life.

Although the effects of psychosocial development on the indirect symptom profile have not been studied, it seems probable that the stages (as outlined by Erik Erikson in Hall and Lindzey, 1978) would influence how individuals deal with the struggle to adapt after a brain insult. Even if one rejects Erikson's eight stages of psychosocial development, people's patterns of emotional and motivational responses at injury correlate with their behavior after injury. Weinstein and colleagues (1956) reported, for example, that the premorbid personality of brain dysfunctional patients with specific delusions about children after their injury differed from that of patients who did not show this phenomenon. They stated that "The most striking and consistent finding in the group described in this study was the great degree to which the patient had structured his life in terms of the parent-child relationship" (p. 294). When the brain is injured, reality is reconstructed based on past modes of thinking and feeling. Thus, upon emerging from a coma, TBI patients describe their environment from the perspective of their prevailing preoccupations in life (Prigatano, 1991b).

Ongoing patterns of interpersonal interaction also seem to influence how patients behave in neuropsychological rehabilitation. A brief example highlights this point. Two patients suffered bilateral frontal lobe injuries—one incurred a TBI; the other had a ruptured aneurysm of the anterior communicating artery. On magnetic resonance (MR) imaging, both patients had clear orbitofrontal damage, although the latter's injury was more extensive. The first patient was a 19-year-old male with a history of dishonest behavior and manipulation. There was considerable evidence that he was struggling to establish his sense of identity as well as to deal with issues of intimacy. The second patient was an accomplished and productive 50-year-old engineer whose behavior had been quite appropriate before his aneurysm ruptured. At the time of his brain insult, he was interested in contributing ideas at work and showed sincere concern for others in his role as manager.

After their brain injuries, both patients were described as having trouble inhibiting their behavior, which was described as "socially inappropriate." The teenager's socially inappropriate responses, however, were expressed sexually. The patient often touched his crotch in the presence of female therapists and gave a sly, childlike smile when caught. He seemed to delight in irritating the female therapists, who were frustrated because they could not get him to behave more honestly and less childishly.

The second patient appeared confused and mildly distressed when his behavior frustrated his therapists. Neither his remarks nor his behavior was ever sexually inappropriate. Rather, his behavioral difficulties consisted of unpredictable and intensely angry outbursts that were always directed at his mother, who asked a variety of essentially unanswerable questions. She also appeared very unsympathetic to her son's changed circumstances. She spoke to him as if he were a child rather than a once accomplished engineer who had suffered a brain injury. Her authoritarian manner obviously irritated him, and he responded angrily because he no longer knew how to respond verbally to her comments.

The behavior of both patients was disinhibited, presumably as a direct result of frontal lobe damage. The expression of that disinhibited behavior, however, partially reflected their individual stage of development and preinjury patterns of emotional and motivational responding.

Although an oversimplification, one concept that emerges when considering Goldstein's work (1952) is that brain injury seems to reduce a person's existing coping strategies. If an injury to any part of the brain lowers coping skills, it is reasonable to assume that premorbid adjustment problems and issues would be more difficult to handle after brain injury than before. Therefore, a person's stage of psychosocial development would appear to be crucial to understanding the symptom profile.

Size, location, and type of brain injury, however, might be equally important and, in some instances, more important than premorbid factors in influencing the symptom picture. The work of Chapman and Wolff (1959) and Kiev and colleagues (1962) bears on this problem. In an attempt to describe the rich variety of behavioral disturbances associated with brain insults, they studied patients with focal and diffuse losses of cerebral tissue (30 to 150 gm):

> The subject's prevailing premorbid defenses were preserved in general form and were exhibited, especially during periods of stress. However, after loss of cerebral hemisphere tissue the defensive and compensatory reactions were less well organized, less well sustained, and less effective in maintaining tranquility and permitting continued fulfillment of social and interpersonal responsibilities. This led to behavior that was less acceptable socially, more highly personalized, and sometimes bizarre. The degree of impairment in the capacity to maintain effective defenses, although linked to the mass of the tissue loss, was not related to the site of the tissue loss within the cerebral hemispheres (p. 384).

They suggested that the less the tissue loss, the more preserved premorbid coping strategies would be. Clearly, more work is needed on this important topic.

Education

Unlike age, an individual's educational level may buffer the effects of brain dysfunction. This possibility was suggested by a study that measured change in cognitive functioning for a large group of elderly individuals with different educational backgrounds (Evans et al., 1993). Persons in either of two age ranges (65 to 74 and > 75 years) with less education showed a greater decline in memory and mental status over time than persons with higher levels of education (Fig. 3-1). Level of

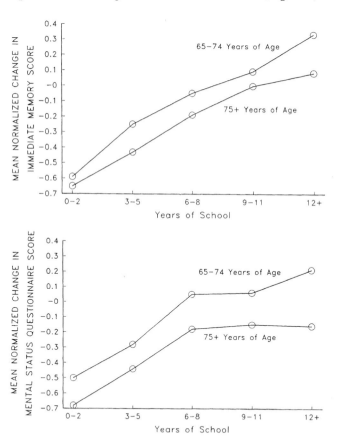

Figure 3-1. Mean normalized change in (top) immediate memory test scores and (bottom) mental status according to years of education for those aged 65 to 74 years old and those 75 years and older. Reprinted from *Annals of Epidemiology*, Volume 3, Evans, D. A., Beckett, L. A., Albert, M. S., Hebert, L. E. Scherr, P. A., Funkenstein, H. H., and Taylor, J. O., Level of education and change in cognitive function in a community population of older persons, pp. 71–77, 1993, with permission from Elsevier Science.

education may therefore serve some protective function, at least in normal aging.

Although age often correlates negatively with level of performance on neuropsychological tests, education tends to correlate positively (i.e., the higher the level, the better the performance). Both the effects of age and education, however, seem to be attenuated by brain injury. For example, in a recent standardization study of the BNI Screen for Higher Cerebral Functions, the correlation between education and performance was +0.50 ($n = 52$, $p = .001$) in normal people. In brain dysfunctional persons, the correlation decreased to +0.22 ($n = 122$, $p = .01$) (Prigatano et al., 1991). Thus, educational level still related to the level of performance, but the relationship was less robust.

Clinically, persons with advanced education are often sensitive to changes in higher cerebral functioning, particularly in our culture. For those with advanced degrees, academic accomplishments are very important to their sense of self. They value academic and intellectual achievements, and the effects of brain dysfunction may be especially threatening because it touches the core of a major source of their self-esteem.

By virtue of their advanced academic training, such persons may also be (and rightfully so) more questioning about neuropsychological rehabilitation programs. For example, one university professor with a TBI was especially skeptical and asked many penetrating questions about a particular program of rehabilitation. His questions were insightful and legitimate. The patient was about the same age as his therapists, and his advanced degree intimidated some of the therapists. Such a scenario has been neglected in the clinical literature. That is, how do therapists deal with the rehabilitation of higher cerebral dysfunction in a patient who has achieved more academically than they have and who may even be at a higher intellectual level than they are? This issue is discussed in later chapters. Little has been written on this important topic.

Satz's (1993) concept of brain reserve capacity suggests another interesting way in which education could relate to symptoms, at least to their development. Satz (1993) suggested that educational level may be an indirect measure of this interesting construct. The higher the person's level of education, the greater the resistance may be to the development of symptoms. Satz (1993) has proposed that this relationship is demonstrated in patients with HIV symptoms as well as in those with Alzheimer's disease. No studies have adequately assessed how educational level relates to recovery of higher cerebral functioning after acquired brain injury. In clinical practice, however, this relationship often seems to be present.

Intellectual Level

The construct of intelligence is complicated. It refers to both cognitive and noncognitive skills in solving problems, in adjusting to environmental changes to aid survival, and in accomplishing various goals (Mata-razzo, 1972). From the perspective of cognitive science, Simon and Kaplan (1990) make the same point about the meaning of intelligence:

> Although no really satisfactory intentional definition of intelligence has been proposed, we are ordinarily willing to judge when intelligence is being exhibited by our fellow human beings. We say that people are behaving intelligently when they choose courses of action that are relevant to achieving their goals, when they reply coherently and appropriately to questions that are put to them, when they solve problems of lesser or greater difficulty, or when they create or design something useful or beautiful or novel. We apply a single term, "intelligence," to this diverse set of activities because we expect that a common set of underlying processes is implicated in performing all of them (p. 1).

Certainly, premorbid intelligence quotient (IQ) level is a crucial variable in the interpretation of neuropsychological test performance after brain injury (Prigatano et al., 1993) and in the evaluation of patients and their symptom profiles.

A recent study by Alexander and colleagues (1997) demonstrated an inverse relationship between cerebral metabolism and estimates of premorbid intellectual ability in Alzheimer patients. Persons with less cerebral metabolism (a measure of impaired brain function) were cognitively more intact if they had higher demographic-based IQ estimates. This study demonstrated that premorbid factors clearly can influence the degree to which a cognitive deficit is observed.

During rehabilitation, persons with above-average intellectual ability often maintain a fund of information and show relatively good abstract reasoning skills even though they have sustained significant brain injury. For example, a computed tomography study of the university professor mentioned above showed left temporal and inferior parietal hemorrhagic contusions with mild mass effect but no evidence of hydrocephalus. About 3 months later, his verbal IQ was measured at 111, his performance IQ was 117, and his full scale IQ was 116. On the Halstead-Reitan Neuropsychological Test Battery, however, his performance was impaired. He made 54 errors on the Halstead Category Test and had a memory score of 9 and a localization score of 3 on the *Tactual Performance Test*. His Halstead Impairment Index Score was 0.7, which produced a *t*-score of 19 for his age and education (Heaton et al., 1991).

Six months later (about 7 months after injury), the professor's performance was much improved. For example, the total number of words he recalled on the *California Verbal Learning Test* (CVLT) produced a *t*-score of 67. His score on long-term free recall was 1 standard deviation below the mean. Subtle language difficulties appeared to be present but were not revealed by psychometric tests. The patient subjectively reported having difficulties in rapidly retrieving words and in communicating his ideas as clearly as before his injury, despite above-average performance on neuropsychological measures.

These impairments, however, did not seem to interfere substantially with his ability to perform his duties as a university professor. It appeared that he could fulfill his duties but perhaps would not achieve promotions as readily as he would have before his injury. His level of recovery was outstanding given the findings on his early diagnostic studies. His case emphasizes that premorbid intellectual abilities interact with the type and severity of injury to produce different levels of neuropsychological outcome.

Persons with a high level of intelligence after brain injury are often, but not always, more easily engaged in the psychotherapeutic process than less gifted patients. Much depends on the therapists' level of intellectual functioning as well as on their life experiences. A substantial mismatch between the intelligence level of a patient and the treating therapist can produce significant tensions during rehabilitation and may influence the manifestation of certain symptoms. A highly intelligent patient may feel that the therapist does not comprehend the complexity of his or her comments; conversely, the therapist may interpret the patient's behavior as rigid or as a sign of premorbid psychiatric problems if the patient fails to follow the therapeutic guidelines.

In my experience, most persons with high levels of intelligence are willing to listen to feedback from others who have achieved similar levels of accomplishment in life. Although intelligence should not be identified as the only important variable in the recovery and rehabilitation process, its importance is undeniable.

Psychosocial Setting

The example of the Norwegian businessman with Alzheimer's disease who began to show significant behavioral problems as his psychosocial environment changed readily demonstrates that cognitive impairment interacts with a patient's perception of the social environment either to accentuate or reduce the expression of certain symptoms. Clinicians often encounter this interaction in the course of neuropsychological rehabilitation. Patients described as behaviorally out of control begin to "settle down" and "behave" more appropriately if others in their environment can anticipate their neuropsychological disturbances and offer adequate structure and support. If removed from a supportive environment, their behavior often deteriorates. Patients made anxious because no one seems to understand the nature of their disturbance tend to become calm and feel considerably less isolated when they recognize that their therapist can enter their phenomenological field and sense what is bothering them (see Chapter 2).

No studies have yet focused on how adjustment to new psychosocial situations either accentuates or diminishes various symptoms. It seems, however, quite obvious that this effect is real. Placing patients in an appropriate milieu can greatly diminish many of the indirect effects of brain injury. A major challenge for the field of neuropsychological rehabilitation, therefore, is to determine systematically how various premorbid and environmental factors influence the neuropsychological symptom profile.

Cultural Milieu

Patients' cultural milieu of origin can influence how they report symptoms after brain injury. Gainotti (1975), for example, showed that Northern Italians with Alzheimer's disease described their symptoms differently than Alzheimer's patients from Switzerland. Although their geographical location was similar, the cultural differences between the groups seemed to have a profound influence on whether the patients denied the existence of various memory and cognitive impairments.

Prigatano and Leathem (1993) also have shown that New Zealanders of English ancestry differ from New Zealanders of Maori ancestry in how they report behavioral disturbances after TBI. Although this issue is discussed in more detail later, cultural variables greatly influence how patients discuss their symptoms not only with family members but with health care providers. Weinstein also noted this relationship (Prigatano and Weinstein, 1996).

Premorbid Personality and Symptoms After TBI

Premorbid personality refers to the psychological descriptors that could reliably and validly be applied to a person before the onset of a disease state (i.e., brain insult). The term *personality* (see Chapter 6) is a construct used to summarize the patterns of emotional and motivational responses that develop over the life of an organism and that reflect individual affective and cognitive modes of coping with internal (i.e., personal and subjective) and external (i.e., interpersonal and objective) demands or conflicts. Premorbid personality represents a mode of adaptation (or lack thereof) before a disturbance of brain function renders a person less effective in coping.

This concept is especially important to rehabilitation, which has as its goal adaptation or habituation to permanent changes in bodily conditions. Consequently, the history of individual adaptation styles is important in understanding how patients should be approached and what adaptation techniques or philosophy is needed in their care.

Clinical Manifestations of Premorbid Personality

Luria (1948/1963) recognized the tremendous role of premorbid personality in the process of recovery. Before him, Goldstein (1942) had also emphasized this point. Although this concept is familiar and well accepted, few studies have pursued it. The following example illustrates relevant clinical manifestations of this issue. Two middle-aged men suffered ruptured aneurysms of the right middle cerebral artery in the right parietotemporal region. Both showed initial problems of hemi-inattention and neglect. Initially, both were unaware of their higher order visuospatial disturbances and were surprised, when asked to do simple puzzles, that they had difficulties performing these tasks.

One became quiet and withdrawn when confronted with his higher-order visuospatial disturbance; the other became irritated and aggressive. The first patient's premorbid intelligence was estimated to have been average, and he ran a small business. His role in life seemed to be one of resolving conflict between others, and he was jokingly referred to as a "peacekeeper." The second patient was an accomplished attorney who was a partner in a major law firm. He was known for his aggressive and angry tactics when frustrated by those around him. Premorbid personality characteristics seemed to greatly influence the manner in which these men interacted with others, particularly when their neuropsychological deficits were at issue. The contrast in their responses, given the similarity of their injuries, suggests that an individual's coping strategies after brain injury partially reflect preexisting personality characteristics.

Related Research

As reasonable as the proposition is that premorbid personality is expressed in the patient's clinical profile after brain injury, it is difficult to find supporting studies in the literature. Kozol (1945) attempted to relate broad diagnostic psychiatric categories to various "mental" symptoms after head injury. In his initial study, 200 individuals with a history of primarily mild-to-moderate TBI (according to today's standards) were classified as having either a "normal personality" or a range of disorders based on diagnostic descriptor categories that included such statements as "psychopathic personality" and "neurotic personality." Kozol (1945) failed to find a relationship between these broad descriptors of patients' preinjury personalities and their complaints of disturbed function afterward.

In a follow-up study, Kozol (1946) further evaluated 101 of his original patients using his "historical/biographic method of personality study" (p. 247). In this study, he identified a list of 60 possible personality descriptors of "traits, tendencies, or characteristics" and attempted to relate these variables to outcome. Again, his results were discouraging. Regardless of how patients were described before their injury, the descriptions failed to relate systematically to their mental symptoms after injury. Kozol (1946) did note, however, that "a substantial number of patients presented certain traits after trauma which had not been present in their personality *before* head injury" (italics added) (p. 256). These patients typically had exhibited "prolonged disorientation" after their injury. He concluded, however, that "There was no close correlation between the severity of the acute injury of the brain and the severity of the sequelae" (p. 275). At the time Kozol conducted these studies, many patients with severe injuries still died. Thus, survivors typically had mild to moderate injuries. Consequently, it is possible that the mental symptoms exhibited after brain injury are not as easily related to measures of severity if an injury is mild.

Kozol (1945, 1946) found that patients with a variety of "post-traumatic mental symptoms" also had more "complicating psychosocial factors" in their lives. These factors included the presence of litigation, "domestic troubles," and "occupational difficulties." However, we do not know from Kozol's (1945) or any other study how premorbid cognitive, emotional, and motivational factors may have contributed to these "complicating psychosocial factors." That is, do the factors exist independently or were they at least partially caused by premorbid personality difficulties?

Brooks and McKinlay (1983) attempted to relate premorbid personality characteristics to postinjury behavioral disturbances. They asked family members to rate TBI patients on a series of bipolar adjectives and to rate the same patient retrospectively (i.e., premorbidly) to determine which personality changes were common after TBI and how they might have related to premorbid factors. Their findings documented what many clinicians have known for some time: Individuals with severe TBIs are often quick to anger, irritable, less energetic, and more immature than before their injury. Typically, such patients are considered "unreasonable" by many family members.

As noted, the problem has been how to relate these specific changes to premorbid factors. Brooks and McKinlay (1983) showed that the severity of brain injury related to some of these changes, but many of these personality factors were unrelated to severity of injury. Earlier, Lishman (1978, p. 207) reported the same finding. In a chapter on the etiology of psychiatric disturbances associated with TBI, Lishman listed a number of factors—including premorbid personality and the patient's psychosocial situation (environmental factors)—that contributed greatly to the symptom profile (Table 3-1).

Brooks and McKinlay (1983) also reported that some of the personality disturbances seemed to emerge several months after injury instead of immediately. This finding supports the model that categorizes personality disturbances associated with TBI as reactionary, neuropsychologically mediated, or characterological. The latter group of problems predates brain injury (Prigatano et al., 1986, pp. 44–45).

There is a growing appreciation that premorbid or characterological problems are important determinants of the behavior of brain dysfunctional persons (Prigatano et al., 1995). Glenn and colleagues (1993) found that self-reported symptoms of childhood behavioral disorders predicted

Table 3-1. Etiological factors in psychiatric disturbances after head injury

Mental constitution
Premorbid personality
Emotional impact of injury
Emotional repercussions of injury
Environmental factors
Compensation and litigation
Response to intellectual impairments
Development of epilepsy
Amount of brain damage incurred
Location of brain damage incurred

From Lishman W. A., *Organic Psychiatry: The Psychological Consequences of Cerebral Disorder*, p. 207, 1978, published by Blackwell Scientific Publications.

verbal and visuospatial neuropsychological test performance in adult male and female alcoholics as well as in normal subjects. The percent of variance accounted for by this factor was modest but nevertheless exerted an important and statistically reliable effect. Robinson and colleagues (Jorge et al., 1993a,b) have also shown that 24% of TBI patients with major depressive illness had a history of premorbid psychiatric disturbances (see Chapter 6, Table 6-4).

In clinical practice, it is difficult to escape the conclusion that premorbid personality characteristics influence various behavioral problems associated with brain injury. How certain personality characteristics seem to accentuate the behavioral disturbances associated with brain injury is especially impressive. This tendency is frequently apparent in individuals who are described as either "perfectionistic" or "narcissistic" (Klonoff and Lage, 1991) before their injury. They often have an extremely negative emotional response to any deficit in higher cerebral functioning that they confront. When they fatigue (as do most brain dysfunctional patients), they are more prone to respond with angry verbal outbursts. If "pushed," they can also become physically violent. These patients seem to have an exceptionally difficult time coping with their residual cognitive disturbances. Their emotional outbursts are difficult to classify as being purely neuropsychologically mediated or reactionary/characterological. This subgroup needs to be assessed more thoroughly because they pose a major diagnostic and therapeutic challenge to clinical neuropsychologists.

Summary and Conclusions

Brain injury is always imposed on a preexisting cognitive structure and methods for coping that have emotional and motivational features. The neuropsychological symptom profile after brain injury must reflect this interaction (Principle 2). All too frequently, the study of brain-behavioral relationships acknowledges this fact and then summarily dismisses it as irrelevant, uninteresting, or inaccessible to scientific study. Consequently, the influence of premorbid factors on symptom profiles has been neglected in research relevant to clinical neuropsychology (Prigatano et al., 1995). In neuropsychological rehabilitation, however, the role of premorbid influences is obvious immediately (Prigatano et al., 1986).

This chapter attempts to demonstrate that patients' neuropsychological symptoms should only be attributed to the direct effects of brain injury with great caution. Some of a patient's neuropsychological characteristics may have existed premorbidly or, more commonly, may reflect the interaction of premorbid cognitive and personality variables with postmorbid-induced disturbances in cerebral function. Approaching the patient's symptom profile from the perspective of premorbid factors helps guide the assessment process. When patients are treated in a manner that reflects this complicated interaction of premorbid and postmorbid features, they are more likely to feel understood and treated in a professional manner. Therapist can then use the information obtained from the neuropsychological examination to help guide patients into appropriate rehabilitation activities. Neuropsychological rehabilitation efforts are more successful when this interaction is understood and acted upon appropriately.

References

Alexander, G. E., Furey, M. L., Grady, C. L., Pietrini, P., Brady, D. R., Mentis, M. J., and Schapiro, M. B. (1997). Association of premorbid intellectual function with cerebral metabolism in Alzheimer's disease: Implications for the cognitive reserve hypothesis. *Am. J. Psychiatry* 154(2): 165–172.

American Psychiatric Association (1994). *Diagnostic and Statistical Manual of Mental Disorders* (4th ed). American Psychiatric Association, Washington, D.C.

Angevine, J. B., and Cotman, C. W. (1981). *Principles of Neuroanatomy.* Oxford University Press, New York.

Benson, D. F. (1988). Classical syndromes of aphasia. In F. Boller and J. Grafman (eds), *Handbook of Neuropsychology* (Vol. 1, pp. 267–280). Elsevier Science, Amsterdam.

Benson, D. F. (1993). Aphasia. In K. M. Heilman and E. Valenstein (eds), *Clinical Neuropsychology* (3rd ed) (pp. 17–36). Oxford University Press, New York.

Bisiach, E., and Vallar, G. (1988). Hemineglect in humans. In F. Boller and J. Grafman (eds), *Handbook of Neuropsychology* (Vol. 1, pp. 195–222). Elsevier Science B. V., The Netherlands.

Brooks, D. N., and McKinlay, W. (1983). Personality and behavioural change after severe blunt head injury—a relative's view. *J. Neurol. Neurosurg. Psychiatry* 46: 336–334.

Chapman, L. F., and Wolff, H. G. (1959). The cerebral hemispheres and the highest integrative functions of man. *Arch. Neurol.* 1: 357–424.

Dian, L., Cummings, J. L., Petry, S., and Hill, M. A. (1990). Personality alterations in multi-infarct dementia. *Psychosomatics* 31(4), 415–419.

Evans, D. A., Beckett, L. A., Albert, M. S., Hebert, L. E., Scherr, P. A., Funkenstein, H. H., and Taylor, J. O. (1993). Level of education and change in cognitive function in a community population of older persons. *Ann. Epidemiol.* 3(1): 71–77.

Frederiks, J. A. M. (1985). Clinical neuropsychology: The neuropsychological symptom. In P. J. Vinken, G. W. Bruyn, and H. L. Klawans (eds) *Handbook of Clinical Neurology* (Vol. 45 Revised Series 1, pp. 1–6). Elsevier Science, New York.

Gainotti, G. (1975). Confabulation of denial of senile dementia. *Psychiatric Clinics* 8: 99–108.

Geschwind, N. (1967). The varieties of naming errors. *Cortex* 3, 97–112.

Gilbert, J. G. and Levee, R. F. (1971). Patterns of declining memory. *J. Gerontol.* 26(1): 70–75.

Glenn, S. W., Errico, A. L., Parsons, O. A., King, A. C., and Nixon, S. J. (1993). The role of antisocial, affective, and childhood behavioral characteristics in alcoholics' neuropsychological performance. *Alcohol. Clin. Exp. Res.* 17(1): 162–169.

Goldstein, F. C., Levin, H. S., Presley, R. M., Searcy, J., Colohan, A. R. T., Eisenberg, H. M., Jann, B., and Bertolino-Kusnerik, L. (1994). Neurobehavioural consequences of closed head injury in older adults. *J. Neurol. Neurosurg. Psychiatry* 57: 961–966.

Goldstein, K. (1942). *Aftereffects of Brain Injury in War*. Grune and Stratton, New York.

Goldstein, K. (1952). The effect of brain damage on the personality. *Psychiatry* 15: 245–260.

Hall, C. S., and Lindzey, G. (1978). *Theories of Personality* (3rd ed). John Wiley and Sons, New York.

Heaton, R. K., Grant, I., and Matthews, C. G. (1991). *Comprehensive Norms for an Expanded Halstead-Reitan Battery*. Psychological Assessment Resources, Odessa, Fla.

Jenkyn, L. R., Reeves, A. G., Warren, T., Whiting, R. K., Clayton, R. J., Moore, W. W., Rizzo, A., Tuzun, I. M., Bonnett, J. C., and Culpepper, B. W. (1985). Neurologic signs in senescence. *Arch. Neurol.* 42: 1154–1157.

Jorge, R. E., Robinson, R. G., Arndt, S., Forrester, A. W., Geisler, F., and Starkstein, S. E. (1993a). Comparison between acute- and delayed-onset depression following traumatic brain injury. *Journal of Neuropsychiatry* 5: 43–49.

Jorge, R. E., Robinson, R. G., Arndt, S. V., Starkstein, S. E., Forrester, A. W., and Geisler, F. (1993b). Depression following traumatic brain injury: A 1 year longitudinal study. *J. Affect. Disord.* 27: 233–243.

Jung, C. G. (1957). *The Practice of Psychotherapy. Bollinger Series XX* (Vol. 16). Princeton University, Princeton, NJ.

Kiev, A., Chapman, L. F., Guthrie, T. C., and Wolff, H. G. (1962). The highest integrative functions and diffuse cerebral atrophy. *Neurology* 12: 385–393.

Klonoff, P. S., and Lage, G. A. (1991). Narcissistic injury in patients with traumatic brain injury. *Journal of Head Trauma Rehabilitation* 6(4): 11–21.

Kozol, H. L. (1945). Pretraumatic personality and psychiatric sequelae of head injury. *Archives of Neurology and Psychiatry* 53: 358–364.

Kozol, H. L. (1946). Pretraumatic personality and psychiatric sequelae of head injury. *Archives of Neurology and Psychiatry* 46(3): 245–275.

Levin, H. S., Mendelsohn, D., Lilly, M. A., Fletcher, J. M., Culhane, K. A., Chapman, S. B., Harward, H., Kusnerik, L., Bruce, D., and Eisenberg, H. M. (1994). Tower of London performance in relation to magnetic resonance imaging following closed head injury in children. *Neuropsychology* 8(2): 171–179.

Lishman, W. A. (1978). *Organic Psychiatry: The Psychological Consequences of Cerebral Disorder*. Blackwell Scientific, Osney Mead, Oxford.

Luria, A. R. (1948/1963). *Restoration of Function After Brain Trauma* (in Russian). Moscow: Academy of Medical Science (Pergamon, London, 1963).

Luria, A. R. (1966). Kurt Goldstein and neuropsychology. *Neuropsychologia* 4: 311–313.

Matarazzo, J. D. (1972). *Wechsler's Measurement and Appraisal of Adult Intelligence* (5th and enlarged edition). Williams & Wilkins, Baltimore.

Petry, S., Cummings, J. L., Hill, M. A., and Shapira, J. (1988). Personality alterations in dementia of the Alzheimer's type. *Arch. Neurol.* 45: 1187–1190.

Prigatano, G. P. (1991a). Disordered mind, wounded soul: The emerging role of psychotherapy in rehabilitation after brain injury. *Journal of Head Trauma Rehabilitation* 6(4): 1–10.

Prigatano, G. P. (1991b). Science and symbolism in neuropsychological rehabilitation after brain injury. *The Tenth Annual James C. Hemphill Lecture*. Rehabilitation Institute of Chicago, Chicago.

Prigatano, G. P. (1992). Personality disturbances associated with traumatic brain injury. *J. Consult. Clin. Psychol.* 60(3): 360–368.

Prigatano, G. P. (1996). Neuropsychological testing after traumatic brain injury. In R. W. Evans (ed), *Neurology and Trauma* (pp. 222–230). W. B. Saunders, Philadelphia.

Prigatano, G. P., Amin, K., and Rosenstein, L. D. (1991). *Manual for the BNI Screen for Higher Cerebral Functions*. Barrow Neurological Institute, Phoenix, Ariz.

Prigatano, G. P., Amin, K., and Rosenstein, L. D. (1993). Validity studies on the BNI Screen for Higher Cerebral Functions. *BNI Quarterly* 9(1): 2–9.

Prigatano, G. P., and Henderson, S. (1997). Cognitive outcome after subarachnoid hemorrhage. In J. B. Bederson (ed), *Subarachnoid Hemorrhage: Pathophysiology and Management* (pp. 27–40). American Association of Neurological Surgeons, Park Ridge, Ill.

Prigatano, G. P., and Leathem, J. M. (1993). Awareness of behavioral limitations after traumatic brain injury: a cross-cultural study of New Zealand Maoris and non-Maoris. *Clinical Neuropsychologist* 7(2): 123–135.

Prigatano, G. P., Fordyce, D. J., Zeiner, H. K., Roueche, J. R., Pepping, M., and Wood, B. C. (1986). *Neuropsychological Rehabilitation After Brain Injury.* Johns Hopkins University, Baltimore.

Prigatano, G. P., and Parsons, O. A. (1976). Relationship of age and education to Halstead test performance in different patient populations. *J. Consult. Clin. Psychol.* 44: 527–533.

Prigatano, G. P., Parsons, O. A., and Bortz, J. (1995). Methodological considerations in clinical neuropsychological research: 17 years later. *Psychological Assessment* 7(3): 396–403.

Prigatano, G. P., and Weinstein, E. A. (1996). E. A. Weinstein's contributions to neuropsychological rehabilitation. *Neuropsychological Rehabilitation* 6(4): 305–326.

Satz, P. (1966). Specific and nonspecific effects of brain lesions in man. *J. Abnorm. Psychol.* 71: 56–70.

Satz, P. (1993). Brain reserve capacity on symptom onset after brain injury: a formulation and review of evidence for threshold theory. *Neuropsychology* 7(3): 273–295.

Schaiel, K. W., and Zelinski, E. (1978). Psychometric assessment of dysfunction in learning and memory. In F. Hoffmeister and C. Mullen (eds), *Brain Function in Old Age* (pp. 134–150). Springer-Verlag, New York.

Simon, H. A., and Kaplan, C. A. (1990). Foundations of cognitive science. In M. I. Posner (ed), *Foundations of Cognitive Science* (pp. 1–47). Bradford, London.

Squire, L. (1991). Memory and its disorders. In F. Boller and J. Grafman (eds), *Handbook of Neuropsychology* (Vol. 3, Section 5, pp. 3–267). Elsevier Science, Amsterdam.

Storandt, M. (1991). Longitudinal studies of aging and age-associated dementias. In F. Boller and J. Grafman (eds), *Handbook of Neuropsychology* (Vol. 4, pp. 349–364). Elsevier Science B. V., The Netherlands.

Taylor, J. (1931–1932). *Selected Writings of John Hughlings Jackson* (Vols. 1–2). Hodder & Stoughton, London.

Van Zomeren, A. H., and van Den Burg, W. (1985). Residual complaints of patients two years after severe head injury. *J. Neurol. Neurosurg. Psychiatry.* 48: 21–28.

Webster's New Universal Unabridged Dictionary (1983). New World Dictionaries/Simon and Schuster, Cleveland.

Weinstein, E. A. (1995). Why do some patients confabulate after brain injury: an argument for the role of premorbid personality factors in influencing the neuropsychological symptom picture. Presented at the 10th Year Anniversary of the Section of Neuropsychology, Barrow Neurological Institute, Scottsdale, Ariz.

Weinstein, E. A., Kahn, R. L., and Morris, G. O. (1956). Delusions about children following brain injury. *Journal of Hillside Hospital* 5: 290–300.

II

THE PROCESS AND OUTCOME OF NEUROPSYCHOLOGICAL REHABILITATION

4

Statement of the Problem: Why Is Neuropsychological Rehabilitation Needed?

> Should my son survive with some disability then I would expect the family to plan with the remedial therapists and psychologists a rehabilitation programme. I would hope that a psychiatrist skilled in the problems which face the young disabled and their families would be available to counsel both us and him. . . ."
>
> B. Jennett, "If my son had a head injury," 1978, p. 1603

If patients who suffered various brain insults were able to recover adequately with time and/or the help of traditional rehabilitation therapies, neuropsychological rehabilitation would be unnecessary. The sad fact is that in many cases not only is the recovery incomplete but patients and their families still struggle with how to manage residual disturbances of higher cerebral functioning. It is for this primary reason that neuropsychological rehabilitation emerged and continues to be an important part of patient care. Principle 3 of this text asserts: Neuropsychological rehabilitation must focus on *both* the remediation of higher cerebral disturbances and their management in interpersonal situations.

To demonstrate why this is the case, we will begin with a case example.

An Illustrative Case

A 40-year-old woman was seen for a neuropsychological consultation 7.5 years after she sustained a severe traumatic brain injury (TBI). Her story is a classic example of what happens after such injuries.

At the age of 32, she was struck by an oncoming vehicle as she crossed a street. She lost consciousness and was transferred to a hospital for medical and surgical treatment. In addition to her brain injury, she suffered a shattered pelvis and ultimately lost a kidney. No admitting Glasgow Coma Scale (GCS) score was recorded, but her records suggest that she may have been unconscious for at least 6 days.

Upon regaining consciousness, she experienced posttraumatic amnesia and initially was aphasic with complete right-sided spastic hemiplegia. She underwent physical therapy and with time showed extraordinarily good motor recovery. She can now walk although her gait is unbalanced. Her right arm is completely functional, but she has difficulties with grip strength and flexible movements of her right fingers. Her language impairment appears to be almost completely resolved. She seems to understand most questions and can respond fluently and coherently, but she has subtle problems with word retrieval and in comprehending ambiguous statements. A slight dysarthria appears periodically. Her face occasionally grimaces when she does not quite grasp what is said to her, and she may ask the examiner to repeat the question.

The patient was referred for neuropsychological evaluation by a psychologist who was seeing her for depression. The psychologist noted that she had a history of craniocerebral trauma and requested a neuropsychological evaluation to obtain a more recent assessment of her neuropsychological strengths and difficulties. The patient reported that she had become severely depressed after she failed an academic course of study. She related the following story.

After her brain insult she received physical and occupational therapy on an outpatient basis. She greatly appreciated those therapies and felt they were helpful. She also underwent speech and language therapy but was less certain about its effectiveness. After her outpatient treatment, she was referred to a day treatment program for her cognitive problems. She felt frustrated with that environment (a common reaction, see Chapter 2) and eventually left the program convinced that the therapists neither understood nor were interested in her problems.

She decided to study to be a certified occupational therapy assistant because she had been so impressed with the work the occupational therapist had done with her. She applied to a university and was accepted. She requested funds from a state vocational rehabilitation agency to support this educational venture but initially was denied on the basis that she was unable to meet the cognitive requirements of such training. With little insight about her difficulties and a strong desire to become independent and self-sufficient, she fought the decision. With the aid of an attorney, she prevailed and received funding from the state agency.

After 1 year of academic training, however, her professors told her that she would not be able to complete the course of training. Concerns regarding safety, difficulty recalling basic information, lack of concise and timely documentation, difficulty reporting and grading appropriate treatment activities, and "demonstrating emotional responses" when given supervisory feedback were cited as the reasons for her disqualification.

Given this feedback, she was not only perplexed but became extremely depressed. Perhaps the state vocational rehabilitation agency was right; on the other hand, she felt that if she had only worked harder she might have accomplished her goal. Two months after her termination, she returned to Phoenix and sought treatment for her depression and was then referred for the neuropsychological evaluation.

In the course of her initial interview, she was asked to list her present difficulties. She stated that her confidence had decreased after her academic failure. She noted that she had lost her motivation to do things. She did not spontaneously note any cognitive difficulties. When asked whether she had any cognitive impairments, she replied that she was "okay" and felt that she only needed to exert adequate effort to be able to remember things and to accomplish her goals. When asked whether her memory was impaired, she stated "my memory is fine."

Thus, 7.5 years after her severe brain injury and after receiving concrete feedback that she lacked the cognitive and memory skills to complete a training course that she was convinced she could handle, her statements indicated her lack of awareness about her true capabilities. She was clearly depressed and amotivational, but she did not link the nature of her impairment with her affective reaction. Both her impaired awareness and depression needed to be treated.

Can This Scenario Be Avoided?

The argument that as people become more aware of their deficits after severe brain injury they tend to become depressed (Godfrey et al., 1993) has not been my typical experience. In fact, what has most often happened is that patients remain unaware but experience a number of life failures. They do not necessarily connect their failures with their impairments in cognitive functioning, which either they do not perceive or minimize. They often attribute their failures to a lack of effort or to factors external to themselves. Depression emerges as they experience failure after failure.

Whether this type of scenario can be avoided is uncertain, but it is the major goal of neuropsychological rehabilitation to avoid such a sequence of events. This case description highlights Principle 3. Namely, disturbances of higher cerebral functioning have inevitable psychosocial consequences. The focus of neuropsychological rehabilitation is on both the remediation of higher cerebral dysfunction and the management of its interpersonal consequences. Broadly speaking, to accomplish these goals requires three events to happen.

First, the attending physician or neurosurgeon involved in the patient's early surgical and medical care should make it clear that the patient most likely will have residual neuropsychological problems after the brain injury in addition to any obvious motor or language impairments. Physicians should emphasize the importance of neurorehabilitation, not only for physical disabilities, but also for potential disturbances in higher cerebral function that may not be easily identified or perceived.

Second, patients need to be referred to a competent, interdisciplinary, neuropsychologically oriented treatment team. The team's responsibility is to engage patients in rehabilitation with the understanding that many patients will naturally resist the process. A team that attributes a patient's resistance to a lack of motivation rather than a consequence of brain injury betrays its lack of understanding about the nature of higher cerebral deficits after severe TBI. It is the team's responsibility to work through these problems with patients so that the latter ultimately perceive the benefit of becoming involved in the neuropsychological rehabilitation program.

Third, the rehabilitation team should have a close working relationship with the state vocational rehabilitation department. If the state vocational rehabilitation department and their representatives work with the rehabilitation team to provide economic support and to guide patients to appropriate vocational choices, fewer resources would be wasted on tuition or inappropriate job placements. During the past 25 years of clinical practice, I have repeatedly witnessed such waste when these activities have not been coordinated. It is absolutely crucial for the physicians involved in the patient's early care, the interdisciplinary rehabilitation team, and the state vocational rehabilitation department to coordinate their efforts on the patient's behalf to avoid economic waste and to spare the patient years of emotionally painful and perplexing experiences. Ideas for accomplishing this goal are discussed in more detail in Chapters 8, 9, and 10.

It could be argued that this case scenario is unique and an atypical outcome for brain dysfunctional patients. Individual case studies must therefore be placed into the perspective of the group data reported in the scientific literature. What, in fact, are the neuropsychological and psychosocial outcomes after various kinds of brain injuries in young and middle-aged adults as well as in children?

Outcomes After Focal Brain Injury

Relatively focal brain injuries can cause significant neuropsychological impairments. This fact was demonstrated dramatically by the famous case of H.M., who became densely amnestic after bilateral removal of the hippocampus for seizure control (Scoville and Milner, 1957; Penfield and Milner, 1958). Even when small lesions do not directly impinge on key neuronal circuits responsible for memory or language, higher cerebral functioning can be disturbed.

If the focal brain disruption is from an elective surgery to clip a cerebral aneurysm or to remove a noninvasive brain tumor such as a meningioma, the higher cerebral dysfunction is often short-lived or minimal. For example, Maurice-Williams and colleagues (1991) reported that 24 of 27 patients (88.8%) who underwent an "uncomplicated aneurysm surgery" and who had a good neurological status before surgery (Grade 1 or 2) returned to their premorbid level of function. Patients without complications during or after surgery had equivalent neuropsychological test scores before and after surgery. Interestingly, however, 11 of the 27 patients (40.7%) complained of some change in their higher cerebral functioning that their neuropsychological test findings failed to corroborate. Psychological symptoms included complaints of memory, concentration, depression, and irritability. Although the authors dismissed these disturbances as likely being functional rather than organic, some of the individuals may have suffered subtle neuropsychological sequelae that were not detected by the measures used for evaluation.

When focal lesions invade the parenchyma of the cerebral hemispheres or when a serious complication such as a subarachnoid hemorrhage (SAH) or vasospasm occurs, cognitive and behavioral disturbances can and often do persist (Prigatano and Henderson, 1996). A recent review of the rehabilitation of patients with cerebral aneurysms and arteriovenous malformations touches on the cognitive, behavioral, and emotional changes associated with such lesions (Clinchot et al., 1994). An earlier study (Chapman and Wolff, 1959), however, better documents how the extent of a lesion influences neuropsychological functioning. In this study, patients whose lesions were estimated to have destroyed as little as 30 gm of brain tissue showed some disturbance in the "highest integrated" brain functions. These patients were described as being slow in their responses, as exhibiting less energy or drive, and as being less able to adapt to frustrations and disruptions in routine. As lesion size increased, so did the number or magnitude of neuropsychological disturbances. Using an aggregate measure of "mentation and behavioral" disruption, the size of the brain lesion was proportionally related to disturbances along this dimension. These findings were interpreted as supporting Lashley's (1938) Principle of Mass Action. Using the original Halstead Battery, Chapman and Wolff (1959) also demonstrated a significant positive correlation (+0.77) between grams of tissue removed from the brain during surgery and neuropsychological test performance. This variable accounted for approximately 59% of the variance in patients evaluated 1 to 7 years after surgery.

Focal brain lesions appear to affect cognition and behavior permanently and negatively. What, however, are the psychosocial consequences of such focal lesions? No simple body of literature answers this question. However, a few studies suggest answers that coincide with my clinical experience. Säveland and colleagues (1986) reported psychosocial and cognitive outcomes after aneurysmal SAH. At a 1-year follow-up examination, one in five patients with a good physical recovery was "incapacitated by persistent psychosocial and cognitive disturbances" (p. 193). In a slightly later study (Sonesson et al., 1989), patients with SAH of unknown origin often had persistent problems with verbal learning and memory as well as impairments in abstract reasoning and judg-ment. Most of these patients were considered to have good neurological recoveries—that is, they were free of physical disabilities.

In a study of long-term psychosocial adjustment after SAH (Ljunggren et al., 1985), most patients experienced persistent difficulties with mental energy and memory. Such individuals are often described as having re-stricted patterns of interests and activities, and the disturbances appear to be permanent in as many as 83% of the patients. It should be noted that these patients had focal lesions in various locations throughout the brain, but the outcomes associated with specific focal lesions are un-known. One study (Stenhouse et al., 1991), however, has suggested that 59% of patients with ruptured aneurysms of the anterior communicating artery have permanent neuropsychological impairments. Nor are precise statistics available on the percentage of individuals who return to pre-vious levels of employment. But Logue and colleagues (1968) investi-gated the quality of life after rupture of an anterior cerebral artery an-eurysm and found that 44 of 79 patients (55.6%) returned to their "former jobs or a job at the same level." The remainder—still a large percentage—did not.

There is an absence of literature on the long-term consequences of specific focal and regional injuries to the brain. The neuropsychological disturbances associated with such brain lesions have been well studied (e.g., Heilman and Valenstein, 1993), but their psychosocial outcomes have not been properly investigated.

Outcomes After Nonfocal Diffuse Brain Injury

Nonfocal or diffuse cerebral damage, particularly in cases of severe TBI, is often associated with poor psychosocial outcomes. To better under-stand the nature of cognitive and personality disturbances associated with severe TBI, a summary of associated pathological changes is useful.

Zimmerman and Bilaniuk (1989) reviewed the common computed to-mography and magnetic resonance imaging findings of patients with a moderate to severe TBI: hemorrhagic contusions, contusional hemato-mas, and diffuse axonal injury (DAI). These space-occupying lesions of-ten affect the anterior tips of the frontal and temporal lobes (see Miller, 1991). The lesions tend to be bilateral and their size and distribution tend to be asymmetrical. DAI is found throughout the white matter and can be assessed indirectly from the relative size of the ventricles in relation-ship to brain mass (Johnson et al., 1994). In more severe injuries, lesions in the splenium of the corpus callosum are common, possibly reflecting shear effects from the brain rotating within the skull. In addition to these primary lesions, a variety of secondary insults can cascade (Fig. 4-1) to damage the brain further (Miller, 1991; Pang, 1985).

Although frontal lobe injuries are common, subdural hematomas have

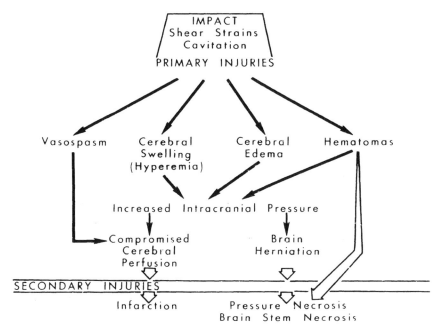

Figure 4-1. Paradigm of head injury lesions. Primary impact injuries result in epiphenomena (i.e., edema, hematoma, cerebral swelling, vasospasm) that lead to increased intracranial pressure and brain herniation. The results are the secondary lesions of cerebral infarction and pressure necrosis, which usually dictate the patient's outcome. From Pang, D. (1985). Pathophysiologic correlates of neurobehavioral syndromes following closed head injury. In Ylvisaker, M. (ed), *Head Injury Rehabilitation: Children and Adolescents* (pp. 3–70). College-Hill, San Diego. With permission from College-Hill.

a propensity for the temporal lobe (Jamieson and Yelland, 1972). Severe compression of the brain stem is reflected in oculomotor disturbances (Levin et al., 1990) and in problems of somnolence, hyperarousal, and probably later sleep disturbances (Prigatano et al., 1982; Manseau, 1995).

Methods of managing early medical and surgical needs have been developed (Jennett and Teasdale, 1981) and refined (Teasdale, 1995). Consequently, a large number of these brain-damaged persons now survive their injuries. Patients with moderate (admitting GCS score of 9 to 12) or severe (admitting GCS score of 3 to 8) TBIs are likely to have an opportunity for inpatient neurorehabilitation even though the length of stay is shortening. The focus of this early rehabilitation is almost always on physical disabilities (Prigatano et al., 1997). Typically, patients are discharged to home or other facilities with a minimal plan for dealing with their inevitable cognitive and behavioral disturbances and the long-term psychosocial consequences of their brain injury. The emergence of the National Head Injury Foundation in 1980 was largely a reflection of the frustration of family members in dealing with the long-term care of their brain dysfunctional relatives and their lack of preparation for doing so.

As the quote introducing this chapter indicates, experienced neuro-surgeons such as Bryan Jennett have long recognized the long-term psychosocial consequences of brain injuries. Yet few programs are equipped adequately to deal with such patients. The emerging collective database supports a convincing argument that traditional rehabilitation focusing primarily on physical disabilities with minimum attention to cognitive impairments is inadequate for the care of these persons.

Again, a sampling of studies clearly makes this point and argues that neuropsychological rehabilitation is needed because these patients too often have persistent cognitive and personality disturbances. Thomsen (1984) reported a 10- to-15-year follow-up study of patients who suffered "very severe blunt head trauma" during adolescence and young adulthood. Most patients lived with their parents. The rate of development of posttraumatic psychosis was as high as 20%, and social isolation was common. Many cognitive and behavioral problems persisted. For example, 2 to 5 years after injury, 80% of the patients were described as having poor memories; 10 to 15 years after injury, the percentage was still 75%.

Alarmingly, some behavioral problems seemed to increase with time. For example, "sensitivity to distress" increased from 23% 2.5 years after injury to 68% 10 to 15 years after injury. Between these two time periods, irritability increased from 38% to 48%. A more recent follow-up (Thomsen, 1995) documented the continued social isolation and deteriorating psychiatric status of many of these patients.

Other workers (Oddy et al., 1985; Livingston et al., 1985a, b; van Zomeren and van Den Burg, 1985) also have documented the relative persistence of cognitive and personality disturbances in this patient group. For example, Oddy and colleagues (1985) asked a group of patients with severe TBIs what problems they experienced 7 years after injury and asked relatives to document their perceptions of the patient's persistent problems.

Approximately 50% of the patients reported persistent memory problems (Table 4-1) and continued difficulties with sustaining attention and concentration. About 28% of the patients reported difficulties in becoming interested in activities and in following conversations. What is striking, however, is that the relatives reported a much higher incidence of memory impairment (79%) than the patients did. Compared to the patients' self-reports, relatives also reported that the patient had a higher incidence of difficulty becoming interested in activities. They also described many patients as becoming easily tired and often impatient. Forty percent of the relatives described the patient as continuing to behave "childishly" and as refusing "to admit to difficulties" 7 years after injury.

Table 4-1. Symptoms reported by patients and relatives 7 years after head injury

Patients	Percent	Relatives	Percent
Trouble remembering things	53	Trouble remembering things	79
Difficulty concentrating	46	Difficulty concentrating	50
Easily affected by alcohol	38	Difficulty speaking	50
Often knocks things over	31	Easily affected by alcohol	43
Often loses temper	31	Difficulty becoming interested	43
Difficulty becoming interested	28	Becomes tired easily	43
Likes to keep things tidy	28	Often impatient	43
Sometimes loses way	28	Sometimes behaves childishly	40
Eyesight problems	28	Likes to keep things tidy	40
Difficulty following conversation	28	Refuses to admit difficulties	40

From Oddy et al. (1985). Reprinted with permission.

These findings document two important problems associated with severe TBI. First, patients may lack insight about the extent of their residual deficits and therefore report fewer problems than they actually demonstrate. Second, patients continue to exhibit poorly defined disturbances in higher cerebral functioning that appear to create substantial problems with social interaction and integration. These findings strongly argue that TBI patients need additional help if they are going to resume a productive lifestyle and learn to cope with their persistent higher cerebral deficits. These findings are the basis of Principle 3: Neuropsychological rehabilitation must focus on both the remediation of these disturbances and their management in interpersonal situations.

One very important interpersonal situation is the work setting. After TBI, many patients have a difficult time maintaining satisfactory interpersonal relationships as well as performing adequately on the job. The few studies available indicate that without the help of neuropsychological rehabilitation, many brain-injured patients are unable to maintain work.

In an investigation of return to work after severe TBI conducted in the United Kingdom (Brooks et al., 1987), 86% of 96 patients had been working at the time of their injury. During the first 7 years after their injury, only 29% had returned to work. Persistent cognitive and personality disturbances clearly separated those who were working from those who were not. Problems with controlling anger and emotional lability figured prominently into the symptom profile of these nonworking patients. Patients with persistent verbal memory deficits also tended to be unemployed.

A study on psychosocial outcome conducted at the Barrow Neurological Institute (Prigatano, et al., 1987) revealed similar findings. Patients completed a questionnaire derived from the Traumatic Coma Data Bank project. Only 23% of patients with severe TBI (admitting GCS score between 3 and 8) were working 2 to 4 years after injury. No patients with admitting GCS scores of 3, 4, or 5 were gainfully employed during that time frame. Many of these patients with severe TBIs required ongoing supervision and were not living independently. Cognitive and behavioral disturbances rather than physical disabilities seemed to underlie these poor outcomes.

Collectively, what do these data suggest? Patients with focal, but invasive, brain injuries, as well as those with diffuse cerebral damage, have permanent neuropsychological sequelae. Inevitably, these sequelae affect the patients' ability to function in interpersonal situations and to maintain work. Precise statistics of the frequency or incidence of the various types of permanent disabilities are unavailable. The data reviewed in this chapter, however, suggest that 20% to 83% of these individuals experience permanent sequelae with major problems in psychosocial adjustment. Evidence also suggests that as time passes, many of these patients remain disabled and are unable to regain a productive lifestyle. Thomsen's (1984) data, for example, suggest that less than 10% of severe TBI patients may actually maintain work 10 to 15 years after a brain injury. This finding coincides with my clinical impression as well. These data clearly emphasize the need for neuropsychological rehabilitation. The question, of course, is whether this rehabilitation substantially improves a patient's quality of life and productivity.

The Need for Neuropsychological Rehabilitation

In planning rehabilitation activities for brain dysfunctional patients, the question of whether any type of therapy substantially improves their cognitive status, emotional and motivational disturbances, and overall psychosocial adjustments inevitably arises. Fifty years ago, Oliver Zangwill (1947) asked this and related questions. Yet, systematic answers to these questions are still lacking, even though Ben-Yishay and colleagues (1982) have reported the usefulness of certain techniques for dealing with the disabilities associated with brain injury. In 1984, Prigatano and colleagues also reported preliminary findings that suggested that patients' psychosocial and emotional status could be improved by intensive neuropsychologically oriented neurorehabilitation. Subsequently, methods of rehabilitating these persons were outlined (Prigatano et al., 1986).

Since these studies appeared, others continue to report that TBI patients experience persistent neuropsychological deficits (Levin et al., 1990) and associated problems of psychosocial adjustment (Klonoff et al., 1986). The problems are not limited to adults but extend to the long-term consequences of brain injury in children as well (Costeff et al., 1985). More recent investigations document a relationship between the initial brain injury and residual neuropsychological impairments (Dikmen et al., 1995). Furthermore, the most common long-term psychosocial problem after brain injury is social isolation (Kozloff, 1987).

Clearly, traditional rehabilitation programs have failed to deal adequately with the cognitive and personality disturbances associated with focal or diffuse brain injury. Therefore, specialty programs have been developed to attempt to treat, if not the neuropsychologic deficits, at least the psychosocial disabilities associated with them.

Such neuropsychological programs, however, are difficult to locate despite the list of such services published in documents such as the *National Directory of Head Injury Rehabilitation Services* (1985). This problem exists because the understanding of the nature of these patients' higher cerebral disturbances continues to be inadequate. Although many therapists are available to work with these patients, few have extensive experience with or knowledge of how to define these deficits and what the most useful way of approaching them may be. Therefore, we now consider the impact of a brain injury on patient, family, and health care system.

Impact on Families and the Health Care System

When a patient suffers from persistent cognitive and personality disturbances after a focal or diffuse brain injury, the impact on family members is inevitably negative and the situation tends to worsen with time. This trend is illustrated by studies of families who have children or young adults with a severe TBI. Observing the long-term strain on the parent-child relationship when a child or young adult suffers a severe brain injury, Thomsen (1989) suggested that "the father/son relationship was particularly vulnerable" (p. 160). In a 3-year follow-up study of children with TBI, Rivara and Jaffe and their colleagues (Rivara et al., 1994; Rivara, 1994) systematically observed the impact of these injuries on families. They found that the academic and behavioral performances of children with a severe TBI deteriorate, as does the functioning of the global family (Figs. 4-2 and 4-3). Especially prominent 3 to 12 months after injury, this deterioration fails to improve with time and may worsen.

Spouses of brain dysfunctional patients may be especially distressed, and marital life can suffer greatly (Florian and Katz, 1991). Wives of patients with severe TBIs experience more difficulty in reaching joint decisions with their husbands than wives whose husbands have a moderate brain injury (Peters et al., 1990). Husbands with severe TBIs also show less physical and verbal affection toward their wives. The result is often significant alienation.

The financial costs associated with persistent physical, cognitive, and personality disturbances after focal and diffuse brain injury are staggering. No single estimate of these costs is available. Max and colleagues (1991), however, developed an economic model to estimate the costs as-

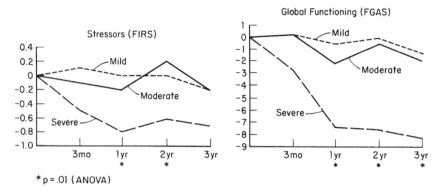

*p = .01 (ANOVA)

Figure 4-2. Change in family functioning from before brain injury to 3 years afterward as a function of the severity of brain injury. Families report more stressors over time and a deterioration in their overall or global functioning. From Rivara, J'M. B. (1994). Family functioning: Its role as a predictor of family and child outcomes in the first 3 years following childhood TBI. Presented at the 4th Conference of the International Association for the Study of Traumatic Brain Injury, St. Louis, Mo. With permission of J'M Rivara.

sociated with head injury in the United States during 1985. Using statistics published in 1991, they estimated that the direct cost of these head injuries in America was approximately 6 billion dollars. When they considered the long-term needs of these persons, which included both medical and psychosocial care as well as lost earnings, the cost increased an additional 42 billion dollars. These estimates reflect only the cost for TBI and do not include patient groups with other cognitive and behavioral disturbances.

Why, then, have adequate specialty programs not been developed and supported by the health care system? The answer is complex. In the United States today, as the twentieth century closes, there is a growing tendency to focus on cost containment as it relates to medical and health care treatment (Cope and O'Lear, 1993). Financial pressures are undoubtedly responsible for part of the failure to support neuropsychological rehabilitation programs. There is, however, another problem that neurorehabilitationists must recognize. As a group, clinicians have failed to do their scientific homework and to demonstrate which forms of neurorehabilitation are helpful for which patients and which forms of neurorehabilitation are not.

As a branch of medicine, rehabilitation is notorious for its failure to study outcomes adequately and to understand mechanisms responsible for recovery. Calvanio and colleagues (1993) have remarked on this topic:

> Some critics have expressed grave doubts about these therapeutic services. Hachinski's editorial comment in the *Archives of Neurology* captures this skepticism well: Few areas in neurology are in greater need

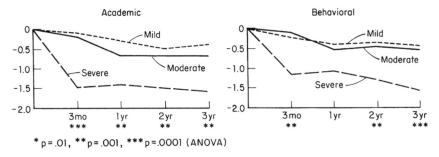

* p = .01, ** p = .001, *** p = .0001 (ANOVA)

Figure 4-3. Change in functioning of children from before brain injury to 3 years after as a function of the severity of the injury. Children with more severe injuries show a clear decline in academic performance over time and a worsening of their behavioral adjustment. From Rivara, J'M. B. (1994). Family functioning: Its role as a predictor of family and child outcomes in the first 3 years following childhood TBI. Presented at the 4th Conference of the International Association for the Study of Traumatic Brain Injury, St. Louis, Mo. With permission of J'M Rivara.

of critical examination than stroke rehabilitation . . . Isaacs lament has not been addressed, "experts in stroke rehabilitation abound, but none of them has ever proven anything about rehabilitation to the satisfaction of anybody else" (p. 25).

This outspoken statement applies to those involved in the rehabilitation of TBI patients. No one would question that activities such as physical therapy and occupational therapy are important in helping patients to improve their stamina, to ambulate, and to cope with the physical consequences of their brain injury. There is, however, a sad lack of systematic studies from speech and language pathology and from psychology that document whether systematic rehabilitation for higher cerebral deficits makes a substantial clinical impact on patient outcomes (not just a statistically reliable finding). Thus, it is important to know what questions to ask in terms of whether neuropsychological rehabilitation programs are needed.

Key Questions

From my perspective, four key questions must be addressed.

1. Is cognitive retraining possible? That is, are certain types of treatment associated with clinically significant improvements in higher cerebral functions—compared to no treatment at all?
2. Can cognitive rehabilitation activities substantially help a person to compensate for persistent cognitive impairment?
3. Does psychotherapy significantly contribute to the adjustment

process after brain injury and, if so, in which patients and by what types of therapies?

____4. Does a holistic (milieu)-oriented neuropsychological rehabilitation program improve social functioning for brain-injured patients? Answers to this question should include direct measures such as the percentage of individuals who can work and live independently (without assistance from others). It should also include measures of the patients' (and their families') continued reliance on the health care system for services. Financial and emotional costs to family members also must be assessed.

Summary and Conclusions

After both focal and nonfocal brain injury, cognitive and personality disturbances often persist. Traditional rehabilitation focuses on the patient's physical disabilities and rarely on the common cognitive and personality sequelae associated with brain-injured persons of all ages. In the United States, the emergence of the National Head Injury Foundation reflected the outcry from family members in response to the lack of adequate rehabilitative care to deal with these long-term problems.

The focus of neuropsychological rehabilitation, therefore, is to better understand the patient's persistent cognitive and personality problems and to help patient and family to manage the problems more efficiently (Principle 4). Failure to do so often exacerbates psychosocial difficulties for patient and family because these problems neither go away nor stabilize. Psychosocial adjustment deteriorates for many patients, who often resurface 5 to 10 years after their injury for evaluation or treatment for depression, inappropriate behaviors, difficulties with the law, failure to maintain a job, and related problems. A convincing body of evidence suggests that neuropsychological consequences are associated with a brain injury regardless of how subtle or obvious the insult may appear to the medical community and family.

The task now is to clarify what the cognitive and personality problems associated with brain injury are. What problems are a direct consequence of brain injury and which are indirect effects?

Armed with a reasonable conceptual model, the clinician can help the patient (and family) observe behavior and associated neuropsychological problems. The patient can be taught to take steps to compensate for persistent disturbances and to avoid choices that increase psychosocial isolation. The patient can also be taught to understand his or her own form of the catastrophic reaction and to manage it properly (Principle 4).

In addition, the study of cognitive and personality problems associated with various types of brain insults helps illustrate Principle 5. Namely, cognition and personality are intimately connected, and the failure to study this interaction leads not only to an inadequate understanding in the cognitive neurosciences but to less effective neuropsychological rehabilitation.

References

Ben-Yishay, Y., Rattok, J., Ross, B., Lakin, P., Ezrachi, O., Silver, S., and Diller, L. (1982). Rehabilitation of cognitive and perceptual defects in people with traumatic brain damage. *New York University Rehabilitation Monograph* 64: 127–176.

Brooks, N., McKinlay, W., Symington, C., Beattie, A., and Campsie, L. (1987). Return to work within the first seven years of severe head injury. *Brain Inj.* 1(1), 5–19.

Calvanio, R., Levine, D., and Petrone, P. (1993). Elements of cognitive rehabilitation after right hemisphere stroke. *Behavioral Neurology* 11(1): 25–56.

Chapman, L. F., and Wolff, H. G. (1959). The cerebral hemispheres and the highest integrative functions of man. *Arch. Neurol.* 1: 357–424.

Clinchot, D. M., Kaplan, P., Murray, D. M., and Pease, W. S. (1994). Cerebral aneurysms and arteriovenous malformations: implications for rehabilitation. *Arch. Phys. Med. Rehabil.* 75: 1342–1351.

Cope, D. N., and O'Lear, J. (1993). A clinical and economic perspective on head injury rehabilitation. *Journal of Head Trauma Rehabilitation* 8(4): 1–14.

Costeff, H., Groswasser, Z., Landman, Y., and Brenner, T. (1985). Survivors of severe traumatic brain injury in childhood. I: Late residual disability. *Scand. J. Rehabil. Med. Suppl.* 12: 10–15.

Dikmen, S. S., Machamer, J. E., Winn, H. R., and Temkin, N. R. (1995). Neuropsychological outcome at 1-year post head injury. *Neuropsychology* 9(1): 80–90.

Florian, V., and Katz, S. (1991). The other victims of traumatic brain injury: consequences for family members. *Neuropsychology* 5(4): 267–279.

Godfrey, H. P. D., Partridge, F. M., Knight, R. G., and Bishara, S. (1993). Course of insight disorder and emotional dysfunction following closed-head injury: a controlled cross-sectional follow-up study.*J. Clin. Exp. Neuropsychol.* 15(4): 503–515.

Heilman, K. M., and Valenstein, E. (1993). *Clinical Neuropsychology* (3rd ed). Oxford University Press, New York.

Jamieson, K. G., and Yellard, J. D. N. (1972). Surgically treated traumatic subdural haematomas. *J. Neurosurg.* 37: 137–140.

Jennett, B. (1978). If my son had a head injury. *Br. Med. J.* 1: 1601–1603.

Jennett, B., and Teasdale G. (1981). *Management of Head Injuries*. F. A. Davis, Philadelphia.

Johnson, S. C., Bigler, E. D., Burr, R. B., and Blatter, D. D. (1994). White matter atrophy, ventricular dilation, and intellectual functioning following traumatic brain injury. *Neuropsychology* 8(3): 307–315.

Klonoff, P. S., Snow, W. G., and Costa, L. D. (1986). Quality of life in patients 2 to 3 years after closed head injury. *Neurosurgery* 19(5): 735–743.

Kozloff, R. (1987). Network of social support and the outcome from severe head injury. *Journal of Head Trauma Rehabilitation* 2(3): 14–23.

Lashley, K. S. (1938). Factors limiting recovery after central nervous lesions. *J. Nerv. Ment. Dis.* 88: 733–755.

Levin, H. S., Gary, H. E., Eisenberg, H. M., Ruff, R. M., Barth, J. T., Kreutzer, J., High, W. M., Portman, S., Foulkes, M. J., Jane, J. A., Marmarou, A., and Marshall, L. F. (1990). Neurobehavioral outcome 1 year after severe head injury: experience of the Traumatic Coma Data Bank. *J. Neurosurg.* 73: 699–709.

Livingston, M. G., Brooks, D. N., and Bond, M. R. (1985a). Three months after severe head injury: psychiatric and social impact on relatives. *J. Neurol. Neurosurg. Psychiatry* 48: 870–875.

Livingston, M. G., Brooks, D. N., and Bond, M. R. (1985b). Patient outcome in the year following severe head injury and relatives' psychiatric and social functioning. *J. Neurol. Neurosurg. Psychiatry* 48: 876–881.

Ljunggren, B., Sonesson, B., Säveland, H., and Lennart, B. (1985). Cognitive impairment and adjustment in patients without neurological deficits after aneurysmal SAH and early operation. *J. Neurosurg.* 62: 273–679.

Logue, V., Durward, M., Pratt, R. T. C., Piercy, M., and Nixon, W. L. B. (1968). The quality of survival after rupture of an anterior cerebral aneurysm. *Br. J. Psychiatry* 114: 137–160.

Manseau, C. (1995). *Severe Traumatic Brain Injury: Long Term Organic Insomnia as a Consequence of Closed Effects on Sleep, Sleepiness and Performance.* Doctoral Dissertation, Carleton University, Ottawa.

Maurice-Williams, R. S., Willison, J. R., and Hatfield, R. (1991). The cognitive and psychological sequelae of uncomplicated aneurysm surgery. *J. Neurol. Neurosurg. Psychiatry* 54: 335–340.

Max, W., MacKenzie, E. J., and Rice, D. P. (1991). Head injuries: costs and consequences. *Journal of Head Trauma Rehabilitation* 6(2), 76–91.

Miller, J. D. (1991). Pathophysiology and management of head injury. *Neuropsychology* 5(4): 235–251.

National Directory of Head Injury Rehabilitation Services (1985). National Head Injury Foundation, Inc., Framingham, Mass.

Oddy, M., Coughlan, T., Tyerman, A., and Jenkins, D. (1985). Social adjustment after closed head injury: a further follow-up seven years after injury. *J. Neurol. Neurosurg. Psychiatry* 48: 564–568.

Pang, D. (1985). Pathophysiologic correlates of neurobehavioral syndromes following closed head injury. In M. Ylvisaker (ed), *Head Injury Rehabilitation: Children and Adolescents* (pp. 3–70). College-Hill, San Diego, Calif.

Penfield, W., and Milner, B. (1958). Memory deficit produced by bilateral lesions in the hippocampal zone. *Arch. Neurol. Psychiatry* 79, 475.

Peters, L. C., Stambrook, M., Moore, A. D., and Esses, L. (1990). Psychosocial sequelae of closed head injury: effects on the marital relationship. *Brain Inj.* 4(1): 39–47.

Prigatano, G. P. (1995). Preparing patients for possible neuropsychological consequences after brain surgery. *BNI Quarterly* 11(4): 4–8.

Prigatano, G. P., Fordyce, D. J., Zeiner, H. K., Roueche, J. R., Pepping, M., and Wood, B. (1984). Neuropsychological rehabilitation after closed head injury in young adults. *J. Neurol. Neurosurg. Psychiatry* 47: 505–513.

Prigatano, G. P., and Henderson, S. (1996). Cognitive outcome after subarachnoid hemorrhage. In J. B. Bederson (ed), *Subarachnoid Hemorrhage: Pathophysiology and Management* (pp. 27–40). American Association of Neurological Surgeons, Lebanon, NH.

Prigatano, G. P., Klonoff, P. S., and Bailey, I. (1987). Psychosocial adjustment associated with traumatic brain injury: statistics BNI neurorehabilitation must beat. *BNI Quarterly* 3(1): 10–17.

Prigatano, G. P., Fordyce, D. J., Zeiwer, H. K., Roueche, J. R., Pepping, M., and Wood, B. C. (1986). *Neuropsychological Rehabilitation After Brain Injury.* Johns Hopkins University Press, Baltimore.

Prigatano, G. P., Stahl, M., Orr, W., and Zeiner, H. (1982). Sleep and dreaming disturbances in closed head injury patients. *J. Neurol. Neurosurg. Psychiatry* 45: 78–80.

Prigatano, G. P., Wong, J., Williams, C., and Plenge, K. (1997). Prescribed versus actual length of stay in neurorehabilitation outcome. *Arch. Phys. Med. Rehabil.* 78: 621–629.

Rivara, J'M. B. (1994). Family functioning: its role as a predictor of family and child outcomes in the first 3 years following childhood TBI. Presented at the 4th Conference of the International Association for the Study of Traumatic Brain Injury, St. Louis, Mo.

Rivara, J'M. B., Jaffe, K. M., Polissar, N. L., Fay, G. C., Martin, K. M., Shurtleff, H. A., and Liao, S. (1994). Family functioning and children's academic performance and behavior problems in the year following traumatic brain injury. *Arch. Phys. Med. Rehabil.* 75: 369–379.

Säveland, H., Sonesson, B., Ljunggren, B., Brandt, L., Uski, T., Zygmunt, S., and Hindfelt, B. (1986). Outcome evaluation following subarachnoid hemorrhage. *J. Neurosurg.* 64: 191–196.

Scoville, W. B., and Milner, B. (1957). Loss of recent memory after bilateral hippocampal lesions. *J. Neurol. Neurosurg. Psychiatry* 20: 11–21.

Sonesson, B., Säveland, H., Ljunggren, B., and Brandt, L. (1989). Cognitive functioning after subarachnoid haemorrhage of unknown origin. *Acta Neurol. Scand.* 80: 400–410.

Stenhouse, L. M., Knight, R. G., Longmore, B. E., and Bishara, S. N. (1991). Long-term cognitive deficits in patients after surgery on aneurysms of the anterior communicating artery. *J. Neurol. Neurosurg. Psychiatry* 54: 909–914.

Teasdale, G. M. (1995). Head injury. *J. Neurol. Neurosurg. Psychiatry* 58: 526–539.

Thomsen, I. V. (1984). Late outcome of very severe blunt head trauma: a 10–15 year second follow-up. *J. Neurol. Neurosurg. Psychiatry* 47: 260–268.

Thomsen, I. V. (1989). Do young patients have worse outcomes after severe blunt head trauma? *Brain Inj.* 3(2): 157–162.

Thomsen, I. V. (1995). What does long-term follow-up tell us about the need for family support? Presented at the First World Congress on Brain Injury, Copenhagen, Denmark.

van Zomeren, A. H., and van Den Burg (1985). Residual complaints of patients two years after severe head injury. *J. Neurol. Neurosurg. Psychiatry* 48: 21–28.

Zangwill, O. L. (1947). Psychological aspects of rehabilitation in cases of brain injury. *Br. J. Psychol.* 37: 60–69.

Zimmerman, R. A., and Bilaniuk, L. T. (1989). CT and MR: Diagnosis and evolution of head injury, stroke, and brain tumors. *Neuropsychology* 3: 191–230.

5

Cognitive Disturbances Encountered in Neuropsychological Rehabilitation

> It is concluded that the degree of impairment of the highest integrative functions is directly related to the total number of inadequately functioning cortical neurons, regardless of whether the defective neurons be aggregated in one area of the homotypical isocortex or diffusely distributed throughout the hemispheres.
>
> A. Kiev, L. F. Chapman, T. C. Guthrie, and H. G. Wolff, "The highest integrative functions and diffuse cerebral atrophy," 1962, p. 393

> A set of distributed brain areas must be orchestrated in the performance of even simple cognitive tasks. The task itself is not performed by any single area of the brain, but the operations that underlie the performance are strictly localized.
>
> M. I. Posner, S. E. Petersen, P. T. Fox, and M. E. Raichle, "Localization of cognitive operations in the human brain," 1988, p. 1627

Given that traditional forms of rehabilitation often do not adequately treat or manage disturbances in higher cerebral functions, it is important that neuropsychological rehabilitation help teach patients the nature of their disturbances in a supportive and effective manner. This teaching process requires that patients be helped to observe their behavior in such a manner that they better understand what is "wrong." Formally, this process involves teaching them about the direct and indirect effects of their brain injury. The therapist must guide this process in order to help patients make choices that aid adaptation and avoid needless complications. This is the heart of Principle 4.

In a way, Principle 4 emphasizes that before patients can be taught about what is "wrong," the therapist must have a good understanding of the disturbances that they face. Armed with this knowledge, the therapist can then help the family and the patient accordingly.

Before this process can occur, however, the neuropsychologist must have a reasonable understanding of higher cerebral functions and the cognitive deficits associated with various forms of brain injury. At first glance, this statement may seem obvious, but interacting with different persons with acquired brain injury reveals that the problem is, in fact, quite complex.

Often, conceptualizing the nature of cognitive function and dysfunction requires many different methodologies and conceptual systems (see Posner, 1990). Interesting experimental findings are often difficult to translate into clinical practice. They may, in fact, result in contradictory theoretical statements, as reflected in the two quotes that introduce this chapter.

The clinician must have a strong theoretical grasp of how brain–behavior relationships are disturbed and how this disturbance may be experienced by persons who have suffered brain injuries. This chapter describes some of the cognitive deficits encountered in neuropsychological rehabilitation, particularly in persons with a traumatic brain injury (TBI). It also attempts to provide a perspective that is useful for the practicing clinician. This perspective can then be used to educate patients and family members. Before exploring what may be a useful perspective, it is helpful to begin with the early observations of Chapman and Wolff (1959).

"Higher Integrative Functions" and How They Are Affected by Brain Damage

Chapman and Wolff (1959) produced an extraordinary analysis of how higher cerebral functions or the "higher integrated functions" of man can be adversely affected by focal and diffuse brain damage. In their scholarly review, they summarized "changing concepts of the brain/ mind relationship" from antiquity through the early twentieth century and what they referred to as "the 'Golden Age' of cortical physiology." They reviewed the neurological findings of soldiers who suffered brain injuries in World Wars I and II as well as the observations of such seminal thinkers as Pavlov, Lashley, Goldstein, Halstead, and Teuber.

Chapman and Wolff (1959) also analyzed several issues by studying 132 patients, in 60 of whom "the amount and site of loss of cerebral hemisphere tissue could be estimated reliably . . ." (p. 377). They used various psychometric and other behavioral measures to help determine how different sizes of brain lesions affected cognition. They were also interested in determining if lesions in the frontal and nonfrontal regions differentially affected behavior and cognition. They (Chapman and Wolff, 1959) reported the following:

A hierarchy of the various components could be discerned in terms of a ranking of the functions impaired as the mass of cerebral hemisphere tissue loss increased, regardless of site. Impairment of imagery, curiosity, pursuit of adventure, new experiences, speed of reaction, spontaneity, rapid learning, abstraction, and ability to resist the disorganizing effects of stress was evident in subjects with small lesions (A and B class), whereas vocabulary, long-utilized skills, and factual information were not significantly impaired until there was a much greater tissue loss (pp. 395–396).

They found striking correlations between overall impaired performance on various neuropsychological tests and the mass of tissue loss (Table 5-1). The larger a lesion was, the greater was the patient's level of impairment, particularly on the *Halstead Battery* (but not limited to it). Even measures of conditioning seemed to be related to the overall size of the lesion if the lesion was in a nonfrontal location. The level of performance on the Digit Symbol, Block Design, Picture Arrangement, and Object Assembly subtests from the Wechsler-Bellevue Scale of Intelligence was significantly influenced by the size of the lesion (not reported in Table 5-1). However, large nonfrontal lesions most notably influenced performance on the psychometric measures. Recent work by Dikmen and colleagues (1995) has also demonstrated a strong relationship between the severity of TBI, as measured by the Glasgow Coma Scale, and the Halstead Reitan Neuropsychological Test Battery (Fig. 5-1). This finding is compatible with the earlier findings of Chapman and Wolff (1959).

Chapman and Wolff's (1959) data are also compatible with the observations of Reitan. Reitan (1986) noted that performance on the Digit Symbol subtest may be a useful indicator of brain dysfunction. He further suggested that Picture Arrangement and Block Design subtest scores may be especially sensitive to right hemisphere dysfunction. Although

Table 5-1. Summary of correlations of impairment scores with mass of tissue loss

Aggregate	Frontal (*r*)	Nonfrontal (*r*)	All Sites (*r*)
Wechsler-Bellevue	0.307	0.510*	0.331†
Halstead (New York Hospital)	0.350	0.771*	0.507*
Halstead (Univ. of Chicago)	0.586*	0.280	0.445*
Halstead (pooled series)			0.530*
Conditioning	0.355	0.655*	0.432*
Rorschach	0.380	0.517†	0.355†

*Significant at 1% level.
†Significant at 5% level.
From Chapman L. F. and Wolff H. G. The cerebral hemispheres and the highest integrative functions of man. *Arch Neurol* 1:357–424, copyright 1959, American Medical Association.

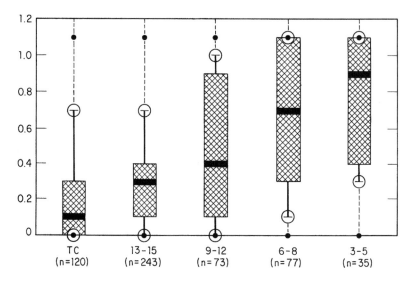

Figure 5-1. Halstead impairment index scores as a function of Glasgow Coma Scale scores in traumatic brain-injured patients 1 year after injury. From Dikmen, S. S., Machamer, J. E., Winn, H. R., and Temkin, N. R. Neuropsychological outcome at 1-year post head injury. *Neuropsychology* 9(1): 80–90. Copyright © 1995 by the American Physiological Association. Adapted with permission.

Chapman and Wolff's observations are important for diagnostic purposes, they are even more important for rehabilitation purposes.

Kiev and colleagues (1962) extended their early analysis to 20 patients with "slowly progressive degenerative disease, resulting in diffuse cerebral atrophy" (p. 385). By interviewing patients, family, friends, and employers, they attempted to assess "behavior and performance in the nonlaboratory setting" (p. 386). This research is especially relevant for the neurorehabilitationist because it is one thing to define cognitive deficits experimentally and another to describe exactly how those deficits affect patients in daily life.

Kiev and colleagues (1962) constructed a list of impairments that were observable in their patients (Table 5-2). Note that many cognitive deficits appear inseparable from affective disturbances (i.e., Principle 5). Their list of behaviors affected by brain dysfunction is not only contemporary in tone but reproduces those behaviors faced by many therapists working with brain dysfunctional patients with a variety of brain disturbances. The list includes behaviors such as decreased tolerance for frustration, decreased capacity to deal with the disorganizing affect of various stressors, impairments in alertness and vigilance, and difficulties with abstract reasoning and flexible problem solving.

Persons with such brain injuries often employ preinjury coping strategies less effectively than they did in the past and have difficulty sustaining appropriate behavior. Inevitably, they have problems with mem-

Table 5-2. Extralaboratory criteria for evaluation of higher integrative functions

1. Reduction of the thresholds for "deprivation" and "frustration"
2. Longer-lasting and more severe disorganization after frustration, deprivation, failure, or conflict
3. Reduced or inappropriate affective response
4. Impaired alertness and vigilance
5. Impaired associative capacity
6. Diminished seeking of the nonadapted state (challenge, adventure, or exploration)
7. Impaired initiation
8. Impaired capacity for abstract thought
9. Impaired capacity to fulfill social, vocational, and interpersonal responsibilities
10. Diminished activity to satisfy appetites and drives
11. Impaired capacity to maintain defensive and compensatory reactions
12. Impaired capacity to develop and maintain appropriate and effective defensive and compensatory reactions
13. Reduction of the intensity of action patterns
14. Reduction of the duration of action patterns
15. Impairment of orientation
16. Memory defects
17. Reduced learning ability
18. Impairment of skilled actions and sensory-motor efficiency
19. Impaired perception of self and self–environment relationship
20. Impaired perception of the environment

Adapted from Kiev et al. (1962).

ory and learning, and their capacity to perceive the meaning of ongoing behaviors objectively is diminished. Any therapist attempting to rehabilitate brain dysfunctional patients in the real world should memorize this list. By addressing these dimensions, therapists are in a much better position to deal with the whole person rather than specific cognitive deficits.

Interestingly, Kiev and colleagues (1962) asserted that "impairment of perception of self and self-environment relationships" was a common sequelae of brain dysfunction in the 20 patients whom they studied. Until recently, this point has been neglected both in the neuropsychological examination and in the experimental literature (Prigatano and Schacter, 1991).

The observations of Kiev and colleagues (1962) underscore the importance of Principle 5. Namely, failure to study the intimate interaction of cognition and personality leads to an inadequate understanding of many issues in cognitive neuroscience and neuropsychological rehabilitation. The problem of initiation after brain injury, for example, could be viewed as a disorder of planning and anticipation. It could also be viewed as a problem of being able to sustain "drive" or "mental tension" (Luria, 1948/1963). When attempting to understand such a problem as a loss of initiative, therapists must constantly recall that cognitive and affective disturbances may underlie this complex problem.

Furthermore, these functions are, by nature, *integrative functions.* Problem-solving skills and personality factors are intimately, intensely, and inseparably connected. Thus, when examining patients, therapists must keep both dimensions in mind.

Consider, for example, the relationship between depression and memory impairment. Prigatano and Wong (1997) documented two cases in which the exacerbation of psychiatric disturbance, including the degree of depression, was paralleled by poor performance on a well-known test of verbal learning and memory. As one patient's psychiatric status improved, so did her long-term free recall and recognition memory. The patient's affective state seemed to influence memory performance on this cognitive task.

As described earlier, the higher cerebral functions appear to be both *convergent* (meaning integrative) and *emergent* (meaning relational) information-processing systems that inherently have an adaptive and problem-solving function (Chapter 2). These information-processing systems do not function independently of an organism's attempt to solve a problem in the social (i.e., real) world. Depending on the problem confronting a given organism, different higher cerebral functions could, theoretically, emerge across time and social situations. They could also be impaired differentially.

A recent experimental finding reflects the interaction of cognition with the social demands of a person's life (Merzenich, 1994). By amplifying high-frequency sounds via cochlear implants, a female patient with a hearing impairment was able to hear sounds that she had never heard before. When this "new information" was presented to her brain, she did not immediately perceive the outside world as persons with normal hearing do. At first the sounds that she heard had no meaning and resembled noise although she could not adequately describe the sounds. With practice, social interaction, and effort, however, the patient's perception of speech sounds improved and now approaches normal limits as evidenced by her subjective reports and by her ability to respond verbally to what she hears.

Merzenich (1994) cited this case as an example of the brain's plasticity. It reflects the basic dynamic quality of higher cerebral functions. These functions develop in concert with environmental inputs and the ability of certain brain structures to process and encode information as well as to transform it in new and different ways. Merzenich suggested that both "bottom-up" and "top-down" central processing occur simultaneously. This characteristic must therefore reflect a fundamental aspect of higher cerebral functioning. Yet, as Mesulam (1990) has suggested, data for describing the nature of these basic mechanisms are inadequate.

These convergent and emergent information-processing systems inherently possess an adaptive problem-solving function, and emotional and motivational features appear to influence directly and to refine these functions. This interaction is often neglected in attempts to understand how mind emerges from brain function (Posner, 1990). Simon (1995) has recently restated this problem, which has always been paramount to clinicians involved in rehabilitation (Prigatano, 1988).

The higher cerebral or integrative functions refer to an exceedingly complex and interactive set of problem-solving abilities that ultimately become more than the sum of their parts. They are heavily dependent on rudimentary activities such as attention and memory as well as on coding and symbolic systems referred to as language. The role of motor functions cannot be underestimated in learning, for action often provides a form of learning distinct from that acquired by reading or thinking. These various components interact in a complex way so that affective components of experience facilitate or impede problem-solving skills, which have a goal-directed component.

Learning Depends on Its Emotional Context

To place these ideas in a practical perspective, let us consider how a 6- to 9-month-old infant actually behaves and how these behaviors seem to influence a complex of higher cerebral functions at the same time. Quite early, infants respond to tone of voice and facial expressions (Scarr et al., 1986). Infants smile or frown depending on the facial feedback that they receive. Certain sounds produce a startle response and crying. Other sounds seem to be comforting and calming. As infants begin to reach out and touch, they explore the outer world. As these motor skills develop, infants not only touch as many objects as possible but put them in their mouths. This behavior is one way in which infants learn what objects are and are not for. The basic biological drive to obtain nurturance (an affective drive) interconnects with the drive to explore the outer world.

As infants begin to hold various objects, they often emit certain sounds. Caregivers or those in attendance often mimic these sounds, which, in turn, the infants mimic. Language seems to emerge as both child and significant others mimic each other's sounds and derive real joy from hearing each other reproduce each other's sounds. By this process, real language develops. The interaction is interpersonal and filled with excitement and joy as well as irritation and frustration. Hearing vowel-consonant sounds is not a purely cognitive task. It is a task also involved with survival and social interaction. As a child makes sounds that are reinforcing to its parents and its parents make sounds that are reinforcing to the child, language acquisition begins to emerge.

Anyone who has watched a toddler for a few days recognizes that during this period of language acquisition, infants also constantly explore the outer world through touch. Interestingly, as infants touch various objects, they also seem to be interested in moving or walking. Despite innumerable falls throughout the course of the day, infants never appear discouraged. The falls seem to be tolerated as inevitable while infants attempt to approximate how to function in the real world. As infants tolerate these falls, they also start to gain a sense of competency in exploring the outer world. In the early stages of the development of higher cerebral functions, children learn to explore the outer world and in the context of that exploration, to meet their biological needs.

Motoric function, language, and problem-solving skills all seem to develop at once. One dimension does not develop in the absence of the other dimensions. This point is important in understanding how to approach patients from a perspective of cognitive retraining. Language is not taught independent of its emotional or motivational quality, and fine motor control cannot be taught divorced from its importance. Nor are memory compensation skills taught for material that is irrelevant to the organism's survival in its daily environment.

The degree to which clinicians can conceptualize the array of cognitive and affective disturbances that can follow brain injury and develop retraining activities that approximate how these functions typically appear in the real world is often the degree to which patients will become engaged in the rehabilitation process. Later chapters focus on this process of engagement.

Cognitive Disorders After TBI

Higher cerebral functions are characterized by this dynamic and constant integration of affect and thinking. Both are brought to bear on problems that concern survival in the outer world. Discussions of localized or distributed brain mechanisms underlying various cognitive functions are of interest but fail to capture the reality of the developing brain. These functions must be distributed because when learning occurs, multiple functions are activated simultaneously. It is naive to think that specific areas of the brain would be responsible for complex higher cerebral functions. Specific neural circuits or patterns of circuits must be crucial to some components of problem-solving as reflected in the introductory quote by Posner and colleagues (1988). Conversely, as Kiev and colleagues (1962) noted, the amount of brain tissue and the complex array that is captured by large regions of brain tissue ultimately must be important to both the development and recovery of higher cerebral functioning. Chapter 13 offers a more complete discussion of recovery and deterioration phenomena. For the purpose of this chapter, however, the reader should keep in mind that cognitive functions are only artificially separated from affective functions. The positive and negative manifestations of cognitive dysfunctions can then better be recognized.

Consequently, it may be helpful to reconceptualize the cognitive disorders that often follow TBI and that have been observed in patients involved in postacute neuropsychological rehabilitation (Prigatano et al., 1986) in terms of their positive and negative manifestations (Table 5-3).

Deficits in Speed of Information Processing After TBI

Pöppel and Von Steinbüchel (1992) have suggested that it may be useful to distinguish two classes of higher cerebral functions. The first determines the content of consciousness or mental activity and the second determines how information actually enters consciousness. In this latter regard, "activation and temporal coordination" (p. 7) of higher cerebral functions are considered the basic logistic functions of brain activity. Earlier, Luria (1973) also suggested that the "first functional unit" of higher brain functions involves activation and a state of vigilance (Caetano and Christensen, 1996). Severe TBI has long been known to result in disorders of arousal, attention, and concentration and to decrease the speed of information processing (Table 5-3 and Prigatano and Fordyce, 1986). These disorders have both positive and negative manifestations.

Let us begin with the negative manifestation of disturbances in the speed of information processing. When asked to perform a task (i.e., the time it takes to wash, shower, shave, dress, and so on), patients with a severe TBI often do so slowly despite encouragement from others to act as quickly as possible. The same behavior is manifested during neuropsychological testing, where, for example, patients may learn new information slowly. Johnson and colleagues (1994) have noted that Performance IQ and scores on the Digit Symbol subtest of the Wechsler Adult Intelligence Scale Performance IQ (WAIS-R) were low (i.e., slow performance) in TBI patients. Moreover, diffuse axonal injury (DAI), as measured by the ventricle-to-brain ratio, positively and significantly correlated with these scores. Interestingly, the correlation was stronger in males than in females.

Dikmen and colleagues (1995) also found that speed of performance correlated highly with estimates of severity of TBI. She and her colleagues noted that "speed, whether involving simple or pure motor skills such as finger tapping or complex problem-solving skills (e.g., Performance IQ), seems to emerge as an important general factor underlying declining performance with increased severity of head injury" (p. 84). Rehabilitation therapists often begin therapy with tasks aimed at improving the speed of information processing (see Chapter 8).

Patients do not automatically accept that they have a deficit in terms

Table 5-3. Common cognitive (and associated behavioral) disorders after moderate to severe traumatic brain injury

Negative Symptoms	Positive Symptoms
Disorders of Speed of Information Processing	
Decreased speed of information processing	Compulsive ordering of information
Slowness in psychomotor activities (i.e., walking, writing, doing mechanical tasks, etc.)	Intolerance for being "rushed" Inability to do two things simultaneously Problems following conversations, with associated signs of irritability
Disorders of Learning and Memory	
Rate of new learning is impaired	Asking the same question repetitively
Free recall of newly learned information with and without cuing is impaired	Confabulation
Material-specific short-term memory deficits (e.g., verbal vs. visuospatial)	Impulsive or "rapid" giving of information to others from apparent fear of forgetting
Amnestic disorder (in some patients)	
Disorders of Arousal, Attention, and Concentration	
Easily "mentally fatigued"	Yawning
Span of immediate attention may be normal with structure (i.e., patient repeats 5 digits upon request) but unable to sustain attention/ concentration without structure	Reports of being bored Intolerance for noise or distractions
Difficulties with selective attention and vigilance (i.e., scanning)	Desire to end cognitively demanding tasks "early"
Poor shifting of attention back and forth so patient may "get lost" in group communication or simple cognitive tasks	Requests for naps or "sleep breaks"
	Reports fatigue when performing any cognitive task
Disorders of Initiation, Planning, and Goal-Directed Activities	
Impairment of the abstract attitude	Prefers "concrete" tasks as opposed to any form of abstract task (which may explain why some patients like cognitive retraining)

(continued)

Table 5-3. —Continued

Negative Symptoms	Positive Symptoms
Disorders of Initiation, Planning, and Goal-Directed Activities	
Impaired ability to initiate action (or sustain drive)	Shows childish behavior
Impaired ability to inhibit action	Reports a lack of interest and may demonstrate blunted affect
Impaired ability to anticipate consequences of behavior	Executes instructions like a computer (i.e., only does as told)
Difficulties monitoring (vigilance) one's own behavior	
Difficulties integrating positive and negative feedback	
Disorders of Judgment and Perception	
Misinterprets actions or intentions of others	Attempts to make sense of confusing happenings
Unable to sequence information and often becomes more confused when multiple bits of information are presented at one time	Reports being able to return to old responsibilities in an effort to regain a sense of normality
Tendency to make socially inappropriate comments	Appears surprised when verbal comments or behavior are described as socially inappropriate
Unrealistic appraisal of self and individual strengths and weaknesses after brain injury	Hallucinations
	Delusions
Disorders of Language Communication	
Articulation difficulties	Hyperverbality/talkativeness
Anomia	Tangentiality in free speech
Paraphasia	Choice of unusual or peculiar words or phrases
Subtle difficulties in auditory comprehension	Asks for clarification of what has been stated
Ineffective word retrieval	
Difficulties maintaining a trend of thought	

Based on Prigatano et al. (1986).

of information processing and thank the therapist for helping them with their obvious impairment. Rather, patients often become irritated for being "rushed." Their threshold for frustration is low when they are asked to handle two tasks at once. They are often irritated when they must follow conversations in which individuals speak quickly. Their irritation can be viewed as a positive manifestation of an underlying disturbance in speed of information processing.

Such individuals are also often compulsive about how they order information. They may insist that individuals speak slowly and that they be allowed to write down information, particularly as they go through rehabilitation exercises. Consequently, clinicians must understand that the underlying disturbance in brain function affecting information processing does not create a purely cognitive deficit. Besides the deficit in rapidly processing information, patients exhibit a series of behavioral and cognitive attempts to cope with the problem as it emerges in the real world.

Van Lehn (1990) observed that typically the relationship between the speed of performance and perceptual motor skills and the numbers of trials of practice can be described as a "power-law" (p. 554). If the time per trial and the number of trials are graphed on a "log-log coordinate basis, a straight line results" (p. 534). After injury, some TBI patients who can perform a given task more quickly after practice often reach asymptote much more quickly than persons without brain injury. This problem can exist despite practice.

In normal children, the speed at which a function is performed often correlates positively with the child's overall cognitive capacity. Kail (1991), for example, noted that reaction time or speed of information processing was linearly related to age. Younger children took a longer time to perform tasks such as mental rotation or name retrieval than older children. The slope of the function was exponential.

Case (1985; personal communication, June 5, 1995) has suggested that this increase in central processing time is inversely related to the level of cognitive development. The implications of this relationship for rehabilitation are obvious. If, in fact, the rate at which information is processed could be improved substantially, then the capacity of the brain to function in a more adaptive manner could also be affected. Cognitive remediation exercises naturally incorporate some activities that attempt to improve the speed of information processing.

Disorders of Arousal, Attention, Concentration

Clinically, damage to almost any area of the brain seems to affect an organism's ability to sustain its arousal level or to show a normal level of alertness. Patients with unilateral focal or bilateral lesions often report less mental energy and have a tendency to fatigue easily when they engage in cognitive work (e.g., Ljunggren et al., 1985; van Zomeren,

1981). This mental fatigue is associated with both mild (Marshall and Ruff, 1989) and severe brain injuries (van Zomeren, 1981).

In their summary of disorders of alertness and attention, Posner and Petersen (1990) suggested that the capacity to maintain an alert state depends on the norepinephrine (NE) system, which arises from the locus ceruleus in the brain stem. Damage to the NE system may partially account for coma and residual disturbances in arousal level after patients emerge from coma.

The process of attention involves the ability to disengage from one stimulus, move to a new stimulus, and then engage the new stimulus (Posner and Petersen, 1990). Impairment of the posterior parietal area, particularly in the right hemisphere, negatively affects the capacity to disengage from a visual stimulus (Posner and Petersen, 1990). Damage to the midbrain seems to affect the actual movement from one stimulus to the next, whereas thalamic lesions (i.e., pulvinar) seem to interfere with the ability to engage a new stimulus (Posner and Petersen, 1990). After TBI, patients often tire rather easily after mental work (Table 5-3). In fact, an interesting aspect of cognitive rehabilitation that has never been adequately explored is whether rehabilitation activities can improve "mental energy" and arousal level. In my clinical experience, patients involved in day-treatment programs often tire quickly during their first few weeks of rehabilitation. Families often report that the patient sleeps several hours at home after working on cognitive retraining tasks 3 to 5 hours a day. With time, patients tolerate increasingly longer efforts. No one, however, has investigated whether cognitive retraining actually improves mental energy or the ability to sustain arousal and attention.

The negative manifestations of impairments of arousal and attention are obvious. Patients complain of being tired, and they sleep more. They also want to terminate tasks because it is difficult for them to maintain a sustained effort. The positive manifestations may be less readily observed but are often present. Patients with arousal or attentional disorders want frequent breaks and want to end a cognitive task early. They also report being "bored" when they cannot sustain the mental energy to perform a task. Many yawn several times throughout the course of the day, even if interested in the task.

When patients' attention and arousal decrease, their tolerance for noise or distractions also decreases. They appear irritable when confronted with distracting noises. The underlying difficulty, however, may be their decreased capacity to sustain their arousal level, attention, and concentration.

Sleep disturbances are also common after TBI, especially in the postacute phase (Cohen et al., 1992; Prigatano et al., 1982). Forty percent to 70% of patients with moderate to severe TBIs often complain of sleep disturbances and an increased need for sleep (von Zomeren, 1981). These early observations have recently been replicated (Manseau, 1995). The

role of helping patients regulate their sleep as an aid to cognitive rehabilitation is also in need of study. Likewise, the effects of cognitive rehabilitation in terms of improving the sleep-wake cycle have never been
assessed. These are natural areas on which to focus during the examination of TBI patients and attempts at their cognitive rehabilitation (see
section below).

Disorders of Learning and Memory

In a recent article, Prigatano and colleagues (1996) reviewed rehabilitation strategies for patients with TBIs and memory impairments. In their
Handbook of Memory Disorders, Baddeley and colleagues (1995) detailed
the various forms of memory impairment that can follow both focal and
diffuse brain injury.

Most, if not all, TBI patients suffer from some form of memory disturbance (Goldstein and Levin, 1995). Episodic memory, however, is affected most dramatically. Patients have trouble learning new information
and errors of intrusion are common, particularly after an injury to the
temporal lobe (Crosson et al., 1993). Intrusion errors on the California
Verbal Learning Test (CVLT), for example, are common after both traumatic and nontraumatic temporal lobe damage. Diffuse brain dysfunction is associated with impairments of semantic and other forms of memory (Goldstein and Levin, 1995). Chapman and Wolff (1959) anticipated
these observations when they argued that the amount of previously
stored and "over-learned" information may deteriorate as the size of a
brain lesion increases.

What are the positive and negative manifestations of memory impairment? The negative manifestations are obvious. Individuals simply
cannot learn new information and often fail to show a capacity to recall
information freely when needed. In some cases, a frank amnestic disorder is present. The positive manifestations (Table 5-3) are reflected by
numerous and repetitive questions, many of which irritate the listener.
In some instances, patients with a memory impairment may confabulate.
The severity of memory impairment per se does not seem to account for
the presence or absence of confabulation. Although patients who confabulate often have a frontal lobe dysfunction (Stuss and Benson, 1986),
not all patients with frontal lobe lesions confabulate. Premorbid personality characteristics also seem to be a part of this symptom picture (Weinstein and Lyerly, 1968; Weinstein, 1995).

Memory impairments have another positive manifestation. During an
examination of a 19-year-old woman with a history of spina bifida and
hydrocephalus, I was impressed that her memory failures led her to become more rigid and impulsive in her problem-solving. Even though she
was able to grasp a concept, when she forgot how that concept could be
applied, her responses became impulsive and rigid. With the anxiety
associated with her memory impairment, she simply responded the same

way each time. She lacked the capacity to stop and observe her own performance. Impulsive and rigid responding is often associated with memory impairments. The development of panic attacks can also be associated with memory disturbances (see Chapter 6). Once again, memory impairment is not isolated from affective impairments. Conversely, the affective aspects of an individual's behavior can surprise clinicians in terms of what patients can remember. For example, patients may remember that they left their lunch in a certain location but find it difficult to remember the name of someone that they just met. How memory and emotion are related awaits further investigation.

Disorders in Initiation, Planning, and Goal-Directed Activities

Van Zomeren (1981) noted that more than 25% of TBI patients report a "loss of initiative." Many patients with moderate to severe TBI have sustained an injury to the frontal lobes (see Chapter 4). Stuss and Benson (1986) have suggested that damage to "frontal functional systems" can disturb "drive," producing various degrees of apathy. Such patients also may have a reduced ability to maintain "cognitive set" and to sequence information properly.

A breakdown of "frontal functional systems" means reduced capacity to anticipate, to select goals, to plan, and to monitor (Stuss and Benson, 1986, p. 244). Stuss (1995) has argued that there is no "central executive" and therefore, no "dysexecutive syndrome":

> The frontal lobes (in anatomical terms) or the supervisory system (in cognitive terms) do not function (in physiological terms) as a simple (inexplicable) homunculus. Monitoring, energizing, inhibition, etc.— these are processes that exist at many levels of the brain, including those more posterior "automatic" processes. Because of their extensive reciprocal connections with virtually all other brain regions, the frontal lobes may be unique in the quality of the processes that have evolved, and perhaps in the level of processing which might be labeled "executive" or supervisory. The different regions of the frontal lobes provide multiple interacting processes (Stuss, 1995, p. 1).

These observations are germane to clinical practice. As noted, moderate to severe TBI is often associated with bilateral asymmetrical injuries to prefrontal and anterior temporal areas of the brain superimposed on DAI (Zimmerman and Bilaniuk, 1989). Figures 5-2 and 5-3 compare common CT and MR imaging findings of hemorrhagic contusions in the frontal and temporal regions of the brain, respectively, after severe TBI. Figure 5-4 reveals a pattern of large ventricles commonly associated with DAI. A wide variety of disturbances in initiation, planning, and goal-directed behavior is possible after such injuries.

These patients seldom seem able to anticipate the consequences of

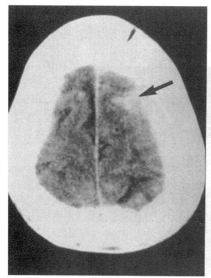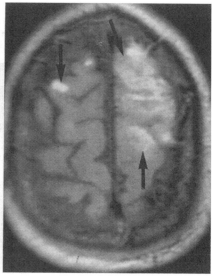

Figure 5-2. Hemorrhagic contusions. A 33-year-old man examined within several days of injury. (A) Axial CT shows a high-density area involving the cerebral cortex on the left (*arrow*). The high density is the same as that of the adjacent bone on these images photographed with a narrow window width. (B) Axial T1-weighted image shows high signal intensity methemoglobin (*arrows*) outlining multiple hemorrhagic contusion of the left frontal gyrus. At least two sites are present on the right. From Zimmerman, R. A. and Bilaniuk, L. T. (1989). CT and MR: Diagnosis and evolution of head injury, stroke, and brain tumors. *Neuropsychology* 3: 191–230. With permission from R. A. Zimmerman.

their actions (Freedman et al., 1987). Negative feedback or negative reinforcement fails to influence their behavior as much as it does that of non-brain-injured individuals. This possibility may explain why working relationships with patients in the context of a milieu-oriented rehabilitation program are often more effective than a straight behavioral modification approach to managing their inappropriate behaviors.

Under this broad category, a wide variety of disorders occurs. Besides difficulties with initiation, patients experience difficulties in planning and organization. They may not only be immobile and fail to initiate action, they also may insist on having precise instructions before they execute an action. The latter behavior is often a positive manifestation of the underlying negative disorder of initiation and planning. Patients also may appear to lack interest in the environment because they do not understand how events relate to one another. Thus, they frequently report being "bored." At such times their behavior may seem childish because they require more supervision than a non-brain-injured individual would need to proceed with a simple task.

The need to separate the positive and negative manifestations of dis-

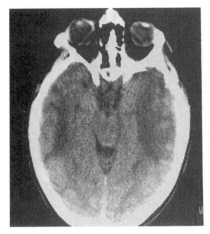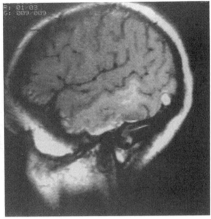

Figure 5-3. Hemorrhagic contusions in a male patient 17 days after being struck by a motor vehicle. (A) Axial CT shows bilateral hypodensities involving the temporal lobes. (B) Sagittal T1-weighted image shows high signal intensity methemoglobin within hemorrhagic contusion of the middle and inferior temporal gyri. From Zimmerman, R. A. and Bilaniuk, L. T. (1989). CT and MR: Diagnosis and evolution of head injury, stroke, and brain tumors. *Neuropsychology* 3:191–230. With permission from R. A. Zimmerman.

orders is important for clinical work. Positive manifestations often are amenable to management, and compensation techniques can be used to help patients behave in a more socially acceptable manner. Negative symptoms are more difficult to treat even though lesion studies have elucidated some of their underlying mechanisms. As the neural circuitry of the frontal and nonfrontal regions is clarified, a greater appreciation may emerge for how specific behaviors are mediated by specific neural pathways.

Disorders in Judgment and Perception

Closely related to difficulties in anticipation, planning, initiation, and self-monitoring are disorders of judgment and perception. This class of disorders, however, is distinguished from the others for at least two reasons. First, the importance of posterior brain structures (i.e., parietal, medial and posterior temporal, and occipital lobes) in registering and integrating somatic, auditory, and visual information (Stuss and Benson, 1986) has long been recognized. Discrete lesions in these regions often disturb perceptions of objects in the outside world (Teuber, 1969). Anterior brain structures (i.e., frontal and anterior temporal areas) are probably less important to the perception of external objects but more important to their contextual perception (Pribram, 1971, 1991). Consequently, damage to posterior areas of the brain can directly disturb

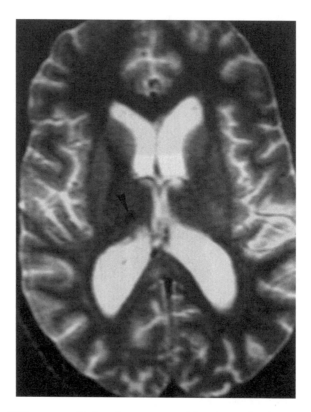

Figure 5-4. Diffuse axonal injury in a 17-year-old male involved in a motor vehicle accident. Follow-up axial T2-weighted image 2 months after injury shows that the ventricles and sulci have dilated in the intervening period. An area of old hemorrhage is seen as a focal hypointensity (*arrowhead*). The angles of the planes of section for the computed tomographic scan and the magnetic resonance image are different. From Zimmerman, R. A. and Bilaniuk, L. T. (1989). CT and MR: Diagnosis and evolution of head injury, stroke, and brain tumors. *Neuropsychology* 3: 191–230. With permission from R. A. Zimmerman.

the perception of reality. Mesial temporal and posterior temporal lesions seem to have an especially negative influence on integrating perceptions with memory, and the world can appear chaotic and unpredictable. Not surprisingly, patients with temporal lobe lesions, particularly in the left hemisphere, tend to exhibit suspiciousness, paranoid ideation, and even frankly psychotic behavior (Prigatano et al., 1988; Falconer, 1973; Cummings, 1985; Prigatano, 1988).

When such disorders exist, the basic building blocks for determining external reality are altered. This situation is qualitatively different from perceiving external reality relatively objectively but not knowing how to act on or interpret that reality. The latter condition is often associated with impairment of the anterior portion of the brain, and the former with more posterior injuries. Patients with TBIs and those with lesions in the temporal and occipital lobes associated with subarachnoid hemorrhage (SAH) or complications from surgery for an aneurysm or arteriovenous malformation (AVM) often experience major difficulties in perceiving the external environment adequately (personal observation). Some of these patients eventually develop hallucinations and delusions. Interestingly, the hallucinations sometimes occur in the hemifield contralateral to the location of the lesion as observed on computed tomography or magnetic resonance imaging.

The second reason for using the term judgment and separating it from the combination of several subcomponents listed above is that the word judgment implies some capacity to integrate disparate pieces of information. This integration often requires combining information from posterior and anterior cerebral centers. Thus, judgment is an emergent function and consciousness and self-awareness are among its key properties. This capacity (discussed in Chapter 11) serves as a metacognitive function and helps individuals to make judgments about the self as well as about others.

Patients who exhibit problems with judgment and perception after TBI often misinterpret the actions or intentions of others (Prigatano and Fordyce, 1986). They often make socially inappropriate comments and appraise themselves unrealistically. They also lack "cognitive flexibility." Vilkki (1992), for example, found that the performance of TBI patients who had nonfrontal parenchymal lesions on a test of cognitive inflexibility was similar to that of patients with anterior cerebral lesions. Thus, lesions throughout the brain could affect the individual's capacity to exercise cognitive flexibility (or judgment).

Flexibility in responding to the varying demands of the environment requires input from multiple brain structures. Consequently, impairments in judgment cannot be attributed to an injury of a specific part of the brain. Different types or subcomponents of problems with judgment may emerge, depending on whether focal lesions are in frontal or nonfrontal areas.

Disorders in Language and Communication

Injury to the brain can produce primary disturbances in language that affect auditory comprehension, naming, sentence repetition, and fluency (Prigatano et al., 1995). Different aphasic syndromes are related to such primary deficits in language (Benson, 1988). Spelling, reading, and writing are also frequently disturbed. Combinations of these impaired functions produce different aphasic syndromes (Benson, 1988). Premorbid cognitive and personality factors do not seem to influence these or the amnestic syndromes substantially (Squire, 1991). Yet different types of naming errors have been linked to premorbid features of the personality (Weinstein et al., 1962).

Various other language difficulties, which have been termed non-aphasic or subclinical language disorders, also occur (Prigatano et al., 1986). For example, Sarno and colleagues (1986) characterized a series of language impairments associated with closed head injuries that did not meet the classical description of aphasia. Such individuals often show problems with anomia, auditory comprehension, efficient and effective word retrieval, and maintaining a trend of thought. Some of these problems could be viewed as the negative manifestations of an underlying language impairment (Table 5-3).

Although the impact of these communication disturbances can be significant, they are difficult to investigate. Patients may become hyper-verbal or talkative in an attempt to communicate (positive manifestations). Their free speech can become tangential, apparently because they experience subtle difficulties in retrieving words and in memory. They often find it hard to follow conversations, particularly when there are more than two speakers (Oddy et al., 1985).

Lackner and Shattuck-Hufnagel (1982) studied the long-term effects of penetrating brain injuries on veterans of the Korean War. Several years after injury, patients with left hemisphere injuries who had initially been aphasic but who showed no obvious impairment of their free speech still demonstrated important but subtle impairments. For example, they had difficulty monitoring messages presented through earphones. When they listened to sentences and word lists, they had an exceedingly difficult time monitoring or shadowing the linguistic inputs compared to non-injured controls. The presence of syntax helped the TBI patients in the process of monitoring. Speed of presentation greatly influenced performance in all patient groups—left hemisphere patients with aphasia as well as other patients who never demonstrated aphasia, either initially or postacutely. Again, brain damage reduced the speed of information processing, even in language-related tasks.

Despite their apparent clinical recovery, children who have experienced aphasia have persistent language deficits that affect their school performance negatively (Alajouanine and L'Hermitte, 1965; Woods and Carey, 1978). Recovered aphasic children perform significantly worse in determining whether a sentence read to them is correct. They also perform poorly on picture-naming and sentence-completion tasks. These findings suggest that the higher integrative functions of language are often compromised even when apparent aphasic syndromes disappear.

Finally, Aram and colleagues (1985) studied children who had sustained lesions of the left and right hemispheres between the ages of 18 months and 8 years. Syntactic production was impaired in the children with left hemisphere lesions whereas children with right hemisphere lesions had difficulties with lexical comprehension and production. The verbal fluency of both groups was decreased. All children, including normal children, experienced difficulties with articulation. Interestingly,

children with left hemisphere lesions produced the most errors of articulation. These findings indicate that important residual nonaphasic language disturbances can persist after an aphasic syndrome has resolved
as well as after almost any injury to the brain. Language impairments
can be associated with both right hemisphere lesions and bilateral lesions
that do not produce a frank aphasic disturbance. The study of language
in non-brain dysfunctional persons also highlights the importance of
both cerebral hemispheres and even the cerebellum. Using cerebral blood
flow as a measure of local brain activity, several studies have demonstrated that different aspects of language seem to involve multiple brain
regions. Roland (1993) has summarized many investigations using regional changes in cerebral blood flow and language tasks.

Bilateral Blood Flow Changes Associated with Speech and Planning to Speak: a Case Example

To highlight how both cerebral hemispheres can be engaged in the act
of speaking and planning to speak, Figure 5-5 is presented. This figure
reveals cerebral blood flow changes that occurred when I was asked to
construct mentally what I would say if giving a lecture to colleagues on
neuropsychological rehabilitation. Blood flow increased in both cerebral
hemispheres, particularly anteriorly. The greatest amount of blood flow
is in the left hemisphere and in the region thought to represent Broca's
area. This area is activated by the *intention* to present ideas and by organizing those ideas but not actually by speaking.

In contrast, when I actually spoke (giving a brief lecture to colleagues),
a different pattern of blood flow was observed (also Figure 5-5). The right
parietal region was more activated. Verbal communication thus seems
to involve visualization as well as articulating vowel-consonant sounds
and generating meaningful words. During an interaction that involves
speech, speakers constantly visually scan each other's reaction to what
is being said. Consequently, language develops in relationship to both
cerebral hemispheres. This fact is important to both neuropsychological
assessment and rehabilitation, as discussed in Chapter 8.

Cognitive Disorders and Focal Brain Lesions

Since at least the early work of Paul Broca (1861), interest in relating
specific anatomical deficits to specific disturbances in higher cerebral
functions has been keen. The history and study of aphasia reflect this
enduring interest. Although size of brain lesion or some overall measure
of severity of injury reliably relates to an individual's overall adaptive
capacities (Chapman and Wolff, 1959; Kiev et al., 1962; Johnson et al.,
1994; Dikmen et al., 1995), focal lesions also can have a traumatic impact
on certain higher integrative functional systems. Recall, for example, that
bilateral lesions of the hippocampus can produce a profound amnestic

disorder (Scoville and Milner, 1957; Penfield and Milner, 1958). A ventromedial lesion of the frontal lobe underlies disturbances in "social cognition" when the consequences of immediate versus delayed decision making may be crucial (Damasio et al., 1991). Focal lesions involving the splenium of the corpus callosum and affecting the left occipital lobe produce difficulties in reading (alexia) without disturbing writing (agraphia) (Benson and Geschwind, 1985).

These and other cognitive impairments are summarized in many neuropsychology and behavioral neurology texts (Heilman and Valenstein, 1993; Mesulam, 1985). In particular, McCarthy and Warrington (1990) provide an in-depth and scholarly analysis of specific cognitive disturbances that are correlated with specific anatomical defects.

In clinical practice, however, a specific cognitive deficit is usually associated with other disturbances in higher cerebral functioning. This observation reflects that higher cerebral functions are integrated rather than isolated. For example, a patient with a SAH was later found to have an AVM that was fed by branches of the left middle and left posterior cerebral arteries. He demonstrated the classic syndrome of alexia without agraphia (O'Brien and Prigatano, 1991). He also had visual and memory difficulties, a mild disturbance in right-left orientation, and persistent but mild bilateral finger agnosia. His scores on tests of abstract reasoning, general fund of verbal information, vocabulary, and speed of finger movement were within normal limits and compatible with his educational background. Yet, several months after his focal injury, both specific and nonspecific changes in higher cerebral functioning could be identified.

In another example, a 26-year-old man suffered a gunshot wound to the left occipital area. He showed an imperfect but complete homonymous hemianopsia with an interesting form of alexia. If words were presented horizontally, he could only read one letter at a time and often was unable to read the entire word. If the letters were arranged vertically, he could read them easily. He frequently turned a book from a horizontal to a vertical position in order to read it. With some practice, he actually became proficient at reading in this manner.

Did this man show only this unique form of alexia? The answer is no. Although his syndrome was striking and supports the concept that a high degree of organization underlies operations for performing such tasks, as Posner and colleagues (1988) have suggested, his clinical profile revealed a number of cognitive and related difficulties. He had trouble with verbal memory. His speed of information processing, particularly verbal information, was slow. On formal psychometric testing, his verbal

Figure 5-5. Cerebral blood flow of the author while (top) preparing a speech and (bottom) during the act of giving a speech. Courtesy of Jarl Risberg, Ph.D.

RESTING
(PREPARING A LECTURE)

CASE 5006.01   REST

F1 %

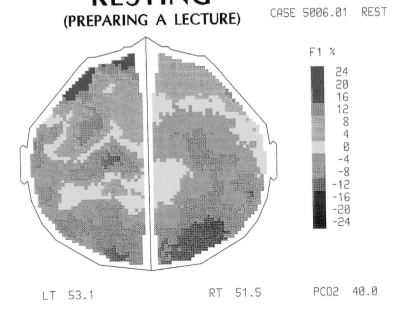

24
20
16
12
8
4
0
-4
-8
-12
-16
-20
-24

LT 53.1   RT 51.5   PCO2 40.0

LECTURING

CASE 5006.02   TEST

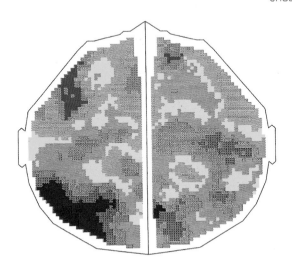

LT 58.1   RT 57.4   PCO2 0.0

fluency was reduced. His approach to different tasks was also slightly rigid (the problem of cognitive flexibility noted earlier). Overall, his abstract reasoning or problem-solving capacity was within normal limits, particularly his ability to solve visuospatial tasks. Although he was cooperative, he described himself as more irritable and belligerent, particularly toward females. Although he had a unique and specific form of alexia, he experienced other disturbances in higher integrative functions.

Thus, even relatively focal brain lesions are often associated with disturbances other than those reported by theoreticians whose primary interest is to correlate specific anatomical areas with specific neuropsychological deficits. This point has important theoretical and clinical implications, as working with patients in neuropsychological rehabilitation makes abundantly clear. Clinicians who examine patients only briefly or who study them only from the perspective of an experimental paradigm and rarely observe patients in more naturalistic environments can often miss these important behavioral disturbances.

Strict localization-oriented theorists who try to reduce higher cerebral functions to circuit diagrams often fail to consider these important clinical phenomena. Henry Head (1926), for example, referred to the so-called "diagram makers" who attempted to parse the complex phenomenon of aphasia into neat little boxes. Although flow diagrams are heuristic for the field of cognitive psychology (McCarthy and Warrington (1990), they are also inaccurate representations of the complex processes of the brain.

Luria's (1966) conceptualization of the higher cerebral functions as reflecting the interactions of functional systems and subsystems explains this phenomenon. A lesion, even a very small one, will often have both distal and regional effects. The larger the lesion or the more diffuse the injury is, the greater will be the overall neuropsychological impairment. Associated systems are always disrupted even if lesions are small and focal. Both Luria's (1966) and Lashley's (1929/1964) ideas must be remembered during attempts to comprehend the effects of brain injury and to develop theoretical and clinical approaches to neurorehabilitation.

Summary and Conclusions

Disturbances of brain function, whether related to focal or diffuse bilateral injuries, have predictable consequences for cognition. Moderate to severe TBIs often disrupt the speed of information processing, learning and memory, alertness and attention, initiation, planning, and a variety of goal-directed activities. Disorders of judgment that affect patients' subjective awareness as well as their perception of reality can be pervasive. Subtle language disturbances, both aphasic and nonaphasic, can exist. These disturbances can wreak havoc on a person's capacity to cope and adjust to life after a brain injury.

From a perspective of neuropsychological rehabilitation, it may be useful to conceptualize these disturbances as negative (i.e., the direct consequences of brain injury) or positive symptoms (i.e., an attempt to cope with the environment given disturbed brain function), as Hughlings Jackson initially suggested. Approaching cognitive symptoms in this way may lead to more effective rehabilitation programs.

The nature of the higher cerebral functions has not yet been defined adequately. They appear to have both convergent and emergent functional properties (see Chapter 2). They seem to depend on both basic sensory inputs ("bottom-up" processes) and "top-down" processes that modulate or influence inputs to the system. Various models have been proposed to explain the emergent and convergent qualities of higher cerebral functioning. However, the role of emotion and motivation in influencing the development and practical functionality of higher cerebral functioning has been neglected. Perhaps using the term integrated rather than cerebral to describe these functions would help remind us of the important interconnections between cognition and personality. Unless these two components are studied in conjunction with one another, the resulting view of higher cerebral functions is distorted (i.e., Principle 5). This produces, at best, a pale reflection of human nature, particularly of people struggling to cope with the effects of brain injury.

References

Alajouanine, T. H., and L'Hermitte, F. (1965). Acquired aphasia in children. *Brain* 88: 635–662.

Aram, D. M., Ekelman, B. L., Rose, D. F., and Whitaker, H. A. (1985). Verbal and cognitive sequelae following unilateral lesions acquired in early childhood. *J. Clin. Exp. Neuropsychol.* 7(1): 55–78.

Baddeley, A. D., Wilson, B. A., and Watts, F. N. (1995). *Handbook of Memory Disorders*. John Wiley & Sons, West Sussex, England.

Benson, D. F., and Geschwind, N. (1985). Aphasia and related disorders: a clinical approach. In M-M Mesulam (ed), *Principles of Behavioral Neurology* (pp. 193–238). F. A. Davis, Philadelphia.

Benson, D. F. (1988). Classical syndromes of aphasia. In F. Boller and J. Grafman (eds), *Handbook of Neuropsychology* (Vol. 1, pp. 267–280). Elsevier Science, Amsterdam.

Broca, P. (1861). Remarques sur le siege de la faculté du language articulé suivie d'une observation d'aphemie. *Bulletin de la Societé de Anatomie de Paris* 6, 330. Translated in R. Herrnstein and E. G. Boring (1965). *A Source Book in the History of Psychology*. Harvard University Press, Cambridge.

Caetano, C., and Christensen, A-L. (1996). The design of neuropsychological rehabilitation: the role of neuropsychological assessment. In J. León-Carrión (eds), *Neuropsychological Rehabilitation* (pp. 63–72). GR/St. Lucie, Delray Beach, Fla.

Case, R. (1985). *Intellectual Development. Birth to Adulthood.* Academic Press, San Diego, Calif.

Chapman, L. F., and Wolff, H. G. (1959). The cerebral hemispheres and the highest integrative functions of man. *Arch. Neurol.* 1: 357–242.

Cohen, M., Oksenberg, A., Snir, D., Stern, M. J., and Groswasser, Z. (1992). Temporally related changes of sleep complaints in traumatic brain injured patients. *J. Neurol. Neurosurg. Psychiatry* 55: 313–315.

Crosson, B., Sartor, K. J., Jenny, A. F., Nabors, N. A., and Moberg, P. J. (1993). Increased intrusions during verbal recall in traumatic and nontraumatic lesions of the temporal lobe. *Neuropsychology* 7: 193–208.

Cummings, J. L. (1985). Organic delusions: phenomenology, anatomical correlations, and review. *Br. J. Psychiatry* 146: 184–197.

Damasio, A. R., Tranel, D., and Damasio, H. (1991). Somatic markers and the guidance of behavior: theory and preliminary testing. In H. S. Levin, H. M. Eisenberg, and A. L. Benton (eds), *Frontal Lobe Function and Dysfunction.* Oxford University Press, New York.

Dikmen, S. S., Machamer, J. E., Winn, H. R., and Temkin, N. R. (1995). Neuropsychological outcome at 1-year post head injury. *Neuropsychology* 9(1): 80–90.

Falconer, M. A. (1973). Reversibility by temporal-lobe resection of the behavioral abnormalities of temporal-lobe epilepsy. *N. Engl. J. Med.* 289(9): 451–455.

Freedman, P. E., Bleiberg, J., and Freedland, K. (1987). Anticipatory behaviour deficits in closed head injury. *J. Neurol. Neurosurg. Psychiatry* 50: 398–401.

Goldstein, F. C., and Levin, H. S. (1995) Post-traumatic and anterograde amnesia following closed head injury. In A. D. Baddeley, B. A. Wilson, and F. N. Watts (eds), *Handbook of Memory Disorders* (pp. 187–209). John Wiley & Sons, West Sussex, England.

Head, H. (1926). *Aphasia and Kindred Disorders* (2 vols.). Cambridge University Press, London.

Heilman, K. M., and Valenstein, E. (1993). *Clinical Neuropsychology* (3rd ed). Oxford University Press, New York.

Johnson, S. C., Bigler, E. D., Burr, R. B., and Blatter, D. D. (1994). White matter atrophy, ventricular dilation, and intellectual functioning following traumatic brain injury. *Neuropsychology* 8(3): 307–315.

Kail, R. (1991). Developmental change in speed of processing during childhood and adolescence. *Psychol. Bull.* 109(3), 490–501.

Kiev, A., Chapman, L. F., Guthrie, T. C., and Wolff, H. G. (1962). The highest integrative functions and diffuse cerebral atrophy. *Neurology* 12: 385–393.

Lackner, J. R., and Shattuck-Hufnagel, S. R. (1982). Alterations in speech shadowing ability after cerebral injury in man. *Neuropsychologia* 20(6): 709–714.

Lashley, K. S. (1929/1964). *Brain Mechanisms and Intelligence: A Quantitative Study of Injuries to the Brain.* Hafner, New York. Originally published (1929) by the University of Chicago.

Ljunggren, B., Sonesson, B., Säveland, H., and Lennart, B. (1985). Cognitive impairment and adjustment in patients without neurological deficits after aneurysmal SAH and early operation. *J. Neurosurg.* 62: 273–679.

Luria, A. R. (1966). Kurt Goldstein and neuropsychology. *Neuropsychologia 4*: 311–313.

Luria, A. R. (1948/1963). *Restoration of Function After Brain Trauma* (in Russian). Moscow: Academy of Medical Science (Pergamon, London, 1963).

Luria, A. R. (1973). *The Working Brain. An Introduction to Neuropsychology.* Allen Lane Penguin Books, Middlesex, England.

Manseau, C., (1995). *Severe Traumatic Brain Injury: Long Term Effects in Sleep, Sleepiness, and Performance.* Doctoral Dissertation, Carleton University, Ottawa.

Marshall, L. F., and Ruff, R. M. (1989). Neurosurgeon as victim. In H. S. Levin, H. M. Eisenberg, and A. L. Benton (eds), *Mild Head Injury* (pp. 276–280). Oxford University Press, New York.

McCarthy, R. A., and Warrington, E. K. (1990). *Cognitive Neuropsychology: A Clinical Introduction.* Academic Press, London.

Merzenich, M. (1994). *The Adapting Brain* [video]. James S. McDonnell Seminar Institute in Cognitive Sciences. Perpetual Productions, Eugene, Ore.

Mesulam, M-M. (1985). *Principles of Behavioral Neurology.* F. A. Davis, Philadelphia.

Mesulam, M-M. (1990). Large-scale neurocognitive networks and distributed processing for attention, language, and memory. *Ann. Neurol.* 28(5): 597–613

O'Brien, K. P., and Prigatano, G. P. (1991). Supportive psychotherapy with a patient exhibiting alexia without agraphia. *Journal of Head Trauma and Rehabilitation* 6(4): 44–55.

Oddy, M., Coughlan, T., Tyerman, A., and Jenkins, D. (1985). Social adjustment after closed head injury: a further follow-up seven years after injury. *J. Neurol. Neurosurg. Psychiatry* 48: 564–568.

Penfield, W., and Milner, B. (1958). Memory deficit produced by bilateral lesions in the hippocampal zone. *Archives of Neurology and Psychiatry.* 79: 475.

Pöppel, E., and Steinbüchel, N.v. (1992). *Neuropsychological Rehabilitation.* Springer-Verlag, Berlin.

Posner, M. I. (1990). *Foundations of Cognitive Science.* MIT, Cambridge, Mass.

Posner, M. I., and Petersen, S. E. (1990). The attention system of the human brain. *Annual Review of Neuroscience* 13: 25–42.

Posner, M. I., Petersen, S. E., Fox, P. T., and Raichle, M. E. (1988). Localization of cognitive operations in the human brain. *Science* 204: 1627–1631.

Pribram, K. H. (1971). *Languages of the Brain: Experimental Paradoxes and Principles in Neuropsychology.* Prentice-Hall, Englewood Cliffs, NJ.

Pribram, K. H. (1991). *Brain and Perception: Holonomy and Structure in Figural Processing.* Lawrence Erlbaum, Hillsdale, NJ.

Prigatano, G. P. (1988). Emotion and motivation in recovery and adaptation to brain damage. In S. Finger, T. LeVere, C. Almli, and D. Stein (eds),

Brain Injury and Recovery: Theoretical and Controversial Issues, (pp. 335–350). Plenum Press, New York.

Prigatano, G. P., Amin, K., and Rosenstein, L. D. (1995). *Administration and Scoring Manual for the BNI Screen for Higher Cerebral Functions*. Barrow Neurological Institute, Phoenix, Ariz.

Prigatano, G. P., and Fordyce, D. J. (1986). Cognitive dysfunction and psychosocial adjustment after brain injury. In Prigatano et al. (eds), *Neuropsychological Rehabilitation After Brain Injury* (pp. 1–17). Johns Hopkins University Press, Baltimore.

Prigatano, G. P., Glisky, E., and Klonoff, P. (1996). Cognitive rehabilitation after traumatic brain injury. In P. W. Corrigan and S. C. Yudofsky (eds), *Cognitive Rehabilitation of Neuropsychiatric Disorders* (pp. 223–242). American Psychiatric Association, Washington, D.C.

Prigatano, G. P., O'Brien, K. P., and Klonoff, P. S. (1988). The clinical management of delusions in postacute traumatic brain injured patients. *Journal of Head Trauma Rehabilitation* 3(3): 23–32.

Prigatano, G. P., Fordyce, P. J., Zeiner, H. K., Roueche, J. R., Pepping, M., and Wood, R. C. (1986). *Neuropsychological Rehabilitation After Brain Injury*. Johns Hopkins University Press, Baltimore.

Prigatano, G. P., and Schacter, D. L. (1991). *Awareness of Deficit After Brain Injury: Clinical and Theoretical Issues*. Oxford University Press, New York.

Prigatano, G. P., Stahl, M., Orr, W., and Zeiner, H. (1982). Sleep and dreaming disturbances in closed head injury patients. *J. Neurol. Neurosurg. Psychiatry* 45, 78–80.

Prigatano, G. P. and Wong, J. L. (1997). Depression and performance on the California Verbal Learning Test (CVLT): Two case examples (abstract). *Archives of Clinical Neuropsychology* 4: 380–389.

Reitan, R. M. (1986). Theoretical and methodological bases of the Halstead-Reitan Neuropsychological Test Battery. In I. Grant and K. M. Adams (eds), *Neuropsychological Assessment of Neuropsychiatric Disorders* (pp. 3–30). Oxford University Press, New York.

Robertson, I. H. (1994). Persisting unilateral neglect: compensatory processes within multiple-interacting circuits. *Neuropsychology Rehabilitation* 4(2): 193–197.

Roland, P. E. (1993). *Brain Activation*. Wiley-Liss, New York.

Sarno, M. T., Buonaguro, A., and Levita, E. (1986). Characteristics of verbal impairment in closed head injured patients. *Arch. Phys. Med. Rehabil.* 67: 400–405.

Scarr, S., Weinberg, R. A., and Levine, A. (1986) *Understanding Development*. Harcourt Brace, San Diego, Calif.

Scoville, W. B., and Milner, B. (1957). Loss of recent memory after bilateral hippocampal lesions. *J. Neurol. Neurosurg. Psychiatry* 20: 11.

Simon, H. A. (1995). The information-processing theory of mind. *Am. Psychol.* 50 (7): 507–508.

Squire, L. (1991). Memory and its disorders. In F. Boller and J. Grafman (eds),

Handbook of Neuropsychology (Vol. 3, Section 5, pp. 3–267). Elsevier Science, Amsterdam.

Stuss, D. (1995). What frontal lobe dysfunction tells us about the nature of higher cerebral functions. Presented at *Neuropsychological Assessment and Rehabilitation After Brain Injury: Empirical and Theoretical Foundations.* Scottsdale, Ariz.

Stuss, D. T., and Benson, D. F. (1986). *The Frontal Lobes.* Raven Press, New York.

Teuber, H-L. (1969). Neglected aspects of the posttraumatic syndrome. In A. E. Walker, W. F. Caveness, and M. Critchley (eds). *The Late Effects of Head Injury* (pp. 13–34). Charles C Thomas, Springfield, Ill.

Van Lehn, K. (1990). Problem solving and cognitive skills acquisition. In M. I. Posner (ed), *Foundations of Cognitive Science* (pp. 527–579). MIT, Cambridge, Mass.

van Zomeren, A. H. (1981). *Reaction Time and Attention After Closed Head Injury.* Swets & Zeitlinger B. V., Lisse, The Netherlands.

Vilkki, J. (1992). Cognitive flexibility and mental programming after closed head injuries and anterior or posterior cerebral excisions. *Neuropsychologia* 30(9): 807–814.

Weinstein, E. A. (1995). Why do some patients confabulate after brain injury: an argument for the role of premorbid personality factors in influencing the neuropsychological symptom picture. Presented at the 10th Year Anniversary of the Section of Neuropsychology, Barrow Neurological Institute, Scottsdale, Ariz.

Weinstein, E. A., and Lyerly, O. G. (1968). Confabulation following brain injury: its analogues and sequelae. *Arch. Gen. Psychiatry* 18: 348–354.

Weinstein, E. A., Marvin, S. L., and Keller, N. J. A. (1962). Amnesia as a language pattern. *Arch. Gen. Psychiatry* 6: 17–28.

Woods, B. T., and Carey, S. (1978). Language deficits after apparent clinical recovery from childhood aphasia. *Ann. Neurol.* 6(5): 405–409.

Zimmerman, R. A., and Bilaniuk, L. T. (1989). CT and MR: diagnosis and evolution of head injury, stroke, and brain tumors. *Neuropsychology* 3(4): 191–203.

6

Personality Disturbances and Brain Damage: Theoretical Perspectives

... emotion may not really be a state of disorganization, but rather one of reorganization with special significance with the totality of behavior.

K. Goldstein, "On emotions: considerations from the organismic point of view," 1971, p. 461

People have both motives and reasons for what they do. The motives define their goals, and the reasons connect those goals with particular courses of action for realizing them. Thinking begins with goals and cannot move without them. Emotions, when aroused from memory, interrupt action and redirect it to alternative motives that have become more pressing than the current one.

H. A. Simon, "The bottleneck of attention: connecting thought with motivation," 1994, p. 19

The intent of this chapter, the preceding one, and the one to follow is to help clinicians understand a body of knowledge that is relevant to Principle 4 and that highlights Principle 5. Namely, neuropsychological rehabilitation needs to help patients and families to understand behavior after brain injury so that their confusion and frustration are reduced. In so doing, the intimate connection between cognition and emotions-motivations (i.e., personality) is at once realized.

Patients referred for neuropsychological assessment and rehabilitation exhibit a wide variety of personality characteristics and (in some cases) disorders. Their emotional and motivational characteristics must be considered constantly when they undergo evaluation for disturbances in

Sections of this chapter on direct effects of brain dysfunction and depression and on symptoms of depression after traumatic brain injury have been adapted from Prigatno, G. P. and Summers, J. D. (1997). Depression in traumatic brain injury patients. In M. M. Robertson and C. L. E. Katona, (eds), *Depression and Physical Illness* (pp. 341–358). John Wiley & Sons, New York. With permission of John Wiley & Sons.

cognition and rehabilitation interventions are planned. These characteristics can greatly contribute to patients' overall symptom picture and to
the outcome of neuropsychologically oriented rehabilitation (Prigatano
et al., 1986). Consequently, a perspective on the meaning of the term
personality and familiarity with several bodies of knowledge that help
clarify the nature of human emotion, motivation, and social behavior are
needed. This chapter provides a theoretical perspective that is intended
to complement the more practical and clinically relevant discussion that
follows in the next chapter.

To understand human behavior, an appreciation of animal behavior
and how the evolution of specific brain structures and functional systems
seems to underlie complex activities such as the establishment of territorial boundaries, mate selection, and aggression is helpful. To understand human personality and how it is disturbed by a brain injury requires knowledge beyond the sphere of human neuropsychology. The
role of sociobiological, psychodynamic, environmental, and cultural factors must also be understood as they influence the emotions and motivations of persons attempting to cope in a given environment after sustaining disturbances of their higher cerebral functions.

Animal Behavior and Paul MacLean's View of the "Brain in Evolution"

Ethologists have approached animal behavior from the perspective of
zoology and have attempted to classify the diversity of animal behavior
and to relate it to the evolutionary demands of adapting to environmental changes (Baerends, 1988). This approach has produced many insights
about how complex behaviors emerge in relationship to environmental
demands. It also has helped to clarify the important role of brain structure and function in complex animal behaviors.

Paul MacLean, a neurophysiologist and physician, has attempted to
relate specific changes in brain development to the behavior of animals
(MacLean, 1970, 1973, 1990). In so doing, he has provided a unique perspective for clinical neuropsychologists working with brain dysfunctional people. MacLean (1973) proposed the following:

> In its evolution, man's brain retains the hierarchical organization of
> three basic types, which for purposes of this discussion are referred to
> in ascending order as reptilian, paleomammalian, and neomammalian.
> Despite great differences in structure and chemistry, all three brains
> must intermesh and function together as a triune brain (p. 21).

Figure 6-1 shows the hierarchical organization of these three basic brains.
The reader is referred to Valzelli's (1980) detailed illustrations of these
brain structures to help clarify the discussion of MacLean's contributions.

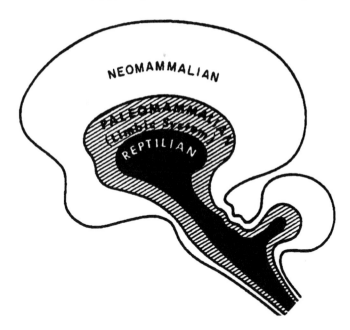

Figure 6-1. Diagrammatic representation of hierarchical organization of three basic brain types, which became part of the inheritance of humans during the evolution of the mammalian brain. For purposes of discussion, they are labeled in ascending order as reptilian, paleomammalian, and neomammalian. The paleomammalian counterpart of man's brain corresponds to the limbic system, which is believed to play a special role in emotional function. From MacLean, P. D. (1985). Brain evolution relating to family, play, and the separation call. *Arch. Gen. Psychiatry* 42:405–417.

MacLean (1973) argued that "the reptilian forebrain is characterized by greatly enlarged basal ganglia which resemble the striatopallidal complex in mammals" (p. 8). In contrast to mammals, he noted "there is only a rudimentary cortex" (p. 8). Reptilian behavior is described as stereotypic, following "ancestral learning and ancestral memories" that greatly aid survival.

Fundamental behavior subservient to establishing territorial boundaries—engaging in display behavior relevant to mate selection and warding off potential competitors—is common. MacLean attributed the tendency to return to home boundaries and to do so compulsively to the reptilian brain. Interestingly, he suggested there may be a connection between what Freud referred to as "man's compulsion to repetition" (p. 10) and his "reptilian brain."

MacLean (1973) also has suggested that during the course of evolution lower mammals were blessed (cursed?) with a "thinking cap" for the reptilian brain. Primitive cortex, in the form of the cingulate gyrus, provides lower mammals with a better "picture" of the outer world and enables the first integration of neural inputs from "inner" reality with "external" reality. This task is accomplished by the limbic lobe (Mac-Lean, 1973).

The first sensory input to the "limbic lobe" is the sense of smell provided by the olfactory tubercle. It is the first representation of the outer world. The sense of smell is important not only for eating but also for selecting a mate. It thereby guides primitive sexual behavior and social behavior helpful to mate selection. These functions are important for the preservation of both self and species.

MacLean suggested that from the olfactory tubercle, two lines of important information emerge and divide in the limbic system [a term he coined in 1954; Fig. 6-2 (in his book, figure 3)]. In describing the function of the two subdivisions, he states the following:

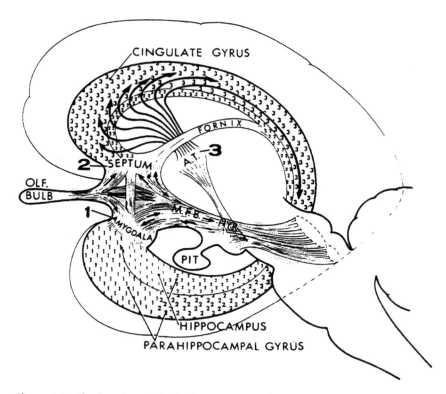

Figure 6-2. The functions of the limbic system are discussed with respect to the three main subdivisions shown in this diagram. The three main cortical regions in the limbic lobe are indicated by the small numerals 1, 2, and 3. [The smaller numerals overlie the archicortex and the larger, mesocortex (i.e., transitional cortex)]. Correspondingly, the principal pathways linking the three cortical regions with the brain stem are labeled by the large numerals. Abbreviations: AT, anterior thalamic nuclei; HYP, hypothalamus; MFB, medial forebrain bundle; OLF, olfactory. Adapted from MacLean, P. D. (1958a). Contrasting functions of limbic and neocortical systems of the brain and their relevance to psychophysiological aspects of medicine. *Am. J. Med.* 25:611–626, illustration reprinted in 1985, *Arch. Gen. Psychiatry* 42: 405–417.

Clinical and experimental findings indicate that the lower part of the limbic brain fed by the amygdala is primarily concerned with emotional feelings and behavior that insure self-preservation (MacLean, 1958a,b; 1959). In other words, there is evidence that its circuits are kept busy with the selfish demands of feeding, fighting, and self-protection (MacLean, 1973, p. 14).

Regarding the second (or septum) input, MacLean wrote the following:

> Several years ago we observed that following electrical or chemical stimulation of the septum and related hippocampus, male cats developed enhanced pleasure and grooming reactions and sometimes penile erection—aspects of behaviour seen in feline courtship (MacLean 1957a, b). These observations suggested that this part of the limbic system was involved in expressive and feeling states that are conducive to sociability and other preliminaries of copulation and reproduction. They were of heuristic value because, curiously enough, there had existed little but indirect evidence from ablation studies that the forebrain was concerned in sexual behaviour. Penfield, for example, who had stimulated the greater part of the cerebral cortex in man apparently never elicited penile erection or erotic sensations (Penfield and Jasper, 1954). The sum total of negative findings seemed paradoxical in view of the highly organized behaviour required for procreation. (p. 15).

MacLean's observations, which he has recently synthesized (MacLean, 1990), suggest that disruption of the amygdala and septum-hippocampal functioning may produce basic disturbances in the "animal" side of human personality. Patients with such impairments may be ineffective in controlling behaviors related to "feeding, fighting, and self-protection." They may also engage in unchecked and crude displays of sexual behavior. Because the limbic system does not "stand alone," disturbances of cortical regions that affect information flow and regulation of limbic system activities can also produce displays of "primitive" classical animal behaviors after brain injury.

Interestingly, many patients with frontal limbic lesions from a traumatic brain injury (TBI) are described as "childish," "insensitive," and quick to display aggressive behavior when provoked. Some are impotent, but most retain a sense of "pleasure" from overeating and sexual arousal. Because they cannot easily "check" or modify these feelings, they may gain large amounts of weight or are grossly indiscriminant in how they approach potential sexual partners.

The third division of the limbic system (MacLean, 1973) develops in primates and reflects a shift in emphasis from the sense of smell to the sense of vision. South American squirrel monkeys, for example, often display their genitals in situations that require either an aggressive or sexual action. The displaying animal may also vocalize or grind its teeth. MacLean (1973) noted examples reminiscent of genital display in man:

> In Italy less than 200 years ago amulets showing an erect phallus are said to have been worn as a protection against the evil eye (Knight, 1865). I have suggested that primitive man may have learnt by covering himself, he reduced unpleasant social tensions arising from his archaic impulse display and that this, rather than modesty has led to the civilized influence of clothing (MacLean, 1962; 1973, p. 51).

In 1973, MacLean also noted that "visual information from the limbic cortex might reach the medial dorsal nucleus through the articulation of this nucleus with the anterior thalamic nuclei" (p. 53). In his more contemporary writings, MacLean (1985, 1987, 1990) further discussed the importance of the thalamic-cingulate division of the limbic system for vocalization and for the development of play. He notes that most reptiles do not vocalize but mammals do. Reptiles also do not engage in anything similar to play behavior but mammals do.

Damage to the thalamic-cingulate division of the limbic system has been implicated in traumatic mutism (Bramanti, et al., 1994). For example, a 10-year-old girl was mute after sustaining bilateral frontal contusions. Her language functions were intact, as evidenced by her ability to follow instructions and to write simple words and answers to questions. Her affect, however, was flat and she showed no apparent distress over her inability to make sounds. When specifically asked if she was frustrated or upset, she shook her head "no" with a rather "deadpan" facial expression.

When she began to make her first sounds several weeks after TBI, they were "mom," "hm" (for home), and "no." These words are interesting because MacLean suggests that the primary role of the thalamic-cingulate connection is to provide the basic vocalization needed to maintain contact between mother and offspring. Damage to "bilateral" anterior cingulate regions could therefore interfere with vocalizations necessary to maintain that contact. In this young girl, the reappearance of vocalizations particularly related to mother and home is interesting, given MacLean's theoretical description of the role of this region of the brain.

MacLean also has detailed the impact of the thalamic-cingulate area in human emotions and the role it may play in feelings of separation as well as in drug addiction. He stated the following:

> As was noted, the reptilian hatchling and new born mammal are at opposite poles with respect to parental dependence. For mammals, any prolonged separation of the sucklings from the mother is disastrous. Because of this, nature appears to have ensured the maternal-offspring separation in mammals results in distress comparable to pain. . . . That

distress of separation continues later in life to affect socially affiliated individuals is evident by the production of separation cries by adult members of a group. In view of the pain of separation and the distressful nature of the separation cry, it is of timely interest that opiate receptors occur in high concentration in the primate cingulate cortex (Wise and Herkenham, 1982) . . . the thalamocingulate division may be implicated in the generation of separation feelings that are conducive to drug addition. Hence it is possible that, 'more than the fleeting effects of euphoria, those suffering from opiate addiction seek release from an ineffable feeling of isolation and alienation (MacLean, 1987, pp. 136–137).

Limbic structures seem crucial to basic appetitive drives and their early affective or feeling correlates. Limbic structures appear crucial to provide the "motivation" to want to vocalize. Limbic structures also appear crucial for the modulation and discharge of basic behaviors necessary for self-preservation and the establishment of social bonds necessary for the preservation of space.

When the amygdala is bilaterally ablated as part of anterior temporal lobectomies in animals, aggressive and sexual behavior changes (Heilman et al., 1993). The Klüver-Bucy syndrome of hypersexuality, an apparent absence of fear responses, and visual agnosia dramatically documents the devastating consequences of certain limbic lesions on normal emotional-motivational life.

TBI patients who are verbally or physically aggressive, socially inappropriate, or sexually disinhibited often find themselves socially isolated from their peers after brain injury (Kozloff, 1987). The lesions that produce these abnormal behaviors are not always well understood and may, indeed, be complex. Yet the changes observed in these TBI patients are reminiscent of the behavior of animals with lesions that affect normal limbic activity. By considering MacLean's (1990) insights, the clinical neuropsychologist gains a better appreciation of how brain dysfunctions disrupt behaviors necessary for the preservation of self and species. Many of these patients may have problems in reestablishing "adult-like" or "civilized" behaviors because of basic limbic-cortical dysfunction. The need to understand how various brain injuries affect behavior is obvious, and MacLean's evolutionary brain model may help the process.

Brain Evolution, Cognition, and Personality

MacLean noted that the paleomammalian counterpart of humans' brain has evolved, leading, in turn, to the development of the neomammalian brain or the advanced "thinking cap" of humans. Although the role of cognition in human personality has long been appreciated (Simon, 1967; Prigatano et al., 1986), it has been poorly understood or studied. Herbert

Simon, the well-respected cognitive psychologist, has repeatedly made a plea to study the interactions of emotion and motivation with thinking (Simon, 1967, 1994).

Cantor and Fleeson (1994) recently summarized their (and others') work on the interconnections between cognition and motivation:

> In pursuing personal goals, individuals imagine alternative worlds and alternative selves—and that is a distinctly cognitive process (Bruner, 1986; Markus and Nurius, 1986). The *interpretive* process is at the very core of personality . . . (p. 129).

If individuals cannot imagine alternative worlds or selves, they are often dull, stereotypic in their behavior, and "stimulus bound" or literal in how they approach environmental situations. Goldstein (1952) recognized the same phenomena earlier when he described how disturbances of the abstract attitude influence personality after brain damage.

Figure 6-3 (figure 1 from Cantor and Fleeson, 1994) presents a contemporary view of how "social intelligence" (a new term for personality?) may be conceptualized from the perspective of cognitive psychology. Key to the model are the concepts of self-knowledge, appraisal of life tasks, and the developmental stage of the individual (age-graded tasks). If individuals have impairments related to self-knowledge (e.g., anosognosia or impaired self-awareness), personality changes would be expected. If individuals cannot adequately appraise key life tasks (i.e., problems in judgment), a variety of personality or behavioral disturbances would be expected. Basic disturbances in this area lead to poor interpretations of situations and poor strategic choices for meeting short- and long-term goals (i.e., outcomes). Within the framework of this model, it is apparent that disturbances in cognition can underlie disturbances in personality.

Marlowe (1992) documented the case of a 7-year-old boy who suffered a focal injury in the right prefrontal region. The boy demonstrated "prominent mood swings, emotional lability, agitation, and destructiveness" (p. 206) and his ability to control himself decreased dramatically. He seemed to have extreme difficulty in appraising social situations and in choosing appropriate strategies for coping.

Price and colleagues (1990) reported two adults who suffered damage to the frontal lobes early in life. Both patients were considered "immature" and had difficulties controlling their emotions when frustrated. Their lack of social and moral development was conspicuous.

My own clinical experience with patients who have suffered focal frontal brain injuries early in life is similar to that reported by these investigators. The inability to delay (or inhibit) action when aroused often contributes to poor choices, which in turn, have devastating social

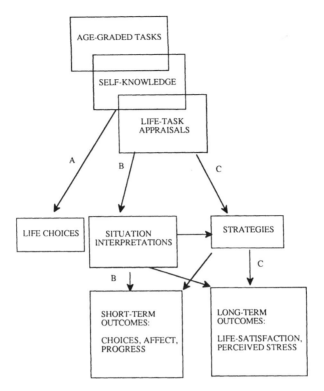

Figure 6-3. Social intelligence and the interpretive process. From Cantor, N. and Fleeson, W. (1994). Social intelligence and intelligent goal pursuit: A cognitive slice of motivation. In W. D. Spaulding (ed), *Integrative Views of Motivation, Cognition, and Emotion* (pp. 125–179). University of Nebraska, Lincoln, Neb.

consequences (Damasio and Anderson, 1993). Children with severe TBIs often apologize for mistakes in judgment more than children with less severe injuries (Papero et al., 1993). Sadly, they may not fully understand where their error in judgment actually occurred.

Although cognitive psychologists can provide useful models for analyzing cognitive dimensions crucial to personality development, they often fail to recognize that persons' basic feeling states can actually mold or modify cognitions, especially during early development. This insight did not escape Freud or Jung.

Disturbances in basic feeling states can adversely affect the development of cognition. The dynamic interplay between these two constructs (cognition and feelings) appears to be constant. It may be useful to examine what Freud and Jung thought about this interplay or interconnection.

Historical Observations of Freud and Jung with Contemporary Implications

More than a hundred years ago, Freud (1895) developed his ideas on how biological changes within the brain can lead to psychological development in a document subsequently referred to as his *Project for a Scientific Psychology*. Pribram and Gill (1976) have reviewed this work. Key to Freud's early thinking were two concepts: the "neuron doctrine" and the concept of inertia. Pribram and Gill (1976) stated that "the concept of inertia became developed into a host of regulatory principles; the neuron doctrine provides the mechanisms of the metapsychology" (p. 23).

Freud wanted to understand human behavior from the perspective of the neurophysiology of his day. He was struck by "the general irritability of protoplasm" (Pribram and Gill, 1976, p. 29) and noted that neurons discharged electrical impulses. The cells of the body thus give rise to the needs of hunger, respiration, and sexuality. Freud only guessed at the mechanism (or mechanisms) that would regulate the conditions that excite (discharge) or inhibit (nondischarge) neurons. He believed, however, that the basic tension caused by excitation and inhibition was the main factor responsible for how psychological processes develop from biological ones.

He used the term "primary process thinking" to describe how basic images emerged from (biological) need states. Secondary process thinking converted those primary images into action in the real world. Interestingly and paradoxically, such action can mean acting *not* to act (or inhibiting).

Freud also struggled with the concept of energy and its relationship to inertia. Energy implies some force that can overcome inertia. He argued that shifts in energy, not necessarily information, could influence behavior. Pribram and Gill (1976) noted that this concept could be related to the modern notion of feedback systems.

Feedback systems, for example, can control temperature in a room as well as the trajectory of a missile. They might also influence whether an animal approaches an object or avoids an object. Pribram and Gill (1976) suggest that Freud's (1895) early concept anticipated the important regulatory function that energy plays in developing and guiding human behavior and personality. Disturbances in mental energy, detected by feedback mechanisms, could alter thinking as well as mood and behavior. This concept, as we will see, might be applied to understanding certain personality disturbances following brain injury.

Additionally, Freud argued that the basic "tension," which produced the "energy," needed to overcome inertia derived from the production of an unpleasurable state. He regarded the production of this unpleasurable state as key to problem solving. Tension was derived from somatic sources while pleasure was derived from solving the problem (i.e., effectively discharging the tension to achieve a solution). This "pleasure principle" argued that human mental processes evolved from the sexual energy necessary to maintain life. The source of this life energy-pleasure continuum was called the *libido* (Dollard and Miller, 1950).

Jung, however, challenged this basic tenet and in so doing engendered an irreparable break with Freud. His book *Transformations and Symbols of the Libido* (originally published in 1912 in German) was translated as *Symbols of Transformation* (Vol. 5 of the collected works of C. G. Jung). In this text, Jung questioned whether sexual energy was the only mechanism underlying the development of cognitive or psychological processes. He argued that there may be many sources of this life energy principle other than sexual. He believed that certain recurring psychological experiences were reflected in symbols seen across cultures. These symbols exerted a powerful influence on the development of human behavior, thinking, and personality. He was furthermore struck by humans' apparent need to create symbols to help deal with aspects of life that they could only partially understand. Jung thus considered symbols to be important sources of information about mental processes at both the conscious and unconscious levels.

Jung went on to argue that symbols from various cultures often appear in people's dreams and that these symbols helped explain a person's internal struggles or perceptions.

Collectively, Freud and Jung argued that psychological development was intimately connected with energy and this energy in part was reflected by basic feeling states. Some of those feeling states could also be seen across cultures and through the history of humans as reflected in recurring symbols.

If these ideas are considered probable, then damage to the brain will disrupt preexisting patterns of psychological functioning and undercut basic neuromechanisms necessary for behaviors to continue for survival purposes. This disruption is indeed complicated and produces formidable roadblocks to understanding how personality disturbances actually become associated with different types of brain lesions in different types of individuals. This concept led to the model of personality associated with brain injury (Prigatano, 1986) that I now attempt to expand based on clinical observations, experimental findings, and the theoretical perspectives described above.

A Neuropsychological Model for Approaching Personality Disturbances after Brain Injury

Personality can be defined as patterns of emotional and motivational responses that develop over an organism's lifetime (Prigatano, 1986, 1992). *Feelings*, the perceptions of internal bodily states, provide the "building blocks" for the emergence of true emotion and motivation. Feelings can be defined as the most rudimentary, generalized, and differentiated perception of internal bodily states. As noted (Prigatano, 1986), core brain receptors involved in the regulation of the organism's metabolic and endocrine functions probably play an important role in these initial sensations referred to as feeling states.

Emotion is the term used to reflect complex feeling states that parallel an interruption of ongoing goal-seeking behavior or programs (Simon, 1967). In contrast, *motivation* refers to complex feeling states that parallel hierarchical goal-seeking behavior (Simon, 1967). Simon (1967, 1994, 1995) has commented that no true theory of intelligence can be obtained until the problems of emotion and motivation are solved. That is, intelligence involves more than computations; it includes a feeling component.

An impressive literature has emerged identifying basic feeling states communicated by the facial expressions of humans and animals. Darwin (1872), perhaps, first brought this issue to the attention of the scientific community. Izard and Saxton (1988) have summarized the literature that supports Darwin's position. They have suggested that there are nine fundamental emotions: interest, joy (happiness), surprise, sadness, anger, disgust, contempt, fear, and shame or shyness.

The research of Ekman and Friesen (1975) has firmly established the existence of six basic feeling states that have been universally identified (i.e., that exist across cultures) and that often appear early in life. From a clinician's perspective, these feeling states can be described as polar opposites (Fig. 6-4). These *core* or basic feeling states seem to help organisms survive because they are associated with approach or avoidance tendencies. Humans tend to avoid situations that sadden, frighten, or produce disgust. In contrast, humans approach situations or people who tend to evoke happiness, anger, or surprise. Thus, the avoidance and approach dimensions can be superimposed on the core polar affective states (Fig. 6-4). Davidson (1992) has also described different disturbances in emotion (affect) from this perspective.

Disruptions of the normal equilibrium or balance in these feeling

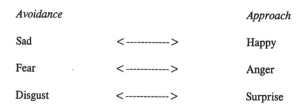

Avoidance		*Approach*
Sad	<------------>	Happy
Fear	<------------>	Anger
Disgust	<------------>	Surprise

Figure 6-4. Six basic feeling states that appear to be universal across cultures. From a clinical perspective, these feeling states form three pairs of polar opposites over which the dimensions of approach and avoidance can be superimposed.

Table 6-1. Regulation or modulation of affective states: Feedback systems and personality disorders

Disturbances of Normal Regulation	Avoidance		Approach	Disturbances of Normal Regulation
Depression	Sad	↔	Happy	Euphoria
				Mania
				Ecstasy
Anxiety	Fear	↔	Anger	Agitation
				Irritation
				Belligerence
				Unexpected acts of violence
Impatience	Disgust	↔	Surprise	Preoccupation and preservation of feelings
				Obsessive/compulsive behavior
				Suspiciousness
				Aspontaneity
				Loss of interest
				Loss of drive

states *or* the approach-avoidance valence disturb feeling states and threaten an organism's adaptation and self-realization (Table 6-1). This model partially explains how disturbances in feedback systems (and energy regulation) can produce the behavioral disorders frequently observed in clinical situations after brain injury.

Disturbances in the regulation of normal energy (Table 6-1) mirror the common personality disturbances associated with TBI (Table 6-2).

Other personality, disturbances are not associated with disturbances in feedback systems, but rather with failures in feedforward systems. These disturbances reflect not so much the correction of an "error" via a feedback loop to maintain adaptive behavior as they do disturbances in the communication of information. They reflect a failure to signal a feedforward system that it should abort its original plan or program. These types of disturbances are the most baffling and difficult to correct. They seem to reflect problems in correctly terminating a program as demanded by an environmental situation. Given this schema, three classic "personality" disturbances or groups of disturbances can be identified: the Klüver-Bucy syndrome, organic delusions and hallucinations (Brown, 1984; Prigatano, 1988), and the classic anosognosias (Table 6-3). Despite "feedback" from the environment, several patients with these disturbances seem to persist in their failure to process new information.

Table 6-2. Emotional and motivational disturbances associated with TBI

Reported Disturbance	Source
Active	
Irritability	Thomsen (1984)
	van Zomeren and van Den Burg (1985)
	Hinkeldey and Corrigan (1990)
Agitation	Reyes, et al., (1981)
	Chandler et al., (1988)
	Corrigan (1989)
Belligerence	Fordyce et al., (1983)
	Hinkeldey and Corrigan (1990)
Anger	Lezak, 1987
	Rosenbaum and Hoge (1989)
Abrupt and unexpected acts of violence or episodic dyscontrol syndrome	Elliott (1982)
	Rosenbaum and Hoge (1989)
Impulsiveness	Goldstein (1952)
	Prigatano et al., (1986)
Impatience	Oddy et al., (1985)
Restlessness	Meyer (1904)
	Schilder (1934)
	Reyes et al. (1981)
	Thomsen (1984)
	Hinkeldey and Corrigan (1990)
Inappropriate social responses	Goldstein (1952)
	Jennett and Teasdale (1981)
	Prigatano et al. (1986)
	Bigler (1989)
Emotional lability (or rapid mood changes)	Thomsen (1884)
	Prigatano et al. (1986)
	Brooks et al., (1987)
Sensitivity to noise or distress	Thomsen (1984)
	van Zomeren and van Den Burg (1985)
Anxiety	Goldstein (1952)
	Levin and Grossman (1978)
	van Zomeren and van Den Berg (1985)
	Lezak (1987)
Suspiciousness (or mistrust of others)	Prigatano et al. (1986)
	Hinkeldey and Corrigan (1990)
Delusional	Lishman (1968)
	Lezak (1987)
Paranoia	Schilder (1934)
	Meyer (1904)

(continued)

Table 6-2.—Continued

Reported Disturbance	Source
Active	
	Lezak (1987)
	Prigatano, O'Brien, and Klonoff (1988)
	Hinkeldey and Corrigan (1990)
Mania or manic-like states	Schilder (1934)
	Shukla et al. (1987)
	Bakchine et al. (1989)
Passive	
Aspontaneity	Ota (1969)
	Roberts (1979)
	Thomsen (1984)
Sluggish	Reyes, Bhattacharyya, and Heller (1981)
Loss of interest in the environment	Thomsen (1984)
	Oddy et al. (1985)
Loss of drive or initiative	Jennett and Teasdale (1981)
	Prigatano et al., (1986)
	Lezak (1987)
	Bigler (1989)
Tires easily	Thomsen (1984)
	Oddy et al. (1985)
Depressed	Schilder (1934)
	van Zomeren and van den Burg (1985)
	Lezak (1987)
Syndromes	
Childishness (self-centered behavior, insensitivity to others, giddiness, overtalkativeness, and exuberance/ euphoric behavior)	Thomsen (1984)
	Oddy et al. (1985)
	Bakchine et al. (1989)
Helplessness (requires supervision or continued cuing to accomplish goals)	Fordyce et al. (1983)
	Hinkeldey and Corrigan (1990)
Lack of insight or awareness of behavioral limitations (also the term denial used)	Goldstein (1952)
	Ota (1969)
	Prigatano et al. (1990)
	Prigatano and Schacter (1991)

Note: TBI = traumatic brain injury.
From Prigatano (1992).

Table 6-3. Feedforward system failures and behavioral disturbances after brain injury*

Classic Personality Disturbances	Symptoms
Klüver-Bucy syndrome dominates	Visual objective recognition disorder Inappropriate sexual behavior
Organic delusions/hallucinations	Paranoid and grandiose perceptions and hallucinations. See or hear objects or events in a damaged perceptual field
Classic anosognosias	Failure to recognize a disorder of information processing

*Basic disturbances not in correcting an error to maintain adaptive behavior but disturbances in information communication.

As a feedforward disorder, it is theoretically not a change in energy that is detected, but a change in redundancy or information.

Brain stem, thalamic, and hypothalamic centers appear to provide the basic neural circuitry for the emergence of core feeling states (Prigatano, 1986; Pribram, 1971). As the cerebral hemispheres develop and cortical and subcortical structures coordinate their activities (e.g., frontal and basal ganglia circuits become established and elaborated), the refinement and conscious experience of these affective states most likely increase in complexity.

The early elaboration and representation of limbic inputs into the cingulate gyrus, as noted earlier, perhaps provide the first true expression of emotion and motivation in humans and animals. Reptiles, deprived of the cingulate gyrus and therefore of the cingulate-thalamic circuits, do not demonstrate the "separation cry" seen in mammals (MacLean, 1985). Nor do reptiles express emotion or motivation in a manner similar to human beings or mammals (MacLean, 1990).

The expression of human emotion and motivation requires the structures of the limbic system and cortex. Disruptions of limbic system activity and its cortical connections undoubtedly disturb personality directly. When the disruption is caused by structural damage to brain (e.g., by contusional hematomas, diffuse axonal injury, or subarachnoid hemorrhage), the problem is often referred to as a *neuropsychiatric* or *neuropsychologically based* disturbance in personality. When the disruption is caused by faulty learning patterns, environmental stresses or deprivation, or even faulty cognitive belief systems, the problem is often called a *psychiatric* disturbance, at least in Western cultures.

Although these two broad approaches have some utility, they often are difficult to distinguish in a daily clinical practice. A patient's behavior is as we find it. Our models simply attempt to fractionate or characterize the behavior in ways that might allow us to understand it and thereby study it.

Consequently, I have found it useful to approach personality disturbances after brain injury in terms of three broad concepts. Some personality disturbances are a direct reflection of brain injury and can therefore be considered to be *neuropsychologically mediated*. Other personality disturbances are an indirect effect of brain injury and therefore might broadly be called *reactionary* problems. A third class of behavioral disturbances seen in brain dysfunctional patients reflects premorbid personality characteristics and can broadly be referred to as *characterological*.

The latter characteristics were the ones recognized by Freud and Jung and are independent of any acquired brain dysfunction. Obviously, characterological features of the personality will be modified by both the direct and indirect effects of brain injury. Yet, when approaching an individual in therapy, it may be useful to conceptualize affective disturbances along these three broad constructs. The problem of depression after TBI briefly highlights the potential usefulness of this approach.

Depression After TBI: An Illustrative Example

Prigatano and Summers (1997) have attempted to relate the above model to depression in TBI patients. Excerpts from that article are repeated here (with the permission of the original publishers) in an attempt to discuss depression as a disturbance in an energetic feedback system.

Depression Independent of Brain Damage

Most people treated for depression have no history that suggests acquired brain damage. According to the DSM-IV (American Psychiatric Association, 1994), patients with depression may demonstrate a major depressive episode, a major depressive disorder, a dysthymic disorder, an unspecified depressive disorder, or several other diagnostic conditions. None of these diagnostic categories includes the criterion of brain damage even though many depressed patients complain of difficulties with memory and concentration that suggest subtle brain dysfunction.

Feighner and Boyer (1991) noted that "depression is an extremely common, debilitating, but treatable psychiatric illness. . . . It is a multifaceted symptom, syndrome and disease which reveals important portraits of itself to those who approach it from different perspectives" (p. xi). When taken from the perspective of traditional psychiatry and clinical psychology, depression seems to have many potential etiologies: neurotransmitter disturbances (Kupfer, 1991), faulty beliefs about the self that seem to develop over several years (Beck et al., 1979), or an abrupt and tragic personal loss.

The DSM-IV (American Psychiatric Association, 1994) fails to provide a single definition for depression under its *Glossary of Technical Terms*.

DSM-IV, however, offers many "descriptive features" that are associated with a major depressive episode: tearfulness, brooding, obsessive rumination, excessive worry, complaints of somatic discomfort, loss of appetite, subjective reports of sadness, and empty feelings. Sleep and eating disturbances are often present and associated with a loss of energy, fatigue, and a decreased ability to concentrate, remember, and think.

Typically, depression can be separated from normal sadness in one important way. Sadness is a normal reaction to a significant loss in life. Yet sadness frequently responds to good news; depression does not. Feedback from the environment that something positive has happened does not seem to shift the energy pattern in a true depressive episode. In practical terms, depressed patients seem to take little if any pleasure in good things that happen to them. They persist in a dysphoric state that has disastrous consequences for their adaptation.

Direct Effects of Brain Dysfunction and Depression

Studies have suggested that a direct relationship exists between brain injury and depression. The work of Robinson and colleagues (Robinson et al., 1983, 1984a,b, 1987; Robinson and Szetela 1981; Robinson and Price, 1982; Starkstein et al., 1987, 1988) has most clearly documented a potential relationship between the location of a brain lesion and the existence of a major depressive episode. For example, they found that a major depressive episode soon after a stroke was frequently associated with injury to the left hemisphere (Robinson and Price, 1982; Robinson et al., 1983, 1984a,b; Starkstein et al., 1987). In particular, left frontal lesions tended to correlate with a major depressive episode in this patient group.

As stroke patients recovered or as time passed, however, depression was less easily correlated with a left anterior cerebral dysfunction. After the first 2 years poststroke, the prevalence of depression remained stable, but the composition of the group changed (Robinson et al., 1987). After 2 years, all patients who were initially depressed improved in terms of depression. The mood of patients who were not initially depressed, however, deteriorated 2 years after stroke. These findings suggest that with time, depression is correlated with factors other than lesion location.

Depression also can exist when multiple areas of the brain are damaged. Studying acute TBI patients, Fedoroff and colleagues (1992) reported that "the presence of left dorsolateral frontal lesions and/or left basal ganglia lesions and, to a lesser extent, parietal-occipital and right hemisphere lesions were associated with an increased probability of developing major depression" (p. 918). As is often the case in TBI patients who suffer brain damage attributable to acceleration or deceleration forces applied to the skull, lesions are typically bilateral and asymmetrical. This pattern precludes an easy correlation between lesion location and specific personality disturbances (Prigatano, 1992), including depression.

Depression as an Indirect Effect of Brain Injury

If depression is an indirect effect of brain damage, it should *not* readily correlate with measures of severity of brain injury or location. Moreover, its frequency and severity should change over time, depending mostly on environmental conditions. Finally, it should be related to premorbid factors. What data support this perspective?

Levin and Grossman (1978) developed a profile of behavioral disturbances in relation to the severity of closed head injury. They reported that depression, as judged by the Brief Psychiatric Rating Scale, was not significantly related to severity of brain injury (Fig. 6-5).

Using a cross-sectional design, Godfrey and colleagues (1993) studied self-reports of depression in TBI patients 6 months, 1 year, and 2 to 3 years after injury. Their reports of depression were compared to those of an orthopedic control group. Six months after injury, the level of depression reported by TBI patients was comparable to that reported by the orthopedic controls. One year after injury, however, TBI patients reported higher levels of depression. This trend was also evident 2 to 3 years after injury.

Finally, Fedoroff and colleagues (1992) noted that of TBI patients who showed evidence of a major depression, 70.6% had a history of premorbid psychiatric disturbance compared to 37% of the TBI patients who did not demonstrate a major depressive disorder. The difference was statistically significant (Table 6-4). Collectively, these findings argue that depression can be an indirect effect of brain injury. Problems with adjustment (including depression) may also have existed premorbidly and be independent of the TBI.

Symptoms of Depression After TBI

Ross and Rush (1981) stated that pathological crying, in the absence of bilateral lesions causing pseudobulbar palsy, is likely to be indicative of depression. Jorge and colleagues (1993a,b) studied specific vegetative and psychological symptoms of depression in 66 TBI patients over 1 year. Initially, 20% of the patients reported a depressed mood. At the 1-year follow-up, the percentage was comparable (26%), but some patients had been lost to follow-up. Vegetative signs of depression varied over time. For example, at the time of initial evaluation, 42% of the depressed patients had sleep disturbances that had disappeared 1 year after injury. In contrast, reports of loss of libido had increased to 60% by the 1 year follow-up examination compared to 32% at the initial evaluation. These findings are reminiscent of an earlier report (Thomsen, 1984) in which TBI patients often were judged to show increased tiredness and sensitiv-

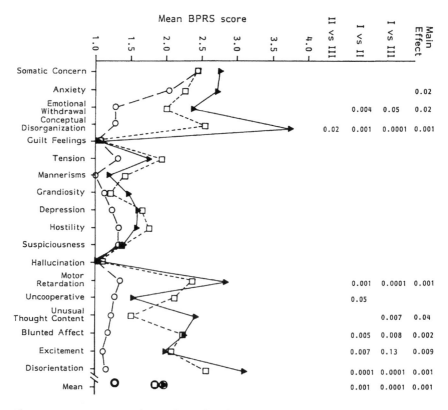

Figure 6-5. Mean score by each grade of injury on individual scales of the Brief Psychiatric Rating Scale (BPRS), with grand mean and results of analysis of covariance. Scale scores were adjusted for effects of variation in the injury-rating interval. Order of scales corresponds to that of published BPRS. Open circles connected by solid lines indicate grade I; open circles connected by dashed lines, grade II; solid triangles connected by solid lines, grade III. From Levin, H. S., and Grossman, R. G. (1978). Behavioral sequelae of closed head injury: a quantitative study. *Arch. Neurol.* 35: 720–727.

ity to stress 10 to 15 years after injury compared to 2.5 years after injury. More information is needed on the relationship between specific symptoms associated with depression and neurophysiological and neuropsychological changes caused by brain injury.

A table constructed by a patient in which he compared his symptoms of depression before and after brain injury is informative (Table 6-5). The lists include symptoms of both depression and brain injury. Before brain injury, for example, the individual reported having a "worry loop." This phrase meant that he often experienced "deep and profound concentration on any problem." After the brain injury, this characteristic was absent. Before the brain injury, he would frequently wake after only 1 to 3

Table 6-4. Characteristics of 64 depressed and nondepressed patients with TBI

Variable	Patients with major depression		Patients without depression	
	Number out of 17	Percent	Number out of 47	Percent
Male	14	82.4	41	87.2
African-Americans	5	29.4	11	23.4
Left-handed	1	5.9	4	8.5
Married	7	41.2	21	44.7
Hollingshead socioeconomic class IV or V	13	76.4	34	72.3
Family history of psychiatric disorder	8	47.1	23	48.9
Personal history of psychiatric disorder*	12	70.6	17†	37.0
Personal history of alcohol and other substance abuse	8	47.1	11†	23.9

TBI = traumatic brain injury.

*Significant difference between groups (χ^2 = 4.38, df = 1, p = 0.04).

†N = 46.

Adapted from Fedoroff J. P., Starkstein, S. E., Forrester, A. W., Geisler, F. H., Jorge, R. E., Arndt, S. V., and Robinson, R. G. Depression in patients with acute traumatic brain injury. *American Journal of Psychiatry*, Volume 147, pp. 918–923, 1992. Copyright 1992 the American Psychiatric Association. Reprinted with permission.

hours of sleep. After the brain injury, he required 10 to 12 hours of sleep and found it extremely difficult to awaken.

The patient also noted a change in his senses of smell, taste, and balance, characteristics that did not exist before his brain injury. Before his injury, he described his mood as unhappy and sad and he tended to retreat. After the brain injury, he used the words frustrated and childish to describe himself and recognized that he had a tendency to lose his temper. This table aptly describes how symptoms can change as a result of brain injury. By interviewing such patients in detail, clinicians can gain insights into which symptoms may be related to brain injury and which symptoms are independent of it.

Depression and Failure of Feedback Systems

Given the above considerations, it is clear that various aspects of depression may be seen as a direct result of brain dysfunction whereas other aspects of depression may be reactions to the injury. The patient's verbal descriptions in Table 6-5 illustrate that depression can exist before a brain injury. These observations support the clinical model of ap-

Table 6-5. Depressed patient's self-assessment before and after brain injury

Characteristic	Depression Before TBI	Depression After TBI
Environmental stress	Generally absent	May be present
Worry loop	Present	Absent
Nervous pulsing pain	Present	Not present
Daily mood cycle	Chronic on waking; at my best in evening	Unpredictable, generally at best in morning
Weight loss	Severe	Overweight
Sleep disturbance	Quick to sleep late evening; wake within 1 to 3 hours	Sleep 10 to 12 hours starting any time, difficult to wake
Follow and understand discussion	Difficult, tend to ignore and act on own	Equally difficult but lack clear vision on what to do
Ability to perform	Enhanced	Reduced
Headaches	Plagued by depression	Nonexistent
Memory	Diary not required	Require comprehensive diary
Concentration	Could read a book	Cannot read a book
Mood	Unhappy and sad, prefer to retreat	Frustrated and childish, likely to lose temper and be violent
Smell and taste	Sensitive	Do not exist
Balance	Satisfactory	Poor
Wife on appearance	Patient has become expert at hiding his feelings, you never know what he is thinking	Patient loses his temper without any warning, says hurtful things

TBI = traumatic brain injury.
From Prigatano, G. P., and Summers, J. D. (1997). Depression in traumatic brain injury patients. In M. M. Robertson and C. L. E. Katona (eds), *Depression and Physical Illness*. Copyright John Wiley & Sons Limited. Reproduced with permission..

proaching personality disturbances after TBI. The description, however, also allows us to focus on the theoretical consideration that depression reflects some disturbance in a feedback mechanism.

As stated earlier in this chapter, sadness is a natural reaction to loss. However, individuals regain energy and become happy when appropriate environmental events occur or they restructure their thought processes regarding the loss. The ability to sense that something "good has happened" implies that individuals have the energy level to experience the affect and that a change in energy can, in fact, be detected. If individuals lack the energy associated with a happy state or cannot perceive internal shifts of energy states, then theoretically they could remain depressed. Cognitive state is important in determining and interpreting these changes in energy states.

The patient who described his depression before and after brain injury noted his need for more sleep. He also noted that his "worry loop" had disappeared after brain injury. His use of the term "worry loop" is interesting given our discussion about feedback systems. The cognitive appraisal of and continual reflection on worries can be assumed to be a form of feedback system. Damage to this "worry loop" would affect some aspects of depression but not others. The characteristics listed in Table 6-5 should be evaluated more thoroughly from the perspective of a failure in a feedback system. Many of the behaviors in this table could be thought of as "detectable" or "not detectable" only if a feedback mechanism were present. Consequently, the individuals can, to some degree, describe which behaviors are absent or present.

Within the context of this model, the potential interaction of variables is obvious. The study of depression after TBI highlights that many of its components are present, some of which are adaptive and some of which are maladaptive. All aspects of depression, however, appear to reflect a disturbance in properly directing energy, permitting the normal balance of sadness and happiness to emerge. In some instances, this disturbance of energy may be caused by brain dysfunction. In other instances, it may reflect individuals' reactions in terms of their attempts to cope with brain dysfunction. In still other cases, the disturbance may be independent of brain dysfunction.

A Tentative Synthesis

The history of psychiatry has suggested that brain damage may release underlying features of premorbid personality. Clinically, it sometimes appears that brain injury "turns up the volume" on certain preexisting personality characteristics. In contrast, the neurological tradition argues that specific brain lesions will produce specific emotional disturbances. The neuropsychological rehabilitation literature suggests that the truth for many patients lies between these two historic extremes.

Working with brain dysfunctional patients day in and day out for weeks to months after injury (and at different time periods after injury) draws different clinical and scientific pictures. What patients reveal about themselves during a 1-to 2-hour interview or while participating in experimental research may differ markedly from what they discuss when they are engaged in frequent therapeutic sessions and the therapeutic relationship is well established. As patients and their families begin to trust the treating clinician, various statements regarding how premorbid factors may be influencing the patient's symptom picture emerge. Certainly, neither patient nor family members are likely to discuss important personal matters until a relationship is established.

As information is revealed in therapy, it often becomes clear that certain features of patients' depression (not all of them) are long-standing. In fact, the accident may even have been an attempt at suicide. The patient may have been progressively depressed and therefore inattentive to details. The consequences may have been decreased self-care and hence the acquisition of a brain injury. Patients may also reveal how an angry outburst was triggered by important pre-existing conflicts or situations.

In contrast, a detailed understanding of the anatomy and physiology of various brain lesions can sober even the most experienced psychodynamically oriented clinician. A child's failure to talk after a brain injury may not be a form of resistance, denial, or depression. Rather, it may reflect a disruption of the thalamic-cingulate connections that has made vocalization impossible (MacLean, 1990) or a cerebellar impairment that interferes with the motor actions necessary for vocalization (Rekate et al., 1985). Clinical neuropsychologists may think parents or other therapists naive if they attribute mutism after brain injury to psychological causes. They too, however, can overstate the role of psychological factors in producing symptom pictures when a biological explanation may be not only more parsimonious but more accurate.

To guard against this problem, treating clinicians must be able to conceptualize and test experimentally what they consider to be the major "causes" of a patient's behavior. Clinical neuropsychologists should be able to state their clinical hypotheses and describe a method for testing them. If the hypothesis cannot be tested, the hypothesis is likely wrong.

In this spirit, I argue that *all* personality disturbances associated with brain injury should be analyzed from this clinical perspective. Which problem or parts of the problem are neuropsychologically (biologically) mediated? What problems or parts of the problem are indirect effects of the brain injury and therefore reflect a reactionary problem? What problem or portions of the problem may have been long-standing or existed premorbidly and in no way involve the brain injury?

Summary and Conclusions

Personality disturbances associated with various brain injuries are poorly understood and have not been the object of rigorous scientific studies (Meyer, 1904; Lishman, 1968; Storey, 1970; Gianotti, 1972, 1993; Derryberry and Tucker, 1992). Animal studies have implicated an important role for the limbic system in the expression and experience of emotions (Papez, 1937). The cerebral cortex, however, is likely important in the interpretation of feeling states. Damage to the cerebral cortex reduces a person's capacity to evaluate and interpret appropriate courses of action to attain different goals or in different social situations. Damage to the cerebral cortex, which is common after TBI, produces predictable personality disturbances that sometimes cannot be separated from underlying cognitive problems.

Conceptualizing these personality difficulties as reflecting changes in feedforward and feedback systems eventually may prove useful. This chapter represents an initial step to describe such disturbances in these terms. However, the important role of premorbid personality characteristics in producing the symptom picture was also emphasized. Recalling this information puts clinicians in a better position to evaluate TBI patients.

Experienced clinical neuropsychologists will easily recognize that contemporary neuropsychological tests and supplemental tests of personality often fail to reveal important affective disturbances associated with brain injury. It is hoped that more innovative and useful measures, driven by both sound theory and empirical observations, will be developed. Careful interviewing of patients and family and observing their behavior in the context of neuropsychological rehabilitation currently are the best ways for clinicians to fully appreciate the role of personality disturbances and their impact on patients' ability to function in the real world.

As clinical neuropsychologists can conceptualize brain dysfunctional patients' emotional and motivational disturbances, they can convey this information to patients and family in a manner that reduces some of the confusion they both experience (Principle 4).

References

American Psychiatric Association (1994). *Diagnostic and Statistical Manual of Mental Disorders* (4th ed). American Psychiatric Association, Washington, D.C.

Baerends, E. P. (1988). Ethology. In R. C. Atkinson, R. J. Herrnstein, G. Lardyey, and R. D. Luce (eds), *Stevens' Handbook of Experimental Psychology* (2nd ed, Vol. 1). *Perceptions and Motivation* (pp. 765–830). John Wiley & Sons, New York.

Bakchine, S., Lacomblez, L., Benoit, N., Parisot, D., Chain, F., and Lehermitte, F. (1989). Manic-like state after bilateral orbitofrontal and right temporoparietal injury: efficacy of clonidine. *Neurology* 39: 777–781.

Beck, A. T., Rush, J. A., Shaw, B. F., and Emery, G. (1979). *Cognitive Therapy of Depression*. Guilford, New York.

Bigler, E. D. (1989). Behavioural and cognitive changes in traumatic brain injury: a spouse's perspective. *Brain Inj*. 3: 73–78.

Bramanti, P., Sessa, E., and Saltuari, L. (1994). Post-traumatic mutism. *J. Neurosurg. Sci*. 38: 117–122.

Brooks, N., McKinlay, W., Symington, C., Beattie, A., and Campsie, L. (1987). Return to work within the first seven years of severe head injury. *Brain Inj*. 1(1): 5–19.

Brown, J. W. (1984). Hallucinations imagery and the microstructure of perception. In J. A. M. Frederiks (ed), *Handbook of Clinical Neurology*, Vol. 1 (45) (pp. 351–372). *Clinical Neuropsychology*. Elsevier Science, Amsterdam.

Bruner, J. (1986). *Actual Minds, Possible Words*. Harvard University Press, Cambridge, MA.

Cantor, N. and Fleeson, W. (1994). Social intelligence and intelligent goal pursuit: a cognitive slice of motivation. In W. D. Spaulding (ed), *Integrative Views of Motivation, Cognition, and Emotion* (pp. 125–179). University of Nebraska, Lincoln.

Chandler, M. C., Barnhill, J. L., and Gualtieri, C. T. (1988). Amantadine for the agitated head-injury patient. *Brain Inj.* 2: 309–311.

Corrigan, J. D. (1989). Development of a scale for assessment of agitation following traumatic brain injury. *J. Clin. Exp. Neuropsychol.* 11: 261–277.

Damasio, A. R., and Anderson, S. W. (1993). The frontal lobes. In K. M. Heilman and E. Valenstein (eds), *Clinical Neuropsychology* (3rd ed) (pp. 409–460). Oxford University Press, New York.

Darwin, C. (1872/1965). *The Expression of the Emotions in Man and Animals*. University of Chicago, Chicago.

Davidson, R. J. (1992). Anterior cerebral asymmetry and the nature of emotion. *Brain Cogn.* 20: 125–151.

Derryberry, D., and Tucker, D. M. (1992). Neural mechanisms of emotion. *J. Consult. Clin. Psychol.* 60(3): 329–338.

Dollard, J., and Miller, N. E. (1950). *Personality and Psychotherapy: An Analysis in Terms of Learning, Thinking and Culture*. McGraw-Hill, New York.

Ekman, P., and Friesen, W. V. (1975). *Unmasking the Face*. Prentice-Hall, Englewood Cliffs, NJ.

Elliott, F. A. (1982). Neurological findings in adult minimal brain dysfunction and the dyscontrol syndrome. *J. Nerv. Ment. Dis.* 170: 680–687.

Fedoroff, J. P., Starkstein, S. E., Forrester, A. W., Geisler, F. H., Jorge, R. E., Arndt, S. V., and Robinson, R. G. (1992). Depression in patients with acute traumatic brain injury. *Am. J. Psychiatry* 149: 918–923.

Feighner, J. P., and Boyer, W. M. (1991). *Perspectives in Psychiatry*, Vol. 2. *Diagnosis of Depression*. Wiley, Chichester, England.

Fordyce, D. J., Roueche, J. R., and Prigatano, G. P. (1983). Enhanced emotional reactions in chronic head trauma patients. *J. Neurol. Neurosurg. Psychiatry* 46: 620–624.

Freud, S. (1895/1966). *Project for a Scientific Psychology*. Standard Edition, Vol. 1 (pp. 281–237).

Freud, S. (1900/1953). *The Interpretation of Dreams*. Standard Edition, Vols. 4–5.

Gainotti, G. (1972). Emotional behavior and hemispheric side of lesion. *Cortex* 8: 41–55.

Gainotti, G. (1993). Emotional and psychosocial problems after brain injury. *Neuropsychological Rehabilitation* 3(3): 259–277.

Godfrey, H. P. D., Partridge, F. M., and Knight, R. G. (1993). Course of insight disorder and emotional dysfunction following closed head injury: a controlled cross-sectional follow-up study. *J. Clin. Exp. Neuropsychol.* 15(4): 503–515.

Goldstein, K. (1942). *Aftereffects of Brain Injuries in War.* Grune and Stratton, New York.

Goldstein, K. (1952). Effect of brain damage on the personality. *Psychiatry* 15: 245–260.

Goldstein, K. (1951/1971). On emotions: Considerations from the organismic point of view. *J. Psychology* 31, 37–49. Reprinted in A. Gurwitsch, E. M. Goldstein Haudek, and W. E. Haudek (eds), *Kurt Goldstein. Selected Papers.* Martinus Nijhoff, The Hague.

Heilman, K. M., Bowers, D., and Valenstein, E. (1993). Emotional disorders associated with neurological disease. In K. M. Heilman and E. Valenstein (eds), *Clinical Neuropsychology* (3rd ed). Oxford University Press, New York.

Hinkeldey, N. S., and Corrigan, J. D. (1990). The structure of head-injured patients' neurobehavioural complaints: a preliminary study. *Brain. Inj.* 4: 115–133.

Izard, C. E., and Saxton, P. M. (1988). Emotions. In R. C. Atkinson, R. J. Herrnstein, G. Lindzey, and R. D. Luce (eds), *Stevens' Handbook of Experimental Psychology* (2nd ed) (pp. 627–676). John Wiley & Sons, New York.

Jennett, B., and Teasdale G. (1981). *Management of Head Injuries.* F. A. Davis, Philadelphia.

Jorge, R. E., Robinson, R. G., and Arndt, S. (1993). Are there symptoms that are specific for depressed mood in patients with traumatic brain injury? *J. Nerv. Ment. Dis.* 181(2): 91–99.

Jorge, R. E., Robinson, R. G., Arndt, S., Forrester, A. W., Geisler, F., and Starkstein, S. E. (1993a). Comparison between acute-and delayed-onset depression following traumatic brain injury. *Journal of Neuropsychiatry* 5: 43–49.

Jorge, R. E., Robinson, R. G., Arndt, S. V., Starkstein, S. E., Forrester, A. W., and Geisler, F. (1993b). Depression following traumatic brain injury: A 1 year longitudinal study. *J. Affect. Disord.* 27: 233–243.

Jung, C. G. (1964). *Man and His Symbols.* Doubleday Windfall, Garden City, New York.

Jung, C. G. (1912/1956). *Symbols of Transformation*, Collected Works, Vol. 5. Bollingen Series XX, Princeton University, NJ.

Jung, C. G. (1927/71). *Psychological Types*, Collected Works, Vol. 6. Bollingen Series, Princeton University, NJ.

Kozloff, R. (1987). Network of social support and the outcome from severe head injury. *Journal of Head Trauma Rehabilitation* 2: 14–23.

Kupfer, D. J. (1991). Biological markers of depression. In J. P. Feighner and W. F. Boyer (eds), *The Diagnosis of Depression* (pp. 79–98). Wiley, Chichester, England.

Levin, H. S., and Grossman, R. G. (1978). Behavioral sequelae of closed head injury: a quantitative study. *Arch. Neurol.* 35: 720–727.

Lezak, M. D. (1987). Relationships between personality disorders, social disturbances, and physical disability following traumatic brain injury. *Journal of Head Trauma Rehabilitation* 2(1): 57–69.

Lishman, W. A. (1968). Brain damage in relation to psychiatric disability after head injury. *Br. J. Psychiatry* 114: 373–410.

MacLean, P. D. (1954). The limbic system and its hippocampal formation. Studies in animals and their possible application to man. *J. Neurosurg.* 11: 29–44.

MacLean, P. D. (1957a). Chemical and electrical stimulation of hippocampus in unrestrained animals. I. Methods and electroencephalographic findings. *AMA Archives of Neurology and Psychiatry* 78: 113–127.

MacLean, P. D. (1957b). Chemical and electrical stimulation of hippocampus in unrestrained animals. II. Behavioral findings, *AMA Archives Neurology and Psychiatry* 78: 128–142.

MacLean, P. D. (1958a). Contrasting functions of limbic and neocortical systems of the brain and their relevance to psychophysiological aspects of medicine. *Am. J. Med.* 25: 611–626.

MacLean, P. D. (1958b). The limbic system with respect to self-preservation and the preservation of the species. *J. Nerv. Ment. Dis.* 127: 1–11.

MacLean, P. D. (1959). The limbic system with respect to two basic life principles. In *Transactions of Second Conference on the Central Nervous System and Behavior.* Josiah Macy, Jr. Foundation, New York (pp. 31–118).

MacLean, P. D. (1962). New findings relevant to the evolution of psychosexual functions of the brain. *J. Nerv. Ment. Dis.* 135: 289–301.

MacLean, P. D. (1970). The triune brain, emotion, and scientific bias. In F. O. Schmitt (ed). *The Neurosciences. Second Study Program* (pp. 336–349). Rockefeller University, New York.

MacLean, P. D. (1973). A triune concept of the brain and behavior. Lecture I. Man's reptilian and limbic inheritance; Lecture II. Man's limbic brain and the psychoses; Lecture III. New trends in man's evolution. In T. Boag and D. Campbell (eds), *The Hincks Memorial Lectures* (pp. 6–66). University of Toronto, Toronto.

MacLean, P. D. (1985). Brain evolution relating to family, play, and the separation call. *Arch. Gen. Psychiatry* 42: 405–417.

MacLean, P. D. (1987). The midline frontolimbic cortex and the evolution of crying and laughter. In E. Perecman (ed), *The Frontal Lobes Revisited* (pp. 121–140). IRBN, New York.

MacLean, P. D. (1990). *The Triune Brain in Evolution.* Plenum, New York.

Markus, H., and Nurius, P. (1986). Possible selves. *Am. Psychol.* 41: 954–969.

Marlowe, W. B. (1992). The impact of a right prefrontal lesion on the developing brain. *Brain Cogn.* 20: 205–213.

Meyer, A. (1904). The anatomical facts and clinical varieties of traumatic insanity. *American Journal of Insanity* LX(3): 25–441.

Oddy, M., Coughlan, T., Tyerman, A., and Jenkins, D. (1985). Social adjustment after closed head injury: a further follow-up 7 years after injury. *J. Neurol. Neurosurg. Psychiatry* 48: 564–568.

Ota, Y. (1969). Psychiatric studies on civilian head injuries. In A. E. Walker,

W. F. Caveness, and M. Critchley (eds), *The Late Effects of Head Injury* (pp. 110–119). Charles C Thomas, Springfield, Ill.

Papero, P. H., Prigatano, G. P., Snyder, H. M., and Johnson, D. L. (1993). Children's adaptive behavioural competence after head injury. *Neuropsychological Rehabilitation* 3(4): 321–340.

Papez, J. W. (1937). A proposed mechanism of emotion. *Archives of Neurology and Psychiatry* 38: 725–743.

Penfield, W., and Jasper, H. (1954). *Epilepsy and the Functional Anatomy of the Human Brain*. Little, Brown, Boston.

Pribram, K. H. (1971). *Languages of the Brain: Experimental Paradoxes and Principles in Neuropsychology*. Prentice-Hall, Englewood Cliffs, NJ.

Pribram, K. H., and Gill, M. M. (1976). *Freud's "Project" Re-Assessed*. Basic Books, New York.

Price, B. H., Daffner, K. R., Stowe, R. M., and Mesulam, M. M. (1990). The comportmental learning disabilities of early frontal lobe damage. *Brain* 113(Pt 5): 1383–1393.

Prigatano, G. P. (1986). Personality and psychosocial consequences of brain injury. In Prigatano et al. (eds), *Neuropsychological Rehabilitation After Brain Injury* (pp. 29–50). Johns Hopkins University Press, Baltimore.

Prigatano, G. P. (1988). Emotion and motivation in recovery and adaptation after brain damage. In S. Finger, T. E. LeVere, C. R. Almli, and D. G. Stein (eds), *Brain Injury and Recovery: Theoretical and Controversial Issues* (pp. 335–350). Plenum, New York.

Prigatano, G. P. (1992). Personality disturbances associated with traumatic brain injury. *J. Consult. Clin. Psychol.* 60(3): 360–386.

Prigatano, G. P., Altman, I. M., and O'Brien, K. P. (1990). Behavioral limitations that brain injured patients tend to underestimate. *Clinical Neuropsychologist* 4: 163–176.

Prigatano, G. P., Fordyce, D., Zeiner, H., Roueche, J., Pepping, M., and Wood, B. (1986). *Neuropsychological Rehabilitation After Brain Injury*. Johns Hopkins University Press, Baltimore.

Prigatano, G. P., O'Brien, K. P., and Klonoff, P. S. (1988). The clinical management of delusions in postacute traumatic brain injured patients. *Journal of Head Trauma Rehabilitation* 3(3): 23–32.

Prigatano, G. P. Fordyce, D. J., Zeiner, H. K., Roueche, J. R., Pepping, M., and Wood, R. C. (1986). *Neuropsychological Rehabilitation After Brain Injury*. Johns Hopkins University Press, Baltimore.

Prigatano, G. P., and Schacter, D. L. (1991). *Awareness of Deficit After Brain Injury: Clinical and Theoretical Issues*. Oxford University Press, New York.

Prigatano, G. P., and Summers, J. D. (1997). Depression in traumatic brain injury patients. In M. M. Robertson and C. L. E. Katona (eds), *Depression and Physical Illness* (pp. 341–358). John Wiley & Sons, New York.

Rekate, H. L., Grubb, R. L., Aram, D. M., Hahn, J. F., and Ratcheson, R. A. (1985). Muteness of cerebellar origin. *Arch. Neurol.* 42: 697–698.

Reyes, R. L., Bhattacharyya, A. K., and Heller, D. (1981). Traumatic head injury: restlessness and agitation as prognosticators of physical and psychologic improvement in patients. *Arch. Phys. Med. Rehabil.* 62: 20–23.

Roberts, A. H. (1979). *Severe Accidental Head Injury: An Assessment of Long-Term Prognosis.* Macmillan, New York.

Robinson, R. G., Bolduc, P., and Price, T. R. (1987). A two-year longitudinal study of poststroke depression: diagnosis and outcome at one and two years. *Stroke* 18: 837–843.

Robinson, R. G., Kubos, K. L., Starr, L. B., Rao, K., and Price, T. R. (1983). Mood changes in stroke patients: relationship to lesion location. *Compr. Psychiatry* 24: 555–556.

Robinson, R. G. and Price, T. R. (1982). Post-stroke depressive disorders: a follow-up study of 103 patients. *Stroke* 13: 635–641.

Robinson, R. G., Starr, L. B., Lipsey, J. R., Rao, K., and Price, T. R. (1984a). A two-year longitudinal study of post-stroke mood disorders: dynamic changes in associated variables over the first six months of follow-up. *Stroke* 15: 510–517.

Robinson, R. G., Starr, L. B., Kubos, K. L., Rao, K., and Price, T. R. (1984b). Mood disorders in stroke patients: importance of location of lesion. *Brain* 197: 91–93.

Robinson, R. G., and Szetela, B. (1981). Mood change following left hemispheric brain injury. *Ann. Neurol.* 9: 447–453.

Rosenbaum, A., and Hoge, S. K. (1989). Head injury and marital aggression. *Am. J. Psychiatry* 146: 1048–1051.

Ross, E. D., and Rush, J. A. (1981). Diagnosis and neuroanatomical correlates of depression in brain-damaged patients. *Arch. Gen. Psychiatry* 38, 1344–1354.

Schilder, P. (1934). Psychic disturbances after head injuries. *Am. J. Psychiatry* 91: 155–188.

Shukla, S., Cook, B. L., Mukherjee, S., Godwin, C., and Miller, M. G. (1987). Mania following head trauma. *Am. J. Psychiatry* 144(1): 93–96.

Simon, H. A. (1967). Motivational and emotional controls of cognition. *Psychological Review* 76: 29–39.

Simon, H. A. (1994). The bottleneck of attention: connecting thought with motivation. In W. D. Spaulding (ed), *Integrative Views of Motivation, Cognition, and Emotion* (pp. 1–21). University of Nebraska, Lincoln.

Simon, H. A. (1995). The information-processing therapy of mind. *American Psychologist* 50 (7): 507–508.

Starkstein, S. E., Robinson, R. G., and Price, T. R. (1987). Comparison of cortical and subcortical lesions in the production of poststroke mood disorders. *Brain* 110: 1045–1059.

Starkstein, S. E., Robinson, R. G., and Price, T. R. (1988). Comparison of patients with and without poststroke major depression matched for size and location of lesion. *Arch. Gen. Psychiatry* 45: 247–252.

Storey, P. B. (1970). Brain damage and personality change after subarachnoid haemorrhage. *Br. J. Psychiatry* 117: 129–142.

Thomsen, I. V. (1984). Late outcome of very severe blunt head trauma: a 10–15 year second follow-up. *J. Neurol. Neurosurg. Psychiatry* 47: 260–268.

Valzelli, L. (1980). *An Approach to Neuroanatomical and Neurochemical Psychophysiology*. John Wright, Littleton, Mass.

van Zomeren, A. H., and van Den Burg, W. (1985). Residual complaints of patients two years after severe head injury. *J. Neurol. Neurosurg. Psychiatry* 48: 21–28.

Wise, S. F., and Herkenham, M. (1982). Opiate receptor distribution in the cerebral cortex of the rhesus monkey. *Science* 218: 387–389.

7

Personality Disturbances
and Brain Damage:
Practical Considerations

> Thus, in this, as in all the other kinds of emotional and behavioral patterns observed in brain damaged patients, a complex interplay between neurological, psychological, and psychosocial factors must be admitted.
>
> G. Gainotti "Emotional and psychosocial patterns after brain injury," 1993, p. 272

Understanding patients' personalities helps in their management during neuropsychological rehabilitation. In this case, the old adage "forewarned is forearmed" is apt because personality disturbances in brain dysfunctional patients seem to be almost as overwhelming to the rehabilitation team (Prigatano et al., 1986) as to family members (Brooks and McKinlay, 1983).

A wide variety of personality disturbances is associated with brain-injured individuals (Prigatano, 1992; also see Table 6-2 in Chapter 6). A given patient's symptom profile reflects the combination of "pre-existing personality characteristics (that) interact with neuropsychologically mediated changes in cognition and affect to yield variable patterns of personality disturbance" (Prigatano et al., 1986, p. 29).

The preceding chapter emphasized that certain patterns of behavior, like establishing territorial boundaries or selecting a mate, may be regulated by brain physiology and anatomy more than is often recognized (MacLean, 1973, 1990). Various forms of display behavior may be associated with biological drives to express sexual and aggressive tendencies. They may emerge rather quickly after traumatic brain injury. Certain behavioral abnormalities appear to be strongly associated with specific brain lesions (Heilman and Valenstein, 1993).

Thus, disturbances in various feedback and feedforward brain mechanisms may affect not only "cognition," but basic and complex feeling states (i.e., emotion and motivation). Conscious and nonconscious response tendencies seem to influence behavior and may be independent of brain damage per se. These latter "characterological features" interact with neuropsychologically mediated changes to shape the reactionary problems brain dysfunctional patients demonstrate. The task now is to demonstrate how this broad model may be useful in assessing and managing personality disturbances associated with brain injury (Principles 4 and 5).

Domains of Information in Assessing Personality after Brain Injury

When choosing among different assessment techniques, clinicians must know what to look for, that is, what class of information would be most useful or clinically relevant for a given patient. In the course of neuropsychological assessment and rehabilitation, clinicians should consider the following six domains of information when formulating opinions about personality disturbances associated with brain injury.

1. Given age, educational background, cultural background, and gender, what are a patient's recurring emotional and motivational response patterns?
2. During the interview, how does a patient communicate about him- or herself verbally and nonverbally?
3. What are the content and manner of self-reports on "objective" measures of personality [e.g., the Minnesota Multiphasic Personality Inventory-2 (MMPI-2)] and various supplementary questionnaires [i.e., the Patient Competency Rating Scale (PCRS)]?
4. What aspects of the patient's personality seem to be "projected" onto the various test stimuli used in the neuropsychological examination and onto questions raised during the interview?
5. What is the person's phenomenological experience as reflected in choice of words, self-descriptions, dreams, choice of music, and artistic expressions?
6. What behavioral or performance characteristics does the patient demonstrate when engaging in neuropsychological testing or rehabilitation?

Methods of Assessment

These six domains of information can be assessed in different ways. Often the first source of information about patients and their recurring patterns of emotional and motivational responding can be obtained from their *history*. Their history can be self-reported or obtained from reliable others. What does the clinician look for?

Premorbidly, what was the patient's manner of adaptation? Did the person choose appropriate goals and complete them once started (e.g., was high school, college, or both completed if initiated)? How were inevitable interpersonal conflicts typically resolved? What were the degree and type of family commitment and support? How did the patient appear to handle intimate relationships and commitments? What is the person's work history and what were his or her vocational choices?

Postmorbidly, what is the patient's manner of adaptation? What changes occurred in the patient's premorbid patterns of responding? How does the patient express frustration and confusion? What steps, if any, has the patient (or family) taken to aid the rehabilitation process? How does the patient (and family) deal with recommendations concerning care?How does the patient (and family) deal with the inevitable problems of anger, anxiety, and depression about the brain injury? How realistic have the patient's choices been about returning to work (or school) and his or her capacity to meet daily demands? How have disturbed interpersonal relationships been handled?

What, if any, behavioral characteristics especially changed after the known or suspected brain injury? In the history obtained from the patient, did he or she emphasize that "they are not the same person as they were before," or did the patient insist that very few changes had occurred? Does he or she describe himself or herself in different terms than before the injury? Do family members agree or have a different perspective? How reliable and "objective" are the family members and the patient?

In addition to the content of the information presented, how does the patient express himself or herself during the interview? This aspect of behavior can be a crucial source of information. Does the patient appear to understand the questions asked? Is she perplexed or usually confused? Can he remember the question asked?

When asked about difficult areas, does the patient become angry, depressed, or show an uncooperative attitude? What is the patient's degree of insight, and does he or she appear to be apathetic about the assessment process? How do these behavioral characteristics compare to what is known about the patient's pattern of emotion and motivational responding before the onset of brain injury?

Based on the interview, what does the examiner perceive to be the strengths and limitations of the patient's personality and are these characteristics long-standing?

What words does the patient choose to describe her phenomenological situation? Does he answer questions clearly? Are the patient's answers to the point or circumstantial and tangential? Is the patient hyperverbal or is it difficult to elicit a verbal response to questions? Does the examiner feel that a sense of rapport can be established with the patient? Does the examiner automatically have a sense of empathy, or does he or she feel any hostility in terms of the patient's response?

Interviewing the patient in the presence of family members can be quite helpful. Can family members inhibit their responses when the patient is asked specific questions? Conversely, can the patient inhibit his or her responses when similar questions are asked of family members? What is the degree of support or nonsupport exhibited between family members and the patient? This general class of information can be quite useful in determining the psychosocial setting, cultural milieu, and environmental circumstances in which the patient must function.

In addition to the information obtained from the history and clinical interview, formal psychometric assessment of personality can be helpful. A patient's self-reports, however, must be interpreted cautiously because patients tend to underestimate certain behavioral characteristics after traumatic brain injury (TBI) (Prigatano et al., 1990). The self-reports of brain dysfunctional patients, however, can be reliable and valid indications of what they are experiencing. Clinicians frequently use the so-called "objective" measures of personality, such as the MMPI-2, to assess TBI patients. The MMPI-2 profile can provide useful information, but its findings must be interpreted cautiously as demonstrated by the case examples to follow.

In addition to these "objective" measures, administering various other questionnaires may be helpful. For example, comparing how a patient completes the PCRS with how relatives rate the patient on the same scale can be quite revealing (Prigatano et al., 1986).

Typically, traditional personality assessments include the use of projective measures, but neuropsychologists seldom use these testing procedures. Roy Schafer (1967) has written insightfully about the role of psychological testing in patient evaluation and the potential usefulness of projective techniques in certain circumstances. When asked later in his career if he still administered the Rorschach, he reportedly commented that he did not. When asked why, he responded that after several years of testing patients he had found that taking a careful history during a clinical interview provides much of the same information as projective measures. Clinical neuropsychologists who have seen a wide variety of patients understand his comments.

For example, when patients are asked to describe facial affect on the *BNI Screen for Higher Cerebral Functions*, patients with Alzheimer's disease often describe a face with a fearful or surprised look as one that is "confused." Certain brain dysfunctional patients, however, describe the same face as "frustrated." These responses seem to reflect the patients' personal experience, which they "project" on the facial stimuli.

Examiners with adequate experience in evaluating brain dysfunctional patients who have listened to patients describe their difficulties will be aware of predictable phenomenological experiences that are associated with various forms of brain damage as well as with experiences that are seldom associated with brain damage. Thus, clinical neuropsychologists who interview patients obviously do so against a background of information that cannot easily be distilled into words or texts. The basic point, however, is that interviewers should be thoroughly familiar with the phenomena that they are attempting to assess. The interviewers will then know what questions to ask as well as what questions *not* to ask at certain points during the assessment or rehabilitation process. Clinicians must have a sense of the phenomenon, the patients' phenomenological field, and the appropriate time when questions should be asked. There are no simple guidelines to outline how to achieve this finesse; it often takes years of training and experience to develop.

Assessing the patients' phenomenological experience is an important task but one that emerges with time. Certainly, the patient's choice of words during the clinical interview gives clinicians the first sense of what the patient's subjective experience might be. Weinstein and Kahn (1955) aptly demonstrated that the words patients choose to describe their disability provide insight into how they view themselves and how premorbid factors may shape their symptom profile. In my experience, a patient's dreams, choice of music, and artistic expressions offer useful insights as well (Prigatano, 1991). After their brain injuries, for example, a number of brain dysfunctional cowboys from Oklahoma preferred music that reflected themes of abandonment and uselessness. Patients who are victims (i.e., their brain injury was caused by the irresponsible actions of someone else) often express this situation artistically in music and drawings that reflect themes of anger and confusion. These are powerful sources of information that help the clinician to construct a working model of the patients' emotional and motivational characteristics (i.e., their personality).

Finally, a patient's behavioral or performance characteristics during the actual testing are important. When given tasks, does the patient appear perplexed by the instructions? Can he engage in the task despite frustration with his poor performance? How does she handle memory failures when performing various tasks of learning and abstract reasoning? The following example highlights the importance of such information as it emerges from a neuropsychological examination.

A 21-year-old woman with a history of hydrocephalus and associated memory impairment was asked to take the Halstead Category Test. Initially, she did reasonably well and grasped the first few concepts with no difficulty. As the test progressed in complexity, however, she began to forget how a previously acquired strategy might be useful. Her responses became impulsive and erratic. This impulsivity and rigidity in her responses emerged only when she experienced a memory failure. In her case, impulsivity appeared to be a reactionary disturbance and secondary to her cognitive deficits. During the interview, she exhibited no evidence of impulsivity or rigidity in her response to questions.

To highlight this general approach and to show how conclusions about personality characteristics associated with brain injury can be reached, several case examples are presented. These cases represent patients who suffered their brain injuries at different times during development.

Brain Injury in Infancy and Personality Disturbances

A 29-year-old man underwent a neuropsychological evaluation for reported "memory" problems observed at work (Case 1; Table 7-1). His history documented that he had suffered a severe craniocerebral trauma at the age of 18 months. He was in a motor vehicle accident and had been ejected from the car at the time of impact. A magnetic resonance (MR) imaging study performed at the time of the patient's neuropsychological evaluation about 27 years later revealed a clear focal area of encephalomalacia, primarily in the left frontal region but also involving the left temporal region (Fig. 7-1).

The patient had obtained a bachelor's degree, but a 4-year program of study had taken him 6 years to complete (Table 7-1). As an adult, he was able to maintain work and eventually married and had a child. His wife noted that he was not easy to engage in conversation, particularly in group settings. Consequently, she felt that he might be depressed. He, however, reported no major disturbances of depression, anxiety, or behavioral dyscontrol. He was clearly a "hard worker" and a devoted father and husband. Nonetheless, his wife complained that he did not spontaneously discuss personal matters, and she was frustrated that he was not as engaged in the relationship as she would have liked. She saw him as aloof even though he did not seem to recognize this behavior in himself.

His job supervisor noted that this patient was a hard worker and dedicated to his job but that he demonstrated significant memory problems. The patient himself recognized no significant memory disturbance. Although his supervisors described numerous examples of memory failure that adversely affected his work performance, the patient felt that the supervisor was needlessly critical. Such perceptions are common among individuals with a severe brain injury.

Neuropsychological testing when this patient was 29 years old revealed a verbal IQ score of 88 and a performance IQ score of 99 on the Wechsler Adult Intelligence Scale-Revised (WAIS-R). On the Rey Auditory Verbal Learning Test (RAVLT), his performance was about one standard deviation below the mean. His recall of short stories on the Wechsler Memory Scale-Revised Form (WMS-R) was at the 25th and 31st percentile for immediate and delayed recall, respectively. His recall of visuospatial information was at the 90th percentile for immediate recall but at the 21st percentile for delayed recall. Memory impairment was evident.

On the PCRS, the patient's total score was 142 of 150 total possible

Table 7-1. Clinical summary of patient who experienced a TBI during infancy

Dimension	Content
Evaluation	
History	TBI at 18 months, examined at 29 years; MR imaging at 29 years revealed clear focal area of encephalomacia in primary left frontal region. Took 6 years to complete a 4-year college education.
Interview	Flat affect; difficult to engage in conversation. Wife feels that he may be depressed, but emphasizes that he is always a "hard worker."
"Objective" personality assessment	No MMPI or MMPI-2 administered.
Self-ratings	On the PCRS, the patient reports only mild memory difficulties. Wife reports more substantial problems with memory, as well as engaging in conversations.
"Projected" information	Exhibits apparent perplexity about the situation.
Phenomenological experience	Patient feels his work supervisor was needlessly critical of him. Believes that he has no substantial problems in doing his job despite considerable evidence to the contrary.
Behavior and emotional/ motivational characteristics during testing	Somewhat shy and reserved. Mildly confused with feedback. Cooperative, hard-working, no affective reaction to failure.
Conclusions	
Reactionary	Social withdrawal and quietness.
Neuropsychological	Flat affect (not depressed); apparent lack of insight or awareness about disability; lacks creativity.
Characterological	Hard working, energetic.

TBI = traumatic brain injury; MR = magnetic resonance.

points. This score indicates that the patient felt that he could perform most activities with ease. His wife, however, reported a total score of 128 for the patient. Although this latter score is "high," it reflects that she perceived her husband as having more difficulties than he reported himself.

What was this young man like as a person? He appeared shy and

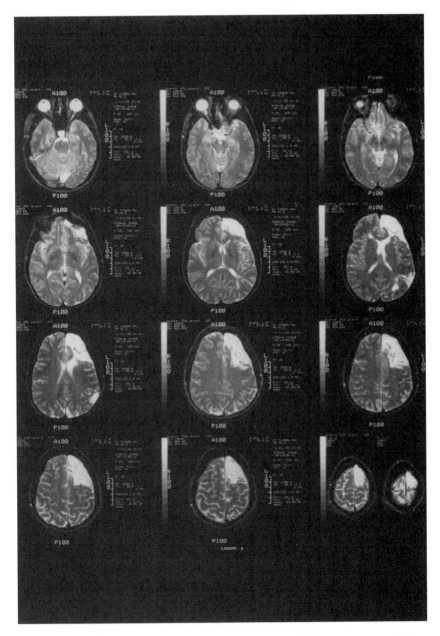

Figure 7-1. Magnetic resonance imaging study obtained from a 29-year-old man approximately 27 years after he sustained a traumatic brain injury.

reserved and often seemed mildly confused when given feedback about his performance. Even with negative feedback, his facial expression often appeared "flat," yet he denied any dysphoric mood. He was hard-working, but the manner in which he approached problems was stereotypic. He could not easily integrate feedback to modify his behavior. He seemed to lack creativity and initiative even though his drive to do a good job was high. Although his behavior was socially appropriate with no obvious disinhibited behaviors, his manner and his ability to interact with others did not appear very sophisticated.

The patient's reactionary problems seemed to center around social withdrawal. He was quiet because he did not know what to say. His apparent depression did not appear to be a true depression but reflected the flat affect often associated with frontal lobe damage. The flat affect appeared to be a neuropsychologically mediated disturbance in personality. The patient's long history of hard work and being energetic and trying to accomplish goals appeared to be independent of his brain injury. These characteristics were fostered by his parents and could be broadly described as characterological. Undoubtedly, they may have been influenced by his early brain injury, but brain injury per se did not contribute to these characteristics.

In a second example, an 8-year-old boy had sustained a severe injury to the left hemisphere at the age of 12 months. He suffered a right hemiparesis that affected his arm more than his leg. This boy also was severely neglected and eventually placed in a foster home. No MR imaging study of his brain has been performed.

The boy was diagnosed as hyperactive. On the playground, for example, he ran back and forth incessantly, exhausting the observer but showing no obvious exhaustion himself. When he was placed on Ritalin, his behavior was calmer although he still did not function at a level that would be considered completely normal arousal or activity.

When given positive news or a message that pleased him, he often grinned widely and jumped up and down as a reflection of his satisfaction. The behavior appeared primitive and childlike and often put the observer at bay. The patient's school speech pathologist considered his language function to be within the normal range and actually recommended discontinuing speech and language therapy. His language skills were considered a strength, with his major problem being "auditory memory." The teachers noted, however, that he had a difficult time developing concepts. It was hoped that this problem would eventually resolve and that he would learn the basic concepts necessary for daily activities (e.g., basic number concepts, the alphabet). The teacher hoped that he would learn more socially appropriate behavior. She did not seem to appreciate fully the extent of his cognitive and linguistic deficits.

A neuropsychological examination revealed that this child had significant anomia with astereognosis. When asked to name objects in his left (or right) hand, he could not do so. He *had* to look at the objects before he could name them. Even when looking at several common objects, he could not name them correctly. When given a picture completion task, he could point to some of the missing objects, reflecting that he knew what was missing but could not produce their names.

In the classroom, he was often asked, along with other children, to describe what he saw in a picture. The teacher was perplexed because the boy often cried out, "I can't," even though he seemed to communicate reasonably well in everyday conversations. His reasonable communication, however, consisted of very brief sentences. It appeared that he had a significant language impairment with prominent anomic features. When asked to describe a picture, he literally could not do so and was obviously frustrated by the task. This type of frustration occurred daily with no one in his environment understanding the nature of his underlying cognitive deficit.

The best word to describe his personality would be "primitive." He displayed a wide grin and a childlike squeal when he was pleased and a quick frown and pulling back when dissatisfied. Basic approach-and-avoidance behaviors were present, but they were exhibited in a disinhibited manner that reflected a low tolerance for frustration.

The boy seemed to lack true communications skills for getting his needs met, yet he displayed the basic emotions described in Chapter 6. He could be happy or angry. He could show sadness or fear. He could even show surprise or disgust. Yet he lacked a communication system that would allow him to approach or avoid situations appropriate to the environments in which he was placed. In his case, basic feedback systems seemed to be essentially unworkable, and his energy component appeared to be completely out of balance. Perhaps his symptom of hyperactivity reflected a disturbance in feedback mechanisms.

When the brain is damaged very early in life, language skills are often compromised. Even though a person can talk, language function is not necessarily normal. These patients often have difficulties understanding exactly what is said to them. They have problems in understanding complicated verbal and written instructions. They often ask that information be repeated over and over again because they are unsure of the actual linguistic message being conveyed. The speakers may respond with irritation at patients' repetitive requests for clarification of a linguistic point.

These patients have reduced problem-solving capacities, which handicap almost every area of their cognitive development. They may be motivated and can complete an educational course of study, but they often do so at a rate slower than their peers. In such cases, the brain injury adversely affects but does not eliminate cognitive strategies for coping.

As their language functions become compromised, brain-injured persons experience more difficulty in defining their experience and communicating their needs. To others they often appear to be perplexed, immature, or childish. Some of these patients can adapt socially even though they become socially withdrawn and often prefer to be by themselves, much like the little boy described above. Others, however, have notable difficulties communicating with the environment. When feedback mechanisms are greatly disturbed, their behavior can indeed veer out of control. An impairment in basic language skills seems to be the basis for many of their behavioral problems.

Interestingly, few of these children are described as sociopathic later in life. Rather, they are described as childlike and immature in terms of the expression of their emotions and motivations. They appear more hedonistic than sociopathic. A different symptom profile prevails, however, when the brain is injured after language function develops.

Brain Injury in Childhood After Language Develops and Personality Disturbance

A 44-year-old man contacted my office to "volunteer for research." He reported suffering a head injury at the age of 7 years (Case 2, Table 7-2). His medical records documented that he was unconscious or at least unresponsive to verbal commands for about 2 weeks. At the time of his injury (1958), neither computed tomography (CT) nor MR imaging was available. A skull radiograph report, however, noted an "extensive left parieto-fronto-occipital fracture and brain contusions."

This highly motivated man completed studies for a bachelor's degree in about 5 years. Yet during the next 20 years of work, he had numerous jobs, none that lasted more than 2.5 years. When asked about his employment record, he felt that people "did not understand him." He often felt harassed by supervisors who did not appreciate his special needs. When asked about these special needs, he focused on the problem of epilepsy, which he had experienced since the accident. He did not spontaneously mention any neuropsychological impairments. If asked if he had specific memory impairments, he replied, "Not really."

About 37 years after his brain injury, he obtained a prorated WAIS-R verbal IQ score of 110 with a prorated performance IQ score of 84. His Digit Symbol Scale score was 6, his Vocabulary score was 12, and his Block-Design score was 8. His recall of short stories read to him was within the normal range on the WMS-R (56th percentile for immediate recall and 59th percentile for delayed recall). In contrast, his recall of visuospatial information was very poor—the 6th and 7th percentile for immediate and delayed recall, respectively. On the California Verbal Learning Test (CVLT), he could only recall 28 words over five trials, producing a t-score of 10 for his age and educational background.

A MR imaging study performed at the time of this neuropsychological evaluation (about 37 years after his trauma) was interpreted as within

Table 7-2. Clinical summary of a patient who experienced a TBI during childhood

Dimension	Content
Evaluation	
History	TBI at 7 years; examined at 44 years. Took 5 years to complete a 4-year college program. History of 25 jobs in 20 years.
Interview	Highly motivated; reports that people do not understand him. Focuses on his physical limitations; does not spontaneously mention cognitive disabilities or difficulties in interpersonal relationships.
"Objective" personality assessment	History of chronic psychological maladjustment with anxiety and depression. MMPI-2 profile suggests "impulsive acting out." This interpretation may be mistaken.
Self-ratings	No major cognitive or behavior problems. No relative available to compare ratings.
"Projected" information	"No one understands me" (versus "I don't understand myself").
Phenomenological experience	"I don't know why I have such a difficult time keeping jobs. I believe people are discriminating against me because I have a head injury. I get easily upset; I know I shouldn't."
Behavior and emotional/ motivational characteristics during testing	Cooperative, quick to make excuses for poor performance on neuropsychological tests.
Conclusions	
Reactionary	Mild depression with moderate anxiety.
Neuropsychological	Immaturity, lack of insight or awareness, long-standing disinhibited behavior.
Characterological	Hard to describe. Appears to be hardworking and motivated but lacks creativity and insight.

TBI = traumatic brain injury.

normal limits. Later inspection of the MR images, however, suggested the possibility of subtle atrophy in the left temporal lobe.

The patient's profile on the MMPI-2 highlights the potential limitations of this inventory for the evaluation of brain-injured people, particularly when an injury occurs in childhood. A computer analysis of his profile stated the following:

Individuals with this MMPI-2 profile tend to show a pattern of chronic psychological maladjustment. The client appears to be quite anxious and depressed at this time. He may be feeling some tension and somatic distress along with his psychological problems and may want relief from situational pressures.

Apparently quite immature and hedonistic, he may show a recent history of impulsive acting out behavior and substance abuse which results in considerable situational stress. He shows a pattern of superficial guilt or remorse over his behavior, but does not accept much responsibility for his actions. He may avoid confrontation and deny problems.

This individual's behavior was indeed immature and he could be described as hedonistic. Although he had a long history of failure, he showed no recent evidence of impulsive "acting out." Acting out implies that an individual has some type of psychological conflict that is not represented fully consciously, and the behavior reflects that underlying conflict. In this case, the patient's "acting out" behaviors reflected long-standing problems of disinhibition.

The individual was anxious and depressed about his situation. However, he perceived no connection between his neuropsychological impairments and his behavioral failures. Thus, to use the terms denial or acting out to describe such persons misses the effect of the brain injury on their personality, particularly when the injury occurred in childhood. This individual was inappropriately evaluated by such an instrument, and clinicians who use these standardized techniques, which were developed for psychiatric patients, risk misidentifying and misunderstanding patients with such personality disturbances.

When language is reasonably well developed before a brain injury occurs, persons often seem to be able to communicate adequately after the injury. They still, however, may show subtle problems in language functioning. For example, the above patient had a normal Verbal IQ and a Vocabulary score of 12. Yet his ability to retrieve words rapidly by letter category was below average. He also had difficulty clearly stating his understanding of his strengths and limitations.

As noted earlier, Weinstein (see Prigatano and Weinstein, 1996) reminds us of Sapir's idea that language not only communicates what has happened but actually defines experience for us. If the brain is damaged in childhood, persons will have difficulties in using language and therefore in defining their experience. Basic approach-and-avoidance tendencies may be present, but the ability to use language to delay gratification or to clarify a feeling state may be altered. Thus, the "second-signal system" described by Freud (1924) or the "executive system" described by modern neuropsychologists and cognitive psychologists is inevitably altered. These cognitive-linguistic disruptions not only impair the ability to inhibit behavior but also impair an individual's ability to represent consciously how he or she has been affected. This impairment leads to statements that can be viewed as reflecting denial when, in fact, they represent disturbances of consciousness (or self-awareness; see Chapter 12).

Brain Injury in Adolescence and Personality Disturbances in Young Adulthood

A 14-year-old girl who suffered a TBI (Case 3; Table 7-3) had an admission Glasgow Coma Scale (GCS) score of 7. Her CT at admission reflected diffuse cerebral swelling, a small left frontotemporal epidural hematoma, and a possible right frontal subdural hematoma. She was evaluated 2 years later at age 16 and then again at age 22. There was little difference between her IQ scores at age 16 and 22, although her vocabulary score decreased as time passed. At age 22 her WAIS-R verbal IQ was 90, her performance IQ was 98. Her Vocabulary subtest score was 8, her Block Design subtest score was 8, and her Digit Symbol subtest score was 9. On the CVLT, the total number of words that she recalled was 47, producing a T-score of only 22. Long-term free recall was one standard deviation below the mean. The patient made only 16 errors on the Halstead Category test. Except for her location score of 3 on the Tactical Performance Test, her performance was within normal limits on the Halstead-Reitan Neuropsychological Test Battery. What cognitive problems did this patient experience, and how did they relate to her personality and psychosocial adjustment?

The patient's mother was concerned about her daughter's ability to maintain employment as well as her continual promiscuous behavior. When asked about both, this very pleasant young woman was nondefensive. She recognized that she had gone through numerous jobs and had loosely connected explanations for why each job ended after a brief time. She had no difficulty discussing her sexual behavior in a straightforward manner and exhibited no embarrassment. Cognitively she recognized that she might not use the best judgment in terms of sexual partners and activities. Yet, while she stated that she often "knew better," she showed no signs of internal distress or worry about such matters. According to Damasio's, Tranel's, and Damasio's (1991) concept of "somatic maker," she seemed to lack the normal autonomic nervous system triggers that warn people that they are engaging in potentially dangerous behavior.

Although the patient's behavior clearly suggested frontal lobe dysfunction, her performance on the Halstead-Reitan Battery, and particularly on the Halstead Category test, was within the normal range. I have seen this pattern many times over the years. That is, patients' medical histories clearly document a moderate to severe TBI, but several years

Table 7-3. Clinical summary of patient who experienced a TBI during adolescence

Dimension	Content
Evaluation	
History	TBI at 14; CT shows small left frontotemporal epidural hematoma and possible right frontal cerebral hematoma; initially seen within 1 month of TBI. Examined at age 16 and again at age 22.
Interview	When patient is age 22, mother voices concern about daughter's difficulty in maintaining work and promiscuous behavior. Patient acknowledges difficulties with work but has loosely connected explanations. Shows no embarrassment in discussing sexual behaviors.
"Objective" personality assessment	MMPI-2 revealed considerable difficulties with interpersonal relations and self-reported anxiety and depression despite how patient presents self during interview.
Self-ratings	On PCRS, patient reports few disturbances in daily functioning.
"Projected" information	None available.
Phenomenological experience	Patient does not understand why her mother is making such a "big thing" out of her behavior. She perceives no major difficulties, though mildly recognizes she might benefit from some "counseling" when it comes to knowing how to handle sexual relationships with young men.
Behavior and emotional/ motivational characteristics during testing	Bland, agreeable, smiles, somewhat flirtatious; no apparent distress over difficulties on various neuropsychological tests.
Conclusions	
Reactionary	No obvious reactionary problems present; possible depression.
Neuropsychological	Lack of emotional distress, lack of insight into difficulties, not denial, per se; disinhibited and inappropriate social behavior.
Characterological	Wants to be independent and live on her own.

TBI = traumatic brain injury; CT = computed tomography.

after the injury the patients may or may not show substantial impairment on neuropsychological tests, at least the standard ones currently in use. Often, however, the patient's personality may be altered in important ways. Sometimes individuals can recognize these changes and sometimes they cannot. Sometimes individuals can logically explain their behavior problems, but most of the time they cannot. These persons often appear to be hedonistic, but they may have retained problem-solving capacities that would result in them being diagnosed as sociopathic.

At the age of 22 years, the above patient had an MMPI-2 profile that was clearly abnormal. Nonetheless, this young woman actually reported very little subjective distress about her daily functioning. The MMPI-2 computer analysis of her profile interpreted this patient as having a great deal of difficulty in interpersonal relationships as well as showing "a long-standing personality disorder." This latter interpretation is questionable. She did not demonstrate difficulties in interpersonal relationships before her injury at the age of 14. It appears that the cognitive-personality disturbances caused by her brain injury account for her present psychosocial adjustment difficulties and much of her MMPI-2 profile.

The MMPI-2 further described this individual as showing behavior indicative of "denial." This denial, of course, must be interpreted cautiously because it may not reflect a true psychological defense mechanism but a disturbance in self-awareness caused by the brain injury.

Brain Damage in Young Adulthood and Later Deterioration of Personality

Many patients who suffer craniocerebral trauma in their early twenties show predictable problems with memory, speed of information processing, impulse control, irritability, and so on as described earlier. Some of these persons eventually adjust reasonably well, recognizing that with time, rehabilitation, or both they can still reconstruct a meaningful life even though they can no longer achieve their previous expectations or goals (Prigatano, 1995). For many of these individuals, the central issue becomes how to deal with the problem of lost normality, as discussed in the chapter on psychotherapy.

The long-term adjustment of persons who are unable to cope with the problem of lost normality is often difficult. Their basic personality structure may deteriorate with time. For example, a 25-year-old man suffered a severe craniocerebral trauma in an airplane crash in February 1977 (Case 4; Table 7-4). When the patient was examined in 1981, his WAIS-R verbal IQ score was 89 and his prorated performance IQ was 85. His Vocabulary scale score was 8, his Block Design score was 9, and his Digit Symbol score was 5.

In January 1996, he was reexamined after his father again brought

Table 7-4. Clinical summary of patient who experienced a TBI during early
adulthood

Dimension	Content
Evaluation	
History	TBI at 25; severe brain injury with severe memory impairment observed 4 years after trauma. Patient evaluated 4 years and then 18.5 years after trauma.
Interview	Seen 4 years after trauma, attributed difficulties in cognitive functioning to headaches. Stated that if he did not have headaches, he would have no difficulties performing cognitive tasks. Twenty-two years later has false memories of what was said to him previously. Blatantly delusional and undisturbed by it.
"Objective" personality assessment	Unable to complete MMPI because of psychiatric state.
Self-ratings	Reports almost no problems in any area. In contrast, family reports considerable difficulties in interpersonal behavior, memory, and social judgment.
"Projected" information	Patient states that I had belittled him years ago with various comments during rehabilitation. The patient appears to feel, in fact, belittled over his brain injury and often told others that he "works with Dr. Prigatano" versus being a patient in a rehabilitation program for which Dr. Prigatano serves as the director.

(continued)

him to my attention. His parents were very concerned about their son's developing paranoid ideation. When I interviewed the man privately, he had false memories of what I had said or done to him during his neuropsychological rehabilitation 14 years earlier. He also described how an attorney who had succeeded in his educational endeavors and whom he described as a Rhodes scholar (a word he could not recall but responded to positively when I provided the phrase) was out to get him. The patient made fragmented statements about ambulances driving around in his neighborhood and about this man constantly following him. He also stated that the physician who had prescribed him medication had moved

Table 7-4.—Continued

Dimension	Content
Phenomenological experience	Appears in less emotional distress than when seen 4 years after injury—yet reports clear delusional ideas as well as hallucinatory experiences. Is unable to handle extensive neuropsychological testing.
Behavior and emotional/ motivational characteristics during testing	Cooperative, but clearly paranoid. Tries very, very hard on tasks, particularly the Halstead Tapping Test where he bangs the key with his finger to get the fastest score possible.
Conclusions	
Reactionary	Initial headaches with associated somatic distress.
Neuropsychological	Lack of awareness ultimately led to delusions, which can be interpreted as a combination of neuropsychological problems and reactionary problems.
Characterological	Very strong need to achieve, to be intellectual, and to have evidence of attaining a bachelor's degree. Also very strong need to achieve in business. Failure to achieve these long-term goals causes psychiatric distress.

TBI = traumatic brain injury.

to the Phoenix area because he was constantly keeping an eye on him. Upon further questioning, the patient described how he had heard people ask him, "Why are you leaving?" when he was about to leave one town to move to his hometown.

The patient had exhibited no evidence of psychotic thinking 14 years earlier. He had, however, shown signs of having difficulty in accepting his limitations, and he had subtle language difficulties and associated problems with memory and speed of information processing. We had worked with this patient to help him pursue work more compatible with his neuropsychological status. For various reasons, however, he (and I believe his parents) did not really believe that it was necessary. He then experienced 14 years of failure without understanding why. What emerged was ultimately a psychotic break with reality (this patient is also discussed in Chapter 13).

Brain Damage in the Second Half of Life and Personality Development

Two cases are presented to highlight common personality disturbances associated with brain injuries that occur during the midforties and early fifties. A successful businessman fell off a horse and sustained a moderate brain injury. He was unconscious for only a few minutes but exhibited posttraumatic amnesia for several hours. After several weeks he had a persistent headache. He finally sought medical attention, and a large subdural hematoma was discovered and surgically evacuated.

The patient and his wife noted that after this accident he appeared much more irritable and short-tempered. Frustrating events that he once could handle now upset him. His reduced tolerance for frustration eventually wore on his wife, who began to think seriously about separating from him.

Before his injury, this patient's history might broadly be described as "risk taking." He was an entrepreneur and had been quite successful in his business ventures. He also engaged in a variety of activities that most people would consider sociopathic, if not reflective of long-term problems with judgment (e.g., alcohol abuse while young, reckless motorcycle riding, a series of sexual relationships with no long-lasting connections till later in life). These behaviors seemed to be long-standing features of his personality and unrelated to his brain injury.

After his TBI, his cognitive functioning seemed less efficient and his tolerance for frustration was reduced. These changes produced a vicious circle. Because he was less able to function cognitively, he became more irritated and frustrated. Others responded to him in a negative way. He could not handle their responses and became more depressed. His difficulties with irritability then escalated to the point that he threatened his wife. This patient is a good example of the psychiatric notion that brain injury reduces "ego defenses" or the ability to cope with internal conflicts. Consequently, certain premorbid characteristics may be manifested in an exaggerated form.

A second patient, a 45-year-old man with a ruptured aneurysm of the anterior communicating artery, experienced considerable marital discord after his brain injury. He became depressed, with suicidal ideation and concern that he would never be able to return to work. After about 6 months in a neuropsychological rehabilitation program, he eventually found work although at a lower level than he had anticipated.

The patient was elated with his accomplishment, but shortly thereafter his wife announced that she was going to leave him. He became extremely angry and bitter. He began to drink heavily but denied alcohol use. He was seen for a series of psychotherapy sessions after rehabilitation. During this time, it was restated that the purpose of neuropsychological rehabilitation was not to make a person "happy," but rather to help a person become independent. The patient was, in fact, independent and confronting some of the major problems that people experience during the second half of life (e.g., the loss of a mate) (Prigatano and Ben-Yishay, (1999).

Within the context of a psychotherapeutic relationship, this patient ultimately was able to deal with his affective reactions and to curb his impulsive behavior. The threats toward his wife diminished. He finally found a level of work that he could accept even though it was, again, less than he had anticipated. As he became productive and reestablished relationships, he managed his cognitive and affective disturbances more adequately. In this particular case, he truly established a sense of meaning in his life after his brain injury.

As discussed in Chapter 3 (and following Eric Erickson's concepts), whatever psychosocial or intrapsychic issue that confronts persons at the time of brain injury becomes crucial to understanding their personality characteristics after brain injury. These brief case scenarios highlight this point. Let us now consider how Freud's and Jung's ideas can improve our understanding of personality problems associated with brain injury.

Dreams and Brain Damage

In 1971, I had an opportunity to work with a young man who had residual aphasic disturbances after a severe TBI. He was the first patient whom I attempted to work with from the perspective of rehabilitation. This young man had wanted to be a librarian, which seemed impossible with his aphasic disturbances. He was depressed and angry. With time, he became suspicious and developed an acute sense of vulnerability. He decided to learn the martial arts to protect himself from future brain injury.

During therapy he recounted a dream in which he was crying, but only from his left eye. When I asked about the meaning of his dream, he stated that people had told him that his inability to remember and speak was a result of his left-sided brain injury. This dream seemed to symbolize in a straightforward manner the sadness that he experienced about his left-brain injury. Dreams of brain dysfunctional patients can reveal long-standing issues in their development as well as current problems with coping with the aftermath of their injury.

Another patient who had suffered a left pontine hemorrhage with right hemiparesis and notable impairment in the motor function of the left arm and leg reported several dreams in which he was walking. Not only was he walking but he was actually moving all his limbs easily, something that he could not do in reality. When he awoke from these dreams, he would become extremely angry. The mental images emanating from his dream state reflect this person's struggles.

By listening to the dreams of patients, clinicians can often obtain useful insights about what they are struggling with but are unable to talk about directly. This concept, of course, was one of the early insights of the psychodynamic theorists, but it is frequently forgotten during the neuropsychological evaluation, rehabilitation, and psychotherapy of brain dysfunctional patients.

After a TBI, the frequency of dreaming (by the patient's subjective report) can be greatly reduced. Several years ago, we demonstrated (Prigatano et al., 1982) that rapid eye movement (REM) sleep was as common in a small group of patients with TBIs as it was in medical controls. The brain dysfunctional patients, however, awoke numerous times throughout the night. The next day they were often fatigued and yawned. A recent study (Manseau 1995) has replicated this finding. Sleep and dreaming are important dimensions in the assessment of brain dysfunctional patients and should be investigated routinely.

Symbols and Personality Adjustment After Brain Injury

Jung (1964) emphasized that people's adjustment to life was represented in their ability to relate to living symbols. The role of symbols in the process of doing psychotherapy with brain dysfunctional patients and their families is discussed in Chapter 9. The goal of this section is only to demonstrate how various symbols influence a patient's behavior.

Let us compare two young men. The first suffered cerebral anoxia from a cardiac arrest in his late teens. The son of a prominent businessman, he had been destined to complete professional training and was anticipating a lifestyle comparable to that of his parents. Before the injury, however, he was an average student and had experienced innumerable frustrations by comparing himself to an older brother who sailed through school easily. Nevertheless, this man's level of achievement would have allowed him to complete studies for a bachelor's degree at a major university.

After the episode of cerebral anoxia, he had notable problems with memory. Initially, he reported verbal recognition of these problems. In reality, he greatly underestimated the impact of these impairments on his daily functioning. When he returned to the university that he had been attending before his brain insult, he was unable to keep up with the academic demands. Almost immediately he developed a variety of somatic complaints, including persistent headache and anxiety attacks. Although he could not make an intellectual connection between his inability to cope in this academic environment and his somatic symptoms, he eventually agreed to attend a university that was much less demanding. As he made this transition, his somatic symptoms decreased substantially.

He completed his training, and his somatic symptoms again increased when he began looking for a position. However, he still saw little connection between his complaints and his job search. Nonetheless, after struggling with his altered functioning and with the fact that he was going to have to function at a lower level than anticipated, he was able to find some meaning in work and satisfaction in completing his bachelor's degree. Several years after brain injury, he has adjusted reasonably well even though some of his behaviors would be considered immature and lacking in insight.

In contrast, another young man of a similar age suffered a severe TBI during college. He also was the son of an affluent businessman and had similar aspirations for achieving lofty business goals and living a financially comfortable life. When seen in neuropsychological rehabilitation, he also showed a number of somatic symptoms. When given a variety of cognitive tests that he could not do, he complained that his headaches prevented him from doing the work but that he would be totally capable of doing the work if he did not have the headaches. After several months of therapy aimed at helping him to understand the connection between his somatic symptoms and his inability to function cognitively, he cautiously accepted that the relationship might be true. He accepted a job in sales—he described himself as a "people person."

While he was successful in this work, he had few somatic complaints. However, he decided to return to his home state to work with his father. He was advised that this was not the best choice because the demands that would be placed on him were beyond his cognitive capacity. Nonetheless, both his father and the young man felt that they wanted to try the arrangement. With time the patient's somatic symptoms again increased, and he was unable to perform the work. His parents supported him financially and encouraged him to do other things. He moved to a resort area where he became socially isolated. Over the years, he developed delusionary thought patterns (see Brain Damage in Young Adulthood and Later Deterioration of Personality, above).

In both cases, these men were motivated by the need to be successful at work. The symbol of work was crucial to their psychological functioning. One adjusted to how he related to this symbol; the other did not. The first continued to pursue work but at a lower level than anticipated. The second could not alter his previous image of what it meant to be successful. It does not require extensive psychoanalytic training to understand the connection between his paranoid ideation and his inability to cope with this symbol. He had failed to complete college and was anything but a Rhodes scholar. He had failed to be a successful businessman and developed fantasies that those who were successful in their lives were somehow the basis of his undoing. These are real and practical examples of the behavior of brain dysfunctional patients and how their personality unfolds after brain injury.

Freud's and Jung's concepts provide useful insights into how brain injury interacts with an individual's normal psychological struggles. Psychological functioning can be reflected in dreams and various living symbols, which motivate behavior and interact with the effects of brain damage to produce the behavior observed in neuropsychological evaluations and psychotherapeutic consultations.

A Return to Goldstein's Insights

As mentioned throughout this book, Kurt Goldstein was one of the first researchers to emphasize how brain injury affected personality, and he wrote insightfully about how brain injury disturbs people's attempts to cope with life's demands and to actualize their potentials. Reconsidering his work refreshes our view about how to approach patients.

Goldstein (1952) made an extremely important observation about the difficulties brain dysfunctional patients experience in binding tension before they respond. He noted that these patients would often respond quickly because they could not function adequately with this tension. Most individuals without brain injury experience tension in their daily life but actually find it helps them to plan and organize their tasks. After brain injury, however, individuals often do not know exactly what should be done. Because of their cognitive deficits, including memory impairments and problems with planning, they tend to act quickly to reduce the pressure associated with an impulse.

In normal daily functioning, the release of tension or pressure produces pleasure, which can be quite reinforcing. That is, when tension is reduced at the right time and place, people experience joy or pleasure. After brain injury, however, a person may reduce the tension prematurely and often experience a negative reaction from others. Negative responses are frustrating and further disorganize the person's behavior.

A 14-year-old girl, for example, with subtle disruption of the left cerebral hemisphere, would tell her parents what was said by her teacher in school as soon as she came home. She was concerned that she otherwise would recall the information inaccurately or forget it. Others would view this behavior as immature, which, in fact, it is. This response, however, misses the point. Namely, such individuals cannot tolerate tension for very long because their cognitive deficits prevent them from using this tension in an adaptive manner. Stated another way, their cognitive deficits are such that they have to act as soon as possible to solve the demands of the environment.

As the quote that introduced Chapter 6 indicates, Goldstein believed that in typical everyday life, emotional reactions may ultimately help an individual to reapproach a problem. In Pribram's (1971) and Simon's (1967) models, emotion serves as an *interrupt* function for behavior. Emotion can stop people from pursuing a potentially destructive course of action. In some instances this tendency turns out to be adaptive; in other instances it is not. Yet Goldstein's holistic approach emphasized that ultimately emotions help people to reassess their situations and therefore to reorganize their approaches to life's events (Goldstein, 1971). This model is not far from the cognitive psychologists' theorizing discussed in Chapter 6. It suggests that an intimate connection between feelings and cognition exists, and this connection determines whether goals are pursued and how people respond to failure to achieve their goals.

Gainotti (1993) has reconsidered the effects of psychodynamic factors and brain injury on the emotional behavior of patients. He emphasized that tests such as the MMPI can be misleading in attempts to understand the behavior of these patients. In citing Goldstein's work, he restated the importance of understanding patients' difficulty in dealing with the environment in terms of their cognitive deficits and the impact their deficits have on their affective reactions.

In the course of doing neuropsychologically oriented rehabilitation with brain dysfunctional patients, seeing them in individual neuropsychological consultation, and listening to their families describe their behavior over several weeks, months, and even years, I have become convinced that psychodynamic factors (as suggested by Freud and Jung), environmental contingencies (as described by Skinner), and the effects of brain damage [as described by numerous authors such Heilman and Valenstein (1993)] are constantly interacting to produce the symptom picture that emerges. Dealing with the personality disturbances of brain dysfunctional patients thus requires an integrated understanding of observations that have emanated from the realms of neuropsychology, clinical psychology, and psychiatry. Unfortunately, most studies with brain dysfunctional patients either take one approach or the other. The failure to integrate these bodies of knowledge in the context of various research designs results in static, unimaginative descriptions of patients' behavior and offers little insight about how to approach them (Principles 4 and 5). Weinstein's work stands as an example of how such an integration can be achieved (Prigatano and Weinstein, 1996).

A Return to Weinstein's Contributions

In studying language and memory impairments, Weinstein demonstrated that patients' premorbid personality characteristics and how they perceive the meaning of their disability relate to the kinds of errors that they make (Prigatano and Weinstein, 1996). He emphasized that patients' ability to describe their impairments or disabilities consciously was influenced by a variety of factors, including the nature and location of the brain injury. He also emphasized, however, that the meaning of the disability for individuals is important. Weinstein also emphasized that the social milieu in which patients' behavior is elicited and observed can have an important influence.

Let us consider some examples of this phenomenon. A young man falls while working as a painter. He suffers a left hemisphere parietal contusion. He shows classic verbal memory deficits as well as subtle problems in understanding higher-order linguistic information. The first thing that he states in the clinical interview is that he does not want to appear "stupid." He quickly related that recently a neurologist made him feel stupid because the neurologist had fired a number of questions at him that he could not answer. He became more withdrawn and somewhat belligerent. The neurologist felt that the patient was experiencing a severe depression. Although the patient certainly was depressed, the manner in which he had been examined contributed to the symptoms that the neurologist had observed and actually had a negative impact on the patient's adjustment. This point would be obvious to many experienced clinicians, but it is seldom stated. That is, how patients are examined can influence the behavioral disturbances that emerge after brain injury.

That patients' preexisting experiences and values will influence their symptom profile after brain injury also is well recognized but seldom adequately discussed or studied. Another patient, a young man who was shot in the left occipital area, had a classic visual field loss with subtle memory impairment. The patient, however, refused to see doctors. With time he developed clear paranoid ideation, feeling that doctors were insensitive to him and only going to force him to return to a job that he did not want. Further exploration of his history revealed that his father had died at an early age from an aneurysm. He viewed the doctors at that time as unwilling to take the need to save his father's life seriously. This long-standing attitude toward physicians was influencing what appeared to be paranoid ideation in the present. This is a clear example of how paranoid thinking does not emerge from a specific brain lesion. The patient's paranoid ideation reflected what he had experienced in the past while he attempted to make sense of the present given his brain injury.

The Neuropsychological Examination and Personality Assessment After Brain Damage

Attempts to assess personality disturbances after brain injury have primarily focused on the use of traditional methods employed in clinical psychology and psychiatry (Prigatano, 1987). Tests such as the Rorschach, the Bender Gestalt, or even the MMPI or MMPI-2 have been used.

One of the major challenges in assessing personality disturbances after brain injury, however, is to consider how cognitive and linguistic deficits actually affect patients' affective disturbances. Understanding how their cognitive deficits interact with the patients' struggles to cope provides helpful insights about the nature of their personality disturbances.

Second, some assessment of individuals' long-standing beliefs about themselves and others seems crucial to understanding personality disturbances after brain injury. To my knowledge, no such measures exist. We never ask people to describe their values, their beliefs, or what gives them a sense of meaning in life. Yet, we ask them to answer a series of questions with yes and no and then draw conclusions about the presence or absence of psychiatric symptomatology. This approach is a major mistake.

Finally, patients' ability to appraise their situation cognitively is crucial in understanding their personality disorders. Goldstein clearly recognized this point, which modern cognitive psychologists now emphasize. Giving patients tests in which they have to make judgments regarding interpretations of different experiences or events would seem crucial to understanding their affective disturbances. We are some distance from achieving such useful methods of personality assessment. It is hoped, however, that clinical neuropsychologists will take this need to develop tests of behavioral and personality disturbances after brain injury seriously. Tests on cognitive dysfunction associated with brain injury are also needed. The recent work of Nelson and colleagues (Nelson et al., 1994) reflects a trend in this direction.

Elsewhere I have attempted to provide specific guidelines for the neuropsychological testing of patients with TBI (Prigatano, 1996) and for those who have suffered subarachnoid hemorrhage (Prigatano and Henderson, 1997). Table 7-5 provides suggested guidelines for interviewing and testing patients. In the context of this set of guidelines, one can see that it is important to inquire what patients experience and to listen to their spontaneous reports. Then specific questions should be asked to highlight areas of difficulty that the practicing clinical neuropsychologist would normally assess. As this table indicates, it is useful to compare a patient's perceptions with those from reliable others. Given the medical information known about a patient (e.g., subjective complaints, lesion size and location), clinicians can form hypotheses that can be tested via the neuropsychological examination. This approach, of course, follows the tradition of Luria (1966).

In assessing personality characteristics associated with brain injury, it is important to remember factors known to influence the results of psychological tests (Table 7-6). A number of these factors relate directly to brain pathology or to the location and size of a lesion. Other factors involve time since injury and the individual's developmental stage at the time the brain injury occurred. The case examples in this chapter have highlighted this point. Finally, the examiner must remember that patients' personal reactions to their deficits will influence how they perform and that the methods used to elicit the disturbances will influence the behavior that emerges. Finally, patients' level of cooperation and motivation to perform and the examiner's sensitivity and sensibility can also influence the behavior observed during the assessment process.

Table 7-5. Suggested guidelines for interviewing and testing patients with subarachnoid hemorrhage

1. Ask patients what problems they experience and note spontaneous replies.
2. If not specifically mentioned, inquire about the presence of the following:
   a. difficulties with mental fatigue
   b. memory problems
   c. problems in planning
   d. difficulties in communicating clearly and concisely
   e. difficulties with visuospatial or mechanical skills
   f. difficulties in speed of information processing (i.e., being slowed down in the ability to perform various tasks)
   g. social judgment
   h. changes in mood or affect.
3. Compare patients' perceptions to perceptions of reliable others who know and observe them.
4. Given information concerning subjective complaints and lesion size and location, form hypotheses regarding what will be observed on neuropsychological testing.
5. Administer standardized tests that sample the following:
   a. primary and secondary language functions
   b. verbal and nonverbal memory
   c. speed of information processing
   d. visuospatial problem-solving skills
   e. ability to shift cognitive set
   f. abstract reasoning skills
   g. speed of finger movement on both hands
   h. patients' perceptions versus perceptions of reliable others

From Prigatano and Henderson (1997). With permission from the American Association of Neurological Surgeons.

Table 7-6. Factors that influence neuropsychological test results after traumatic brain injury

Lesion location
Size (extent) of lesion
Severity of the initial brain injury
Pathological nature of the lesion
Developmental (biological and psychosocial) stage
Chronicity of the lesion
Personal reactions to altered functioning
Materials (methods) used to elicit disturbances in higher cerebral functioning
Cooperation and motivation of the person to perform on the test
Sensitivity and sensibility of the examiner

From Prigatano, G. P. (1996). Neuropsychological testing after traumatic brain injury. In R. W. Evans (ed), *Neurology and Trauma* (pp. 222–230). W. B. Saunders, Philadelphia.

Summary and Conclusions

This chapter has attempted to bridge the theoretical ideas concerning personality disturbances associated with brain injury presented in Chapter 6 with the actual assessment of patients as they enter neuropsychological rehabilitation or are seen for neuropsychological assessment.

Clinicians must attend to different domains of information. Information derived from the patient's history and the clinical interview may be especially important. It is useful to classify personality disturbances as either reactionary, neuropsychologically mediated, or characterological (i.e., independent of brain injury per se). Specific case examples were provided to show how brain injury at different stages of development seems to influence personality. Within the context of this schema, case examples highlighted how different classes of information can be extracted and used to draw clinical conclusions.

The chapter restated the importance of understanding patients' emotional and motivation characteristics in addition to understanding their cognitive deficits to establish a reasonable picture of how they have been affected by their brain injury. Within the context of this picture, the examiner should have a sense of both the direct and indirect effects of the brain injury. The examiner also should have some idea of patients' premorbid personality and how they can be approached most effectively.

The final message of this chapter is the desperate need for appropriate measures to assess emotional and motivational disturbances in brain dysfunctional patients and the need to relate those measures to both empirical and theoretical considerations. Against this background, we now discuss the actual process of neuropsychological rehabilitation and consider a program that incorporates psychotherapy in this endeavor.

References

Brooks, D. N., and McKinlay, W. (1983). Personality and behavioural change after severe blunt head injury—a relative's view. *J. Neurol. Neurosurg. Psychiatry* 46: 336–334.

Damasio, A. R., Tranel, D., and Damasio, H. (1991). Somatic markers and the guidance of behavior: Theory and preliminary testing. In H. S. Levin, H. M. Eisenberg, and A. L. Benton (eds), *Frontal Lobe Function and Dysfunction*. Oxford University Press, New York.

Freud, S. (1924). *A General Introduction to Psychoanalysis* (24th ed). Simon and Schuster, New York.

Gainotti, G. (1993). Emotional and psychosocial problems after brain injury. *Neuropsychological Rehabilitation* 3(3): 259–277.

Goldstein, H. (1951/1971). On emotions: Considerations from the organismic point of view. *J. Psychology* 31: 37–49. Reprinted in A. Gurwitsch, E. M. Goldstein Haudek, and W. E. Haudek (eds), *Kurt Goldstein Selected Papers*. Martinus Nijhoff, The Hague.

Goldstein, K. (1952). The effect of brain damage on the personality. *Psychiatry* 15:245–260.

Heilman, K. M., and Valenstein, E. (1993). *Clinical Neuropsychology* (3rd ed). Oxford University Press, New York.

Jung, C. G. (1964). *Man and His Symbols*. Doubleday Windfall, Garden City, New York.

Luria, A. R. (1966). *Higher Cerebral Functions in Man*. Basic Books, New York.

MacLean, P. D. (1973). A triune concept of the brain and behavior. Lecture I. Man's reptilian and limbic inheritance; Lecture II. Man's limbic brain and the psychoses; Lecture III. New trends in man's evolution. In T. Boag and D. Campbell (eds), *The Hincks Memorial Lectures* (pp. 6–66). University of Toronto, Toronto.

MacLean, P. D. (1990). *The Triune Brain in Evolution*. Plenum, New York.

Manseau, C. (1995). Severe Traumatic Brain Injury: Long Term Effects on Sleep, Sleepiness and Performance. Doctoral Dissertation, Carleton University, Ottawa.

Nelson, L., Satz, P., and D'Elia, L. (1994). *The Neuropsychology Behavior and Affect Profile Manual*. Mind Garden Press, Palo Alto, Calif.

Pribram, K. H. (1971). *Languages of the Brain: Experimental Paradoxes and Principles in Neurospsychology*. Prentice-Hall, Englewood Cliffs, NJ.

Prigatano, G. P. (1987) Psychiatric aspects of head injury: problem areas and suggested guidelines for research. In H. Levin, J. Graftman, and H. M. Eisenberg (eds), *Neurobehavioural Recovery from Head Injury* (pp. 215–231). Oxford University Press, New York.

Prigatano, G. P. (1991). Disordered mind, wounded soul: the emerging role of psychotherapy in rehabilitation after brain injury. *Journal of Head Trauma Rehabilitation* 6: 1–10.

Prigatano, G. P. (1992). Personality disturbances associated with traumatic brain injury. *J. Consult. Clin. Psychol.* 60: 360–368.

Prigatano, G. P. (1995). 1994 Sheldon Berrol, MD, Senior Lectureship: the problem of lost normality after brain injury. *Journal of Head Trauma Rehabilitation* 10(3): 87–95.

Prigatano, G. P. (1996). Neuropsychological testing after traumatic brain injury. In R. W. Evans (ed), *Neurology and Trauma* (pp. 222–230). W. B. Saunders, Philadelphia.

Prigatano, G. P., Altman, I. M., and O'Brien, K. P. (1990). Behavioral limitations that brain injured patients tend to underestimate. *The Clinical Neuropsychologist* 4: 163–176.

Prigatano, G. P., and Ben-Yishay, Y. (1999). Psychotherapy and psychotherapeutic interventions in brain injury rehabilitation. In M. Rosenthal (ed), *Rehabilitation of the Adult and Child with Traumatic Brain Injury* (3rd ed). F. A. Davis, Philadelphia (in press).

Prigatano, G. P., and Henderson, S. (1997). Cognitive outcome after subarachnoid hemorrhage. In J. B. Bederson (ed), *Subarachnoid Hemorrhage: Pathophysiology and Management* (pp. 27–40). American Association of Neurological Surgeons, Park Ridge, Ill.

Prigatano, G. P., et al. (1986). *Neuropsychological Rehabilitation After Brain Injury.* Johns Hopkins University, Baltimore.

Prigatano, G. P., Stahl, M., Orr, W., and Zeiner H. (1982). Sleep and dreaming disturbances in closed head injury patients. *J. Neurol. Neurosurg. Psychiatry* 45: 78–80.

Prigatano, G. P., and Weinstein, E. A. (1996). Edwin A. Weinstein's contributions to neuropsychological rehabilitation. *Neuropsychological Rehabilitation* 6(4): 305–326.

Schafer, R. (1967). *Projective Testing and Psychoanalysis.* International Universities, New York.

Simon, H. A. (1967). Motivational and emotional controls of cognition. *Psychol. Rev.* 76: 29–39.

Weinstein, E. A., and Kahn, R. L. (1955). *Denial of Illness: Symbolic and Physiological Aspects.* Charles C Thomas, Springfield, Ill.

8

Neuropsychological Rehabilitation for Cognitive and Personality Disorders After Brain Injury

> ... I did not have to read books to know that the theme of life is conflict and pain.
>
> C. Chaplin, *Charles Chaplin: My Autobiography*, 1992, p. 210

In the late 1970s and early 1980s, postacute day-treatment rehabilitation programs were established to address the needs of patients with moderate to severe traumatic brain injury (TBI), (Ben-Yishay et al., 1982; Prigatano et al., 1986). Those programs often fostered a holistic approach as initially articulated by Goldstein (see Prigatano and Ben-Yishay, 1999). The influence of Luria's approach was also clear, particularly in Europe (Christensen and Caetano, 1996).

These programs made no claim that the underlying cognitive deficits of severely brain-injured young and middle-aged adults could be substantially reversed by neuropsychological rehabilitation. They did, however, foster the notion that patients might improve certain "generic" or broadly defined skills *and* that their psychosocial adjustment could be substantially helped. For example, many TBI patients showed apparent difficulties in "attention." This broad (and often poorly defined) set of skills might be improved so that residual capacities could be used more effectively. The basic attentional deficits, which were directly caused by a brain lesion, would most likely prove refractory to "attentional training." Skills, not capacities, were being "retrained."

It was argued that by teaching patients to use residual cognitive abilities, one might further help their psychosocial adjustment. In this regard, many postacute TBI patients appear socially isolated and some show enhanced behavioral disturbances with the passage of time (see Chapter 4). It was thought that working with these persons in intensive, day-treatment programs, which included individual and group cognitive exercises, could, in fact, improve patients' psychosocial adjustment.

In the late 1970s and early 1980s, Ben-Yishay and Diller conducted a number of workshops at New York University, Rusk Rehabilitation Institute. They showed videotapes of Israeli soldiers treated with such intensive, holistic approaches. Before-and-after videotapes of these patients' behaviors revealed drastic improvements that encouraged others to develop similar programs throughout the United States and abroad.

One such program began in February 1980 at Presbyterian Hospital in Oklahoma City (Prigatano et al., 1984; Prigatano et al., 1986). Working primarily with postacute TBI patients who demonstrated a variety of cognitive and personality deficits (presented in Chapters 5 and 6), it became clear that *more* than cognitive retraining was needed to help many of these patients. Dealing with these patients' residual disturbances in higher cerebral functioning required nothing less than psychotherapeutic interventions by persons knowledgeable about these patients' cognitive disturbances as well as their particular forms of psychological suffering. It also became clear that many of these postacute TBI patients showed little insight into their impairments, and there was a suspicion that their self-awareness was altered after their brain injuries. This important problem had to be approached via different treatment modalities.

Neuropsychological rehabilitation of postacute TBI patients who show moderate to severe cognitive and personality deficits appeared to require five interrelated activities. Those activities included: efforts at cognitive remediation or retraining; psychotherapy; the establishment of a therapeutic community or treatment milieu; protected work trials; and the active support, involvement, and education of family members (Prigatano, 1992, 1995b).

That program of care has been described earlier (Prigatano et al., 1986), but over the past several years, a series of observations regarding such a treatment program has become clearer. This chapter revisits briefly that postacute neuropsychological rehabilitation program and highlights some of its more important elements. A case example is used to demonstrate how such a program might work and how a given patient can be treated effectively in such a program.

Following that discussion, the problem of cognitive retraining is analyzed briefly. Later chapters detail the efficacy of cognitive retraining and thoughts concerning how this area might be expanded in the future. Chapter 9 specifically discusses in detail psychotherapeutic interventions after brain injury and highlights Principle 7. Chapter 10 discusses issues in working with the interdisciplinary team that attempt to conduct neuropsychological rehabilitation.

Components of a Holistic Neuropsychological Rehabilitation Program

As noted above, holistic neuropsychological rehabilitation consists of five interrelated activities: establishing a therapeutic milieu or community, cognitive rehabilitation or retraining, psychotherapy, the ongoing involvement and education of family members, and a protected work trial.

In the context of such a program of care, therapeutic activities include individual and group therapies aimed at restoring higher cerebral functioning and learning methods of adaptation and compensation. Patients and treatment team members meet regularly (preferably daily) to monitor the course of care and to manage the inevitable misunderstandings, disappointments, and conflicts (perceived and real) that personal needs stimulate. This program of care requires some "insulation" from other treatment or hospital activities so that a true therapeutic community can emerge. This therapeutic milieu, however, has limits. It is a time-limited, protected environment geared toward helping patients achieve a progressively higher level of independence and productivity. It is also aimed at improving their social skills so that they can maintain independence and productivity.

Immediately after brain injury, cognitive and personality deficits are often best revealed in complex, unstructured social situations. Thus, neuropsychological rehabilitation initially provides a semicomplex, structured social situation that progressively and deliberately moves to a more complex, less structured social situation to determine what patients can adapt to and handle.

The social environment can be either therapeutic or punitive. It is the responsibility of the clinical director and the rehabilitation team to foster the former and guard against the latter. Thus, they must begin by establishing a therapeutic milieu.

Establishing a Therapeutic Milieu

As described in Chapter 2, patients with acquired brain injury are often confused and frustrated. To work with them effectively, they must be placed in physical environment that helps reduce their confusion and frustration. This environment includes a designated space for them. It should be protective and foster a sense of security.

The environment also requires distinct social and psychological characteristics. It should be welcoming and encourage frank discussion about neuropsychological and related problems. It should anticipate many of the patients' needs. It should foster a sense of community and community responsibility. The brain dysfunctional patient who enters this program has certain responsibilities that need to be met in order to be maintained in the treatment program. In turn, the therapeutic community, including the rehabilitation therapists, have responsibilities to help the patient improve and adjust to the effects of their higher cerebral dysfunction so that they can, in fact, be maintained in this program of care.

Ultimately, the rehabilitation staff plays a key role in determining whether or not a true therapeutic community is established. Their challenge is to provide a combination of individual and group rehabilitation activities to a heterogeneous group of brain dysfunctional patients. They must provide this treatment in a supportive, cost-efficient, and effective manner. If they do so, this important element of neuropsychological rehabilitation will be established. If they fail to take these responsibilities seriously, this important and elusive aspect of neuropsychological rehabilitation will quickly erode.

When patients first enter a holistic rehabilitation program, they often recognize why other patients are present. Many are convinced, however, that they do not belong in such a setting. Involving them in a therapeutic day program, which includes group work, may help some of these patients to realize progressively their need to be in such a treatment center.

Quickly, many brain dysfunctional patients will experience what other patients report about their own injuries. As they listen to this feedback, they have an opportunity to get multiple perspectives on how brain injury may affect a person and that person's reaction to them. A therapeutic milieu provides an unusual opportunity for feedback that is seldom available in other settings. The feedback always must be given in a supportive but clear and concise manner.

In this regard, I have previously discussed the *sandwich* technique introduced to me by Dr. Ben-Yishay (Prigatano, 1989). While working with brain dysfunctional patients in small group activities, Dr. Ben-Yishay always alerts patients when he needs to bring up a difficult topic. He tells patients that he knows the topic will be difficult but hopes that the patients will consider his points. He then gives patients the news or feedback and quickly compliments them for listening. Alerting patients to forthcoming issues may make it easier for them to attend to problems. By concluding the discussion with a positive comment about their willingness to listen, Ben-Yishay helps patients to "swallow" difficult emotional sandwiches. This technique represents the essence of a milieu program. As previously discussed (Prigatano, 1989), therapists must have considerable skill to be able to deliver such information in a therapeutic rather than a punitive manner.

Cognitive Remediation or Retraining

Cognitive rehabilitation can be defined as a learning experience aimed at either restoring impaired higher cerebral functioning or improving performance in the "real world" using substitution or compensation techniques (Prigatano, 1995a). In the context of a holistic neuropsychological rehabilitation program, cognitive retraining occurs in small-group sessions as well as in individual sessions. Let us consider some of the activities and the underlying rationale.

Small-Group Cognitive Retraining Hour

When doing "mental work," brain dysfunctional patients often fatigue quickly (see Chapters 2, 4, 5, 6, and 7). Their speed of information processing is also often slow (Chapter 5). Small-group cognitive retraining activities often begin the rehabilitation day focusing on this problem. The activities are used to generate alertness or arousal and to be inherently interesting to the patients. These features are crucial for engaging patients in the rehabilitation process—the foundation of all neurorehabilitation.

During these tasks, patients begin to record and observe changes in their speed of processing. Such observations help reduce their "confusion" about why they need to participate in a rehabilitation program. As they begin to observe their behavior in a systematic way, patients may become more realistic about their potential strengths and limitations (i.e., their awareness increases).

If cognitive retraining is conducted in a large room with two or three patients and one therapist to a table (with perhaps three or four tables present), patients can observe their progress compared to others. They can learn to demonstrate their strengths and weaknesses in front of others. They begin to experience themselves as a part of a community. This time has proven immensely valuable, even if repetition exercises per se do not substantially improve cognitive function (Klonoff et al., 1989; Prigatano, 1995a; Prigatano, et al., 1996).

During these cognitive group exercises, therapists have an unusual opportunity to build a working or therapeutic alliance with patients. As I have noted, "the staff first monitors the patient's behavior and then has the patient monitor their performance on the same task. This allows the patients to see that staff is willing to expose their cognitive strengths and weaknesses" (Prigatano et al., 1986, p. 103). Frequently, however, even experienced, competent therapists fail to engage in this activity.

The reasons for this failure are complicated. At times staff may become weary of approaching patients in this manner. Yet I have repeatedly found that if therapists are willing to reveal their personal strengths and weaknesses and to embody the spirit of free dialogue about the nature of a difficulty, patients are more willing to engage in cognitive retraining tasks. If therapists fail to reveal themselves and only give feedback about patients' performances, their comments are often interpreted as intrusive. Patients too easily feel criticized within the context of cognitive retraining.

Cognitive Group Therapy

A second rehabilitation activity that focuses on cognitive deficits is Cognitive Group Therapy. During this time therapists work with patients to improve their communication skills, which are often compromised even when frank aphasia is absent (see Chapters 2 and 5). People who suffer brain injury during early childhood may have inordinate difficulties verbalizing ideas or feelings (Prigatano et al., 1993). Therefore, activities that encourage patients to practice speaking with one another within the context of a small group are imperative.

A variety of activities can be used. Having patients monitor the clarity of their own and others' verbal responses has repeatedly been demonstrated to be a useful technique in the rehabilitation process. Some patients can follow simple cuing techniques while others can monitor themselves when their communications become tangential, inappropriate, or unclear.

In addition to using this time to improve their communication skills, it is often helpful to have patients monitor their own progress throughout the course of neuropsychological rehabilitation. Incorporation of a "wall chart," as used in the program developed in Oklahoma City, can be especially helpful for this task (Fig. 8-1). Using this chart, therapists ask patients to describe their progress in rehabilitation. Their description is applied to the flow chart to help determine their actual stage in the rehabilitation process. This tool helps patients begin to verbalize whether they are actively or passively engaged in the rehabilitation process. It also gives them a chance to discuss difficulties with engagement in a nonthreatening manner.

This cognitive retraining activity also has multiple goals that are dealt with simultaneously: improving verbalization skills and identifying and labeling one's status and progress in rehabilitation. Catrambone (1995) emphasized the importance of verbal labels for individuals to learn subgoals instrumental for novel problem-solving. Although we had not initially conceptualized the techniques this way, patients' ability to verbalize their stage in the rehabilitation process in a clinical setting seems to help them achieve the goal of being actively involved in rehabilitation.

Individual (IZED) Cognitive Retraining

Much has been written about working with patients individually to improve or compensate for their specific cognitive deficits (Sohlberg and Mateer, 1989; Wilson, 1987, 1995). The need to make these interventions practical and to follow up patients over long periods of time to determine their efficacy cannot be overstated.

In the context of a holistic program, patients typically receive individual speech and language therapy, occupational therapy, and "specifically tailor-made" attempts at cognitive rehabilitation. During this time, patients are often taught a method for compensating for their memory deficits (Kime et al., 1996). Direct retraining of underlying cognitive impairments often helps build rapport with the therapist but has not proven to be especially helpful in reversing the underlying impairment (see Prigatano, 1995a). This problem is further discussed below.

Psychotherapy

The role of psychotherapy in the neuropsychological rehabilitation process has become progressively clear and established. After brain injury, patients ask, "Why did this happen to me? Will I be normal again? Is

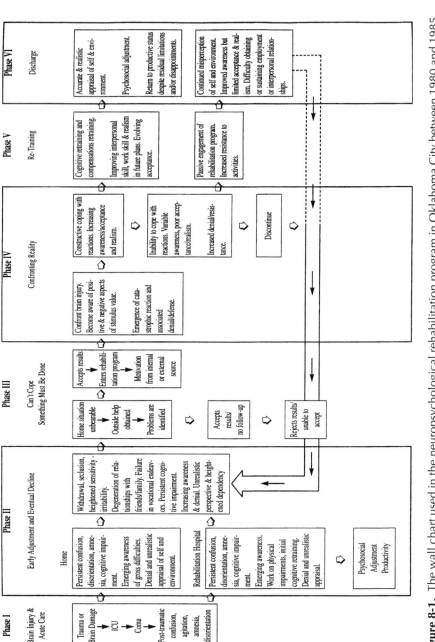

Figure 8-1. The wall chart used in the neuropsychological rehabilitation program in Oklahoma City between 1980 and 1985 (Prigatano et al., 1986).

life worth living after brain injury?" These questions (and their answers) are highly relevant to patients' attitudes toward rehabilitation. If psychotherapists can help patients to struggle with the problem of lost normality (Prigatano, 1995b; 1995c) and engage them in the rehabilitation process, such activities have a greater likelihood of assisting patients (Prigatano et al., 1994).

It must be emphasized, however, that there is nothing "magical" about psychotherapy. It consists of a dialogue between a patient and a therapist. Through this dialogue patients are helped to learn to behave in their own best self-interest. The process is highly individual. As discussed in the next chapter, however, guidelines are available to help facilitate this process.

Ultimately, neuropsychological rehabilitation or any form of training that attempts to return patients to work must deal with the patients' personal and emotional reactions to their impairment and its impact on their ability to work and be independent (Goldstein, 1942). Patients' negative affective reactions do not go away if they are ignored. They are present every time patients experience a failure or are reminded of functioning at a level lower than their previous status. These affective difficulties play a major role in whether patients will maintain a job or work at establishing interpersonal relationships.

In the context of a neuropsychological rehabilitation program, however, both individual and group methods of psychotherapy can be of considerable help to some patients. Previously (Prigatano et al., 1986; Chapter 5), I have attempted to outline the goals of psychotherapy and a strategy for approaching psychotherapy with people after brain injury. For the purposes of this chapter, a few points are restated.

Group psychotherapy can provide an opportunity for patients to hear how others experience their brain injury. This can provide the first step for reducing a patient's social isolation.

Group psychotherapy, however, does not progress on its own. Therapists must be able to direct the discussion in a practical manner that is to the point and that incorporates enough redundancy to overcome the memory difficulties common to this group of patients.

Introducing group psychotherapy to patients is an art. I often begin group psychotherapy by telling the patients that my colleagues have told me that I may be wasting my time working with them because four problems that they have can interfere with the effectiveness of individual and group psychotherapy. First, they have difficulties in remembering things and consequently would not recall what was discussed the previous day. Second, they often have problems with attention and concentration. Therefore, they may not listen to the discussion consistently. Third, they may not always grasp the point of what is being said and therefore may misperceive or misinterpret information stated during a group session. Finally, they have less control of their emotional reactions and therefore can overrespond to disturbing information both during a group session and at home.

Given that these four issues are, in fact, potential problems of TBI patients and others who suffer cerebral lesions, I would tell patients that we have a choice. Either we do not pursue group psychotherapy or we take steps to counteract these problems: First, we repeat each day what we discussed the previous day to compensate for memory problems. We will do this no matter how long it takes, even if it takes most of the group time. Second, if a person is clearly not attending to the discussion, the therapist will politely but regularly bring the person back into the group discussion. Third, each day we will attempt to restate comments to clarify any misunderstanding or confusion. Fourth, if a patient becomes emotionally upset we will not stop the group. The individual will be asked to sit quietly until the group has finished. In the rare instance that a patient becomes so upset that he or she wants to leave the room, the therapist will still maintain the group while another individual outside the group attends to the needs of the disturbed patient. I point out that if a person needs to leave the group several times, the therapist has most likely brought that individual into the group prematurely. Over the years, I have found this format to be very helpful.

The process of individual psychotherapy is more complicated and is discussed in the next chapter. At this point, it only need be emphasized that individual psychotherapy should attempt to enter patients' phenomenological field to help them better understand how their behavior is maladaptive and to use their present strengths to compensate for these maladaptive responses.

Family Involvement and Education

The importance of working with family members cannot be overemphasized. The initial contact with family members is important and can set the tone for the latter working relationship.

Family members are often interviewed with the patient during the first consultation. Both the patient's and family members' perceptions of "what is wrong" are requested and needed. Family members are asked to provide systematic information on how they believe the patient functions in various settings. Using the relative's version of the Patient Competency Rating Scale (PCRS) has been especially helpful in obtaining this information (Prigatano et al., 1986). Family members are given detailed information about the neuropsychological rehabilitation program and encouraged to spend a day (a least once a month) observing and participating in therapies. They are met weekly and sometimes several times a week depending on their needs. Issues concerning the patient's progress or lack of it are openly discussed with family members in both individual and group formats. A relatives' group is an essential treatment activity. When patients' family members stop coming to the relatives' group, it indicates that the family's needs are not being met.

During the course of the rehabilitation program, the staff formally rate their working alliance with both patient and family members, and the family members and patient are likewise asked to rate their working alliance with the staff. These ratings permit an ongoing dialogue about the status of the working alliance (see Prigatano et al., 1994 for details on rating the working alliance between patient and rehabilitation staff and between family members and the rehabilitation staff).

Some guidelines for establishing a good working relationship are as follows:

1. Listen carefully to the family member's perspective. Do not interrupt even if you disagree with part or all of their comments.
2. Approach family members (as well as patients) as consultants—not as people who have control over their decisions. Provide your perspective and rationale about what should be done but do not force it.
3. Be clear about expectations from patient and family members to maintain the patient in the rehabilitation program. Be careful, however, not to be punitive (i.e., do not discharge a patient needlessly because the patient or the family members have not met your expectations). Specific behavioral criteria for maintaining involvement in the program must be developed and communicated to patients and family members.
4. Have frequent discussions that include educational materials on what brain injury is, how higher cerebral functions are affected after brain injury, and what level of recovery can be expected.
5. Recognize that your job is to engage the family member in the therapeutic process.

Sometimes this final goal requires extra effort from the therapist. For example, family members may refuse to attend the relatives' group. Rather than accepting this refusal as the family's unwillingness to become involved, the therapist may need to meet with the family members individually before eventually bringing them into the group. Sometimes family members resist coming for a variety of reasons. In such cases, the therapist must take extra steps to remain in contact with the family member. For example, I find it useful to identify a time, even late in the afternoon, when the family member can be phoned to review progress and concerns about the patient. When family members see that therapists are willing to work beyond a 40-hour week to help the patient, it helps establish a therapeutic alliance.

The Protected Work Trial

Making work a part of rehabilitation is crucial for two reasons. First, how individuals approach work and what they can do outside of rehabilitation activities can be observed. Second, difficulties at work become important areas of rehabilitation focus. That is, if a person has trouble with speed of information processing or with solving a task cognitively, the issue could be addressed within the context of cognitive rehabilitation. If a person is consistently late or has difficulties with inappropriate social behavior, the issue can be focused on during a number of individual and group-oriented therapies. The integration of work as a part of the treatment day provides a more dynamic, real-world sample of patients' behaviors. Rehabilitation becomes a true adjunct, not the center, of a person's existence. The goal is to help patients become independent and productive, and work trials allow the unique opportunity to accomplish these goals.

Within this context, the concept of a *protected work trial* emerged. A protected work trial is defined as a true work experience in which individuals have definite responsibilities to meet but failure to do so does not automatically lead to reprimands or dismissal. Rather, individuals are protected by their status as patients and their involvement in the rehabilitation program. Patients are then helped via rehabilitation activities to meet the demands of the job and to improve behavior that disrupts their performance. Because these work trials are protected, they are frequently voluntary positions.

Patients' receiving payment during their protected work trial has advantages and disadvantages. In my opinion, however, voluntary work suits this model best. Patients give their time and effort to obtain honest feedback and educational experiences that help them to correct disruptive behaviors. This work trial is a *part* of but not the end product of rehabilitation.

Work trials must be practical. They need to be close to the rehabilitation setting so that therapists have frequent contact with patients in their work environment. Therapists doing the actual therapy need to be the individuals who visit the actual job site and work with patients' voluntary supervisor and others. Having a vocational rehabilitation counselor or a job coach do this work is impractical. Therapists who know the details of the patient's higher cerebral deficits and their emotional reactions to frustrations are the individuals who need to be involved in managing patients' work activities. This first-hand information is invaluable when attempting to influence patients positively to improve their chances of regaining independence.

A key element in this process is the extensive evaluation of patients at work. Several years ago my colleagues and I in Oklahoma City developed a questionnaire to evaluate the work trial (Prigatano et al., 1986). The questionnaire includes a number of questions concerning the patient's behavior: promptness, efficiency at work, basic abilities to follow instructions, and so on. The final question is "If a job opening developed, would you hire this individual for a paid position given his or her present performance?"

Many supervisors made glowing comments about the patient's behavior, but then indicated they would not hire the patient. When asked why, the supervisors gave more accurate descriptions of the patients. They might, for example, focus on the patient's extreme slowness, difficulty in grasping concepts, inappropriate behaviors, taking frequent breaks, or making disruptive comments. Or patients might not be malleable or easy to influence and consequently the supervisors would not want them as employees. Answers to this simple but important question were discussed with the patient and work supervisor, again in the spirit of honest dialogue. This piece of information was invaluable in helping patients to understand the level of work responsibilities they could perform.

An "Ideal" Scenario for the Holistic Neuropsychological Rehabilitation of Young Brain-Injured Adults

The preceding sections of this chapter outlined the essential components of a holistic neuropsychological rehabilitation program. Such a program attempts to focus on patients' higher cerebral deficits and their personal reactions to those deficits. It may be useful, however, to describe in more practical terms a typical patient involved with this type of the treatment on a given day. Table 8-1 describes the day-treatment program of the Adult Day Hospital for Neurological Rehabilitation (ADHNR) at the Barrow Neurological Institute, St. Joseph's Hospital and Medical Center in Phoenix, Arizona, as it was practiced in 1993 when I served as Clinical Director.

A hypothetical patient (Tommy) and how he is treated throughout the course of a rehabilitation day are described. One or two scenarios that typically emerge in the treatment of such patients and how they should be handled are also presented. How Tommy's parents should be worked with and approached within the context of this work is also described.

Entering the Program

Tommy has undergone a neuropsychological evaluation and was determined to have memory and speed of information processing deficits associated with a moderate or severe TBI. He lacks insight into his residual disturbances but has failed to return to school or work. He has tried a number of jobs but is "unhappy" with each of them. It is now 3.5 years since his injury. He has undergone multiple forms of inpatient and outpatient therapies but is "lost." His parents recognize that some effort is still needed to assist him.

Tommy passively agrees to a neuropsychologically oriented rehabili-

Table 8-1. Typical weekly work reentry program

	Monday	Tuesday	Wednesday	Thursday	Friday
08:15–08:55	Cognitive retraining	Cognitive retraining	Cognitive retraining	Cognitive retraining	Work trial (optional)
09:00–09:40	Individual therapies	Individual therapies	Individual therapies	Individual therapies	
09:40–09:50	Break	Break	Break	Break	
09:50–10:25	Individual/group	Individual/group	Individual/group	Individual/group	
10:30–11:10	Cognitive group	Cognitive group	Cognitive group	Cognitive group	
11:15–11:45	Group psychotherapy	Group psychotherapy	Group psychotherapy	Group psychotherapy	
11:45–12:00	Milieu	Milieu	Milieu	Milieu	
12:00–01:00	Lunch	Lunch	Lunch	Lunch	
01:00–05:00	Work trial	Work trial	Work trial	Work trial	Work trial (optional)
01:45–02:45		Relatives' group			
03:30–04:30	Staff meeting	Staff meeting	Staff meeting	Staff meeting	
05:00–06:00		Relatives' group			

During the first week of the work trial, patients will work 2 hours per day and increase to 3 to 4 hours during Week Two if they can handle it. By Week Three, the goal is to have patients working 3 to 4 hours four days a week, depending on the needs of the work supervisor and patient. (Generally, months 3 through 6 will be designated for less supervised activities.)

From Prigatano (1988). With permission from Barrow Neurological Institute.

tation consultation. The first step is not to accept him too quickly into the rehabilitation program. A cautious attitude is best taken about whether rehabilitation can help him. Discussions with Tommy and his parents summarize the clinical experiences in working with persons with brain injuries and published data concerning the process and outcome of such rehabilitation efforts. Discussions emphasize that only 50% of the people accepted into this form of care return to gainful employment. That the level of recovery and the ultimate rate for job placement are often less than both patient and family desire is discussed at a time that does not overwhelm Tommy or his parents.

Before entering the rehabilitation program, Tommy and his parents are asked to consider the decision for at least 2 weeks. That time and energy are required on the part of patient, family, and the rehabilitation staff is stressed. They are also advised to proceed cautiously given the cost of the venture.

Beginning the Program

After Tommy and his parents read the neuropsychological report, visit the rehabilitation program, talk with other parents (and family members), and discuss whether they wish to pursue this course, Tommy begins the program. On his first day of treatment, Tommy is welcomed and further oriented to the program. He is introduced to other patients, all of whom wear a name tag to help him remember their names. The name tags are the first tangible evidence that a therapeutic community exists and is willing to take steps to help individuals cope with their memory problems.

Tommy begins the cognitive retraining hour during this first day. For the first one or two days, he listens as others respond to the queries: What is the name of this hour? *Cognitive Retraining.* What is the purpose? *To try to improve speed of information processing or thinking.* Why do we bother to do this activity? *Because after brain injury our thinking and speed of problem solving are slower.*

Tommy begins one of the many tasks. He starts at a level that is moderately challenging but that does not overwhelm him. This level must be predetermined and anticipated by the treatment team. For several weeks Tommy works at these tasks, which are graded according to level of difficulty. He records his responses, begins to observe his performances, and plots a learning curve. The idea of taking steps to compensate for deficits that do not improve with time and practice is gently introduced. Tommy begins to see how he is "doing" compared to other patients who are sitting at the same rehabilitation training table. Tommy begins to see that there are some things he can do better than others and other things that he does more poorly. Slowly, he becomes aware of his strengths and limitations. Because of the pacing of the program, this realization does not overwhelm him; it simply reflects reality.

After a time, the therapist gives Tommy a stopwatch and asks him to monitor his (i.e., the therapist's) performance on various tasks that Tommy has been practicing. Rather than demonstrating that the therapist can perform these tasks better than Tommy, the goal is for Tommy to have an opportunity to see how a person who has not suffered a brain injury performs.

Tommy may do better than the therapist on some tasks and the therapist may do better than Tommy on others. This comparison is an extremely important point. Brain injury does not reduce all problem-solving skills. Thus, therapists must have the courage and clinical sensitivity to demonstrate their own cognitive limitations within the context of this training time. Their willingness to be vulnerable gives Tommy the courage to be honest about his own strengths and limitations. If therapists cannot tolerate revealing their own limitations, patients will be uncomfortable discussing theirs.

Patients may also realize that the therapist performs some tasks much more efficiently than they do despite their intensive practice. Thus, the comparison opens the door for frank discussions about the practical utility of compensatory strategies in rehabilitation. It also provides an opportunity to establish a true therapeutic alliance.

Although they may agree with this concept in principle, many therapists often resist its application. They may be embarrassed if patients perform some tasks better than they do. Yet, if therapists cannot approach the task in this manner, they will fail to establish a true therapeutic environment.

Cognitive Group and Wall Chart

Tommy completes his cognitive retraining hour and moves on to the cognitive group. During this time the tasks are varied. Patients are asked to list their strengths and weaknesses and give feedback to others concerning theirs. They may be asked to condense information from a message and present it in a few words in the form of a telegram.

Tommy is asked to monitor his progress on a wall chart like the one discussed earlier. Tommy can identify that he is in the early stages of his rehabilitation and just beginning to be involved in the therapeutic tasks. Other patients further along in the process discuss their progress or lack of progress with Tommy. During this time, Tommy begins to experience the importance of communicating his ideas as clearly and concisely as possible.

The problem of tangentiality may now reveal itself. Tommy is asked to explain what brought him to the rehabilitation program. He answers as follows:

> I suffered a head injury when I got into a wreck when driving my father's car from Norman, Oklahoma, to Oklahoma City. The car that

I was driving was a '55 Chevy. My father and I really liked that Chevy. We spent a lot of time working on it. We repainted it, we rebuilt the engine, we got new hubcaps, and it was in really mint condition. I really miss that car. My aunt, however, has a Chevy like it although it is not in as good condition. She lives in Wisconsin. I go up to Wisconsin during the summer months and at times work with the animals. There is one particular animal up there, a prize bull, that I enjoy working with.

At this point, the therapist interrupts Tommy and politely states that he had asked Tommy to describe what had brought him to the rehabilitation program and that while Tommy had begun to answer he had ended up talking about bulls in Wisconsin. At that point, Tommy may respond, "Yes, I know that, but I am getting to it." The therapist politely replies that it is difficult to follow Tommy's answer and that many people would tire trying to follow the trend of his thoughts. The therapist turns toward other patients and asks if they could follow Tommy or if it appeared that he was off the point. Often, patients will respond that he was doing a fine job and that the therapist was overstating Tommy's problems. At this point, the therapist would have to involve Tommy and the other patients in the task of monitoring Tommy's verbalizations to determine when he gets off the point.

Dr. Ben-Yishay is a master of this strategy. He often asks one patient to monitor "Tommy" and when Tommy starts to drift from the point, to raise one finger politely. Another patient is asked to monitor the patient who was monitoring Tommy, and a third patient monitors the other two while the therapist monitors all of them. Cognitive group work does not mean working with one patient while other patients observe. It means engaging all patients in a cognitive task that involves communication and thinking processes. In this context, patients start to take the need to help one another seriously and, particularly, the need to help Tommy recognize when he is getting off track.

After these forms of small-group cognitively oriented therapies, Tommy works in a variety of practical therapies that may include physical therapy, occupational therapy, individualized cognitive retraining, or individual psychotherapy.

Group Psychotherapy

Tommy next enters group psychotherapy. Here again he is asked to identify the time (i.e., *Group Psychotherapy*). Someone then asks, "What is the purpose of Group Psychotherapy?" *To discuss one's feelings.* The therapist asks, "Why do we bother to discuss feelings?" *How we feel partially determines how we act and how we act partially determines how people react to us.*

The therapist might say that many people with a brain injury complain that others do not treat them properly but that the brain-injured individuals may not always realize how they contribute to peoples' reactions to them. A variety of topics could be discussed, many of which have been described elsewhere (Prigatano et al., 1986). During this time, Tommy and others begin to discuss their feelings about their brain injury, about being in a rehabilitation program, about the usefulness of work trials, about the reaction of their parents to their brain injury, and many related topics. After group psychotherapy, Tommy proceeds to milieu (Table 8-1).

Milieu

As milieu begins, patients are again asked to name the hour. They are then asked the purpose of milieu, and the answer is to talk about the business of the day in a family manner. The clinical director then asks, "What business do we have today?"

Typically, administrative issues are discussed, but eventually patients talk about their progress in therapy. They discuss what had gone well and what had not gone so well during the day. Both therapists and patients are accountable for how the treatment day went, another point extremely important for establishing a therapeutic alliance. On a "good" day, milieu is often happy and pleasant. On a "bad" day, it can become very tense. Milieu is perhaps the most important time of the treatment day. A typical scenario associated with a bad day follows.

After a month and a half of this form of rehabilitation, Tommy gets very upset with how the cognitive retraining time has gone. One morning he comes in very upset, slams his books and papers on the desk, insults the therapist doing the work, and states that he is tired of this kind of treatment. This point is a crucial crossroads in working with Tommy. If the therapist avoids or does not formally recognize his outburst, Tommy's behavior will continue. If the therapist overresponds and is punitive, Tommy may become more out of control or withdraw from this type of treatment.

Tommy's therapist, however, is skilled and tells Tommy that he sees that Tommy is upset. The therapist indicates that his problem will be discussed during milieu and, if possible, during group psychotherapy. Tommy blurts out that he wants to discuss the problem *now* because he has a memory problem, as the therapist has so often reminded him! Tommy is so upset that he can proceed no further without discussing the issue immediately. The therapist responds that he understands that Tommy has a memory problem and promises that if Tommy forgets to raise the issue in milieu, he will do so. Tommy accepts the therapist's proposal although he is still angry and tension fills the room.

The therapists' capacity and that of the other brain dysfunctional patients to work under tension are a crucial component of daily life. In this way the therapeutic milieu mirrors real-life experiences. At times we all must work under tension or uncomfortable circumstances and cannot leave our worksite because we are unhappy.

The therapist also asked Tommy to stay in the room and did not excuse him. Time-out procedures are not especially helpful when the goal is to return patients to a higher level of social integration. For more severely brain-injured patients, time-out procedures may be useful (Wood, 1987). However, they do not have a reasonable place at this level of neuropsychologically oriented rehabilitation.

So Tommy goes through the other therapy hours. At milieu the therapist begins by stating that he has something to bring up about Tommy that is difficult to discuss. The therapist asks Tommy if he would be kind enough to listen to the feedback that he is going to give Tommy and begins by saying that it was a difficult morning and Tommy became upset. At this point, Tommy explodes with another angry outburst. He states that the therapist is nagging him and cannot drop an issue that is now 2 or 3 hours old.

The therapist is aided by the clinical director, who states that he recognizes that Tommy may not wish to discuss this topic today—all of us have times when we are not ready to discuss an important issue. The clinical director makes it clear that if Tommy does not wish to discuss these issues today, they can be dropped. Tomorrow, however, the clinical director will return and ask Tommy to discuss what happened. This general attitude of allowing Tommy to control when he will discuss a problem but making it clear that ultimately the problem *will* be discussed is an important feature of milieu that teaches patients social responsibility.

Along the same line, therapists sometimes make a mistake and must face the consequences of their mistakes within the context of milieu. Many therapists dread such a scenario, a powerful example of which is discussed in Chapter 10.

The Work Trial

After being involved in the treatment program for 2 months and doing reasonably well, Tommy attempts a work trial. His progress is monitored and feedback is given to the therapists. Difficulties such as compensating for memory problems are integrated into the treatment day. Eventually, Tommy begins to discuss with other patients in group psychotherapy his personal reactions to working at a level less demanding than in the past. He also discusses working in a job with less status and financial reward than before his injury. In the context of these real-world experiences, patients and staff form a clearer view of how brain injury affects an individual and what steps are necessary to compensate for those problems.

Candidates for a Holistic Neuropsychological Rehabilitation Program

Although it may seem paradoxical, not all patients need the type of program outlined above. This program is geared toward individuals who are at the postacute stage following their brain injury and demonstrate moderate to moderately severe cognitive and personality deficits. These patients must have enough resources, however, to return to a productive lifestyle. A productive lifestyle, however, does not always mean gainful employment.

Patients with mild injuries may be worked with in a more parsimonious and less demanding fashion. This text does not discuss this patient population and their treatment needs. Also, patients who are very severely injured and who do not have adequate cognitive and personality resources to return to a productive lifestyle might be treated with alternative forms of care. This book does not address this problem.

The Problem of Cognitive Rehabilitation

Teaching brain dysfunctional patients how to "remediate" or overcome a cognitive deficit is extremely problematic (Ben-Yishay et al., 1982). Because we often do not know the exact nature of the cognitive deficit or how higher cerebral functions are normally organized, little is actually known about how to "retrain" the person properly (i.e., Principle 6). Yet, some guidelines can be offered.

In this chapter, we have described a holistic approach that considers the entire individual when attempting cognitive retraining. More specific things can be said about the cognitive retraining process. In this process, it becomes extremely important that therapists repeatedly try to refine their understanding of the exact nature of the underlying cognitive deficit. This task is not easy. What appears to be a problem of attention (Ponsford and Kinsella, 1988) may actually turn out to be a problem of speed of information processing (Ponsford and Kinsella, 1992). Repeated observations of the patients in testing as well as in unstructured environments may prove useful in this regard. Second, it is important to determine what variables actually influence the functional deficit. Technically, this task is defined as being able to determine the function rule of a higher cerebral function (see Chapter 13). Clinically, the task often translates into being able to determine what components of a cognitive process seem to be specifically affected. For example, is the problem reading per se or the visual perception of letter characters? Is it a problem in pronouncing vowel or consonant sounds? Is it a problem in actually grasping the meaning of single words or phrases? Until we understand what the underlying functional component deficits are, it is extremely difficult, if not impossible, to retrain the individual.

Third, it is important to determine whether there is evidence that the brain of a given patient has the potential for cortical plasticity for the function being retrained. This remains a major area of concern to the field.

Finally, we must have at our disposal a technology for delivering retraining activities in a manner that is cost efficient and effective.

Merzenich and colleagues (1996) and Tallal and colleagues (1996) provided an interesting prototype of how technology can be used with children with languaged-based learning impairments. The function that seemed to be disturbed was identified as the encoding of phonemic aspects of sound. The children were then given auditory stimuli in a manner that required finer and finer temporal discriminations. The tasks were engaging to the children rather than frustrating. The interventions produced greater improvements in different speech and language functions than traditional speech and language therapies.

Summary and Conclusions

This chapter gives an overview of the essential ingredients of holistic neuropsychological rehabilitation programs that have evolved from practice over the past 20 years. Issues important to working with patients and staff are briefly described. The various therapeutic activities focus on both cognitive and personality disturbances. A therapeutic milieu is established when individuals begin to interact with others about the impact of their brain injury on their daily functioning. Patients are given a protected work-trial experience in which they can experience the types of problems they may encounter in competitive employment or a long-term voluntary position.

The principles that guide this work are important. Disturbances in higher cerebral functioning have inevitable psychosocial consequences. Thus, neuropsychological rehabilitation must aim not only at restoration of higher cerebral function but at the management of those disturbances in interpersonal situations.

Guidelines for cognitive retraining can be broadly specified, but little is known about how to retrain systematically a person who has cognitive deficits because the nature of higher cerebral functions has never been adequately defined (Principle 6). This chapter, however, provides broad guidelines for dealing with cognitive deficits but not a microscopic analysis of how patients should be taught specific tasks. Other materials and texts address this issue (Berg, et al., 1991; Luria, 1948/1963; Luria, et al., 1959; Luria, 1972; Milders, et al., 1995; Sohlberg and Mateer, 1989; Wilson, 1987; Ben-Yishay, et al., 1978, 1979, 1980, 1981, 1982, 1983; Prigatano, et al., 1986; von Cramon, et al., 1992).

Finally, guidelines can be developed to help patients adjust to significant changes and loss after their brain injury (Prigatano, 1994). The process, however, is personal and individual. Literature describes the process as the "hero's journey." When psychologists or psychiatrists attempt to help individuals with this path after brain injury, it is referred to as psychotherapy (Boss, 1983).

We now turn to the important topic of providing psychotherapeutic interventions for brain-injured patients and their families. Before doing so, however, the initial quote that introduces this chapter should be recalled. Charlie Chaplin, the accomplished actor and film director, noted in reflecting on his life that he did not have to read books to know that life was filled with conflict and pain. Conflict and pain are present before and after brain injury. After brain injury, however, individuals have fewer cognitive and personality resources for dealing with the conflict and pain. The entire scope of neuropsychological rehabilitation is intended to help these persons grasp this reality. In particular, psychotherapy is geared toward helping individuals make a personal adjustment to this reality.

References

Ben-Yishay, Y. Working approaches to remediation of cognitive deficits in brain damage. New York University Rehabilitation Monographs: No. 59 (1978); No. 60 (1979), No. 61 (1980), No. 62 (1981), No. 64 (1982), No. 66 (1983).

Ben-Yishay, Y., Rattok, J., Ross, B., Lakin, P., Silver, S., Thomas, L. and Diller, L. (1982). A rehabilitation-relevant system for cognitive, interpersonal and vocational rehabilitation of traumatically head injured persons. In *Rehabilitation Monograph No. 64: Working Approaches to Remediation of Cognitive Deficits in Brain Damaged Persons* (pp. 1–15). New York University Medical Center Institute of Rehabilitation Medicine, New York.

Berg, I. J., Koning-Haanstra, M., and Deelman, B. G. (1991). Long-term effects of memory rehabilitation: A controlled study. *Neuropsychological Rehabilitation* 1(2): 97–111.

Boss, M. (1983). *Existential Foundations of Medicine and Psychology*. Jason Arson, New York.

Catrambone, R. (1995). Aiding subgoal learning: effects on transfer. *Journal of Educational Psychology* 87(1): 5–17.

Chaplin, C. (1992). *Charles Chaplin: My Autobiography*. Penguin Books, New York.

Christensen, A-L and Caetano, C. (1996). Alexander Romanovich Luria (1902–1977): contributions to neuropsychological rehabilitation. *Neuropsychological Rehabilitation*, 6(4): 279–303.

Goldstein, K. (1942). *Aftereffects of Brain Injury in War*. Grune and Stratton, New York.

Kime, S. K., Lamb, D. G., and Wilson, B. A. (1996). Use of a comprehensive programme of external cueing to enhance procedural memory in a patient with dense amnesia. *Brain Injury* 10(1): 17–25.

Klonoff, P. S., O'Brien, K. P., Prigatano, G. P., Chiapello, D. A., Cunningham,

M., and Shepherd, J. (1989). Cognitive retraining after traumatic brain injury and its role in facilitating awareness. *Journal of Head Trauma Rehabilitation* 4(3): 37–45.

Luria, A. R. (1948/1963). *Restoration of Function after Brain Injury Trauma* (in Russian). Academy of Medical Science, Moscow (Pergamon, London, 1963).

Luria, A. R., Naydin, V. L., Tsvetkova, L. S., and Vinarskaya, E. N. (1969). Restoration of higher cortical function following local brain damage. In P. J. Vinken and G. W. Bruyn (ed), *Handbook of Clinical Neurology*: Vol. 3. *Disorders of Higher Nervous Activity* (pp. 431–433). North-Holland, Amsterdam.

Luria, A. R. (1972). *The Man with the Shattered World*. Basic Books, New York.

Merzenich, M. M., Jenkins, W. M., Johnston, P., Schreiner, C., Miller, S. L., Tallal, P. (1996). Temporal processing deficits of language-learning impaired children ameliorated by training: *Science* 271: 77–80.

Milders, M. V., Berg, I. J., and Deelman, B. G. (1995). Four-year follow-up of a controlled memory training study in closed head injured patients. *Neuropsychological Rehabilitation* 5(3): 223–238.

Ponsford, J. and Kinsella, G. (1988). Evaluation of a remedial program for attentional deficits following closed-head injury. *J. Clin. Exp. Neuropsychol.* 10(6): 693–708.

Ponsford, J. and Kinsella, G (1992). Attentional deficits following closed-head injury. *J. Clin. Exp. Neuropsychol.* 14(5): 822–38.

Prigatano, G. P. (1989). Bring it up in milieu: toward effective traumatic brain injury rehabilitation interaction. *Rehabilitation Psychology* 34(2), 135–144.

Prigatano, G. P. (1992). Neuropsychological rehabilitation and the problem of altered self-awareness. In N. von Steinbuchel, D. Y. von Cramon, and E. Pöppel (eds), *Neuropsychological Rehabilitation* (pp. 55–65). Springer-Verlag, New York.

Prigatano, G. P. (1994). Individuality, lesion location and psychotherapy after brain injury. In A-L. Christensen and B. Uzzell (eds), *Brain Injury and Neuropsychological Rehabilitation: International Perspective* (pp. 173–199). Lawrence Erlbaum, Hillsdale, NJ.

Prigatano, G. P. (1995a). The current status of cognitive rehabilitation: where we are, where we need to be. Paper presented at a meeting on the Links Between Cognitive Science, Education and Cognitive Rehabilitation, Eugene, Oregon: James S. McDonnell Foundation.

Prigatano, G. P. (1995b). 1994 Sheldon Berrol, MD, Senior Lectureship: The problem of lost normality after brain injury. *Journal of Head Trauma Rehabilitation* 10(3): 87–95.

Prigatano, G. P. (1995c). Strengths and limitations of psychotherapy after brain injury. *Advances in Medical Psychotherapy* 8: 23–34.

Prigatano, G. P. and Ben-Yishay (1999). Psychotherapy and psychotherapeutic interventions in brain injury rehabilitation. In M. Rosenthal (ed), *Rehabilitation of the Adult and Child with Traumatic Brain Injury* (3rd ed). F. A. Davis, Philadelphia.

Prigatano, G. P., Fordyce, D. J., Zeiner, H. K., Roueche, J. R., Pepping, M., and

Wood, B. (1984). Neuropsychological rehabilitation after closed head injury in young adults. *J. Neurol. Neurosurg. Psychiatry* 47: 505–513.

Prigatano, G. P., Glisky, E., and Klonoff, P. (1996). Cognitive rehabilitation after traumatic brain injury. In P. W. Corrigan and S. C. Yudofsky (eds), *Cognitive Rehabilitation of Neuropsychiatric Disorders*, pp. 223–242.

Prigatano, G. P., Klonoff, P. S., O'Brien, K. P., Altman, I., Amin, K., Chiapello, D. A., Shepherd, J., Cunningham, M., and Mora, M. (1994). Productivity after neuropsychologically oriented, milieu rehabilitation. *Journal of Head Trauma Rehabilitation* 9(1): 91–102.

Prigatano, G. P., O'Brien, K. P., and Klonoff, P. W. (1993). Neuropsychological rehabilitation of young adults who suffered brain injury in childhood: clinical observations. *Neuropsychological Rehabilitation* 3(4), 411–412.

Prigatano, G. P., et al. (1986). *Neuropsychological Rehabilitation after Brain Injury*. Oxford University Press, New York.

Sohlberg, M. M., and Mateer, C. (1989). *Introduction to Cognitive Rehabilitation: Theory and Practice*. Guilford, New York.

Tallal, P., Miller, S. L., Bedi, G., Byma, G., Wang, X., Nagarajan, S. S., et al. (1996). Language comprehension in language-learning impaired children improved with acoustically modified speech. *Science* 271: 81–84.

von Cramon, D. Y., Matthes-von Cramon, G., and Mai, N. (1992). The influence of a cognitive remediation programme on associated behavioural disturbances in patients with frontal lobe dysfunction. In N. von Steinbüchel, D. Y. von Cramon, and E. Pöppel (eds), *Neuropsychological Rehabilitation* (pp. 203–214). Springer-Verlag, Berlin.

Wilson, B. A. (1987). *Rehabilitation of Memory*, Guilford, New York.

Wilson, B. A. (1995). Management and remediation of memory problems in brain-injured adults. In A. D. Baddeley, B. A. Wilson, and F. N. Watts (eds), *Handbook of Memory Disorders* (pp. 451–479). John Wiley, Chichester, England.

Wood, R. L. (1987). *Brain Injury Rehabilitation: A Neurobehavioural Approach*. Croom-Helm, London.

9

Psychotherapeutic Intervention with Patients and Family Members

> Three years after the accident psychotherapy was attempted in a psychiatric clinic nearby. Jack's emotional problems were obvious; he was given opportunity to air his resentment and feelings of failure. Therapy did not prove a great success, due to difficulties commonly encountered with children with organic involvement.
>
> E. M. Taylor, *Psychological Appraisal of Children with Cerebral Deficits*, 1971, p. 109

> In our contacts with these families of head injured patients, however, we found relatively negligible movement past denial into anger, bargaining, or mourning losses, even when trained counseling help was available and even when families were engaged in family or group counseling processes. This very persistent family denial was manifested in several trends . . .
>
> (M. Romano, "Family response to traumatic head injury," 1974, pp. 1–2)

Psychotherapy can be one of the most practical types of assistance to offer another human being, or it can be an incredible waste of time, energy, and money. In some cases, it can even affect a patient negatively (Mohr, 1995); in others, it can produce modest to significant benefits. In the context of this book and a previous one (Prigatano, et al., 1986), I have argued that psychotherapy can be a useful component of neuropsychological rehabilitation for *some* patients after brain injury (i.e., Principle 7). The purpose of this chapter is to develop this theme more fully and to discuss my own interpretation of approaches that have been useful in this work. This chapter also describes how and why psychotherapy has emerged as a potentially useful treatment in the rehabilitation of brain-injured patients. The essential ingredients of psychotherapy and various forms of psychotherapeutic interventions are considered. These observations are related specifically to the problem of lost normality after brain injury.

Psychotherapy and Psychotherapeutic Interventions After Brain Injury

Brain damage does not produce only neurological deficits. It can produce a profound state of personal loss, mental confusion, and associated frustration. Patients, sooner or later, experience failures and losses and may or may not understand why. Certainly, the degree and type of "mental confusion" that patients experience vary with the location and nature of the brain insult (Chapters 2 and 5). Patients' understanding is also influenced by their stage of development when the brain injury occurs (Birch, 1964) (see Chapter 7). Finally, patients' social milieu and their personal interpretation of their failures and losses contribute greatly to their symptom picture and how they attempt to deal with their frustrations (Prigatano and Weinstein, 1996).

During the training of clinical neuropsychologists, little, if any, attention is placed on how to help patients with this more personal side of brain damage. However, the broad field of psychotherapy and psychotherapeutic interventions based on various models of psychotherapy can help patients in their personal adjustment. This help can be an important component of patients' neuropsychological rehabilitation.

Despite their technical knowledge about brain-behavior relationships, clinical neuropsychologists are often ineffective as psychotherapists if they cannot apply their insights in a clinically sensible manner. They must have a realistic view of the patient and what they have to offer the patient.

Clinical Sensibility in Psychotherapy After Brain Injury

Years ago Schafer (1967) described the capacity of *clinical sensibility*. It is worthwhile to consider what Schafer (1967) meant by this term and how it applies to the practice of psychotherapy.

Clinical sensibility includes an unobtrusive, empowering recognition of the tragic in life—the life of nonpatients too, the life of the clinician too. This sense of tragic implies that psychic development and organization inevitably have their arduous, painful, and self-limiting aspects; that conflict and subjective distress per se are not pathology, and naming them is not name-calling; that every adaptation has its price and leads into new areas of conflict; that many important experiences are inexpressible or, at best, expressible only indirectly and approximately; and that, as regards therapy and testing, the basic objective is not to unmask each patient or to dispose of him with diagnostic or psychodynamic labels, but to see how, and at what cost, he is trying to make the best of a bad internal situation—and is perhaps compelled to make the worst of a not-necessarily-so-bad external situation. The tragic sense is not despondent, inert, or self-pitying; it does not preclude zest

and humor, and it certainly enhances the observer's interest and ob-
jectivity. (Schafer, 1967, p. 3)

As Schafer (1967) notes, sensible clinicians can recognize the tragic in life
and are not overwhelmed by it. Sensible clinicians attempt to describe
and diagnose, not to "dispose" of the patient, but to help clarify what
is "wrong" and how the patient is attempting to cope. Sensible clinicians
are interested but objective in their description of patients and approaches to treatment.

This perspective takes time to develop and is especially relevant for
clinical neuropsychologists attempting psychotherapy with brain dysfunctional individuals. For years, however, skepticism concerning the
usefulness of psychotherapy, both before and after brain injury, has been
expressed. Goldstein and Luria did not refer to psychotherapy when they
described the rehabilitation of patients with higher cerebral disturbances.

Why then has psychotherapy slowly emerged as an important service
for brain-injured people?

The Emerging Role of Psychotherapy in Rehabilitation After Brain Injury

The development of postacute versus acute brain injury rehabilitation
programs greatly fostered the development of psychotherapy as a potentially useful service. When brain dysfunctional patients are seen soon
after injury, their physical needs clearly overshadow their psychological
needs (Prigatano, et al., 1997). During the early phases after brain injury,
the therapist and family understandably exert considerable effort to
teach patients to walk, to feed themselves, to dress, to communicate, and
to establish basic behaviors necessary for survival and safety. At that
point, many patients and families are not ready to consider the long-
term personal impact of disturbances in higher cerebral functioning.

Only when patients begin to struggle with the consequences of these
disturbances does the potential role of psychotherapy begin to emerge.
As patients start to experience repeated failures at work and/or in interpersonal relationships (but cannot understand why), the potential role
of psychotherapy comes into focus. Only when family members start to
experience anger and resentment toward the patient do they consider
the possibility that their personal needs have been neglected. When the
patient and family begin to consider the meaning of the brain injury as
it impacts both their present life and their future, psychotherapeutic interventions may become useful.

As noted in Chapter 8, this emerging recognition that psychotherapy
may be useful is typically paralleled by three questions that patients ask:
*Why did this happen to me? Will I be normal again? Is life worth living after
brain injury?* When these questions surface, patients have begun to recognize that they may have experienced a permanent loss of higher ce-

rebral functions and adaptive skills. They are not the way they used to be. What was normal for them in the past has been lost (Prigatano, 1995a). They struggle with this issue and ask why (Prigatano, 1989). When patients become anxious or despondent over this loss (Prigatano and Summers, 1997), the role for psychotherapeutic interventions becomes clear.

Attempting to answer these questions with the patient, of course, is an individual process. Each patient has a different preinjury history. Each patient has different neuropsychological impairments. Each patient has different values in terms of what makes life meaningful. Before considering how psychotherapy may help these patients, the meaning of the term must be clarified.

Psychotherapy: What It Is and Is Not

Psychotherapy can be defined in different ways. Ultimately, psychotherapy is teaching patients to learn to behave in their own best self-interest, not selfish interest (Prigatano, et al., 1986; Prigatano, 1991). This process begins by establishing a therapeutic alliance between the therapist and the patient. Within the context of that alliance, the therapist typically helps patients to reduce their personal suffering (e.g., frustration, confusion, anxiety, depression, suspiciousness). This goal can be achieved in many ways. The process reflects the "art" of human interaction and basic knowledge of what will "make sense" to the patient as a "first step" (this awareness is another measure of clinical sensibility). No "formula" exists—the process reflects the clinical sensitivity of the neuropsychologist. Once this understanding has been achieved, the psychotherapist slowly begins to help patients to observe aspects about their behavior that they may not fully recognize. The therapist may continue by providing patients with practical guidelines and suggestions for how to cope with specific problems. The suggestions, however, are offered in the context of a progressively more enlightened or realistic view of the complexity of patients' personalities and their methods of coping.

Not all behavior is consciously driven; conversely, not all behavior is unconsciously driven. The emotions of people are ambivalent, and both positive and negative forces guide behavior (Watzlawick, 1983). Both patient and therapist need to see the big picture of a patient's life before they can deal with the effects of the brain injury in the wisest manner possible. This need refers to the capacity of teaching patients to live "well and wisely" after their brain injury (Hebb, 1974). Psychotherapy after brain injury is predicated on a reasonable understanding of human behavior and a dedication to understanding the fabric of patients' lives.

Thus, psychotherapy also can be defined as the relentless, but humane and gentle, search for truth in a person's life. The emphasis is not just on the search for the truth, but in engaging in the process in a humane but persistent manner. If therapists believe that they must force patients to see something about themselves, the "therapy" is never therapeutic. If therapists have a certain theoretical model that patients must fit into, therapy is seldom, if ever, useful. If, however, therapists can enter the patients' phenomenological world and listen carefully to their stories, the beginning of a therapeutic alliance typically emerges. Within this context, patients often can reveal their struggles either through verbalization or artistic expressions.

Dora Kalff's (1980) excellent work on sandplay highlights the importance of having the patients produce some external representation of what they feel internally. She made the poignant statement that when the "inner problem" is made "exterior," it points to the next stage in development. No psychotherapist should forget this powerful statement. If patients struggling with an issue can express the conflict in an external form such as writing in a diary, describing their feelings in a poem, drawing a picture, or picking a song that reflects what they are experiencing, this "hard copy" can be returned to repeatedly to help clarify what individuals are actually experiencing. Amazingly, as individuals' understanding of what they are experiencing improves, the next step in their psychological development often becomes clear. Other authors have also made this point (Brun, et al., 1993). Psychotherapy is thus a process that helps individuals to face their own psychological development (or lack of it).

I have been impressed with the work of Carl Gustav Jung because he emphasized the importance of a patient's individuality and the role that individuality can play in the psychotherapeutic process. Jung appreciated psychodynamic concepts and applied them in his analytic psychology. Yet his work and the work of his followers recognized that patients must help therapists to understand what they, as patients, are experiencing. That process then points the way to patients' continued psychological development.

In this regard, it is important to recognize that psychotherapy is not about happiness. Psychotherapy is about achieving a greater understanding of one's self and one's behavior. With this information, individuals are better able to make choices that do not complicate their adjustment to life. An analogy shared with me years ago by our consulting psychiatrist in Oklahoma City (Dr. Robert Werenike) has continued to ring true. He defined psychotherapy as the process of slowly turning the lights up in a dark room that was filled with bear traps. As the light comes on, the bear traps do not go away. Psychotherapy allows individuals to see the bear traps in their lives. It offers patients an opportunity, or better stated, a choice about whether they will or will not step into the bear traps. Offering this choice is no small contribution to a human's life. If patients can avoid further complications, the results can range from improved physical health to avoiding suicidal behavior. Although psychotherapy cannot promise happiness, effective psychotherapy can help patients to avoid pain and suffering by making appropriate choices. This potential is why psychotherapy can be important and valuable.

Freud observed that even though people may see "bear traps" in their life, they may still step in them. There are many examples of this phenomenon. Individuals may know that smoking will increase their likelihood of future medical problems, but they still smoke. Individuals may fully appreciate that drinking alcohol will not solve their problems, but they continue to drink when overwhelmed. Individuals may recognize that multiple affairs are not a solution to their suffering and yet still engage in affairs. This basic fact of life, that is, human beings seeing a "bear trap" but still choosing to step into it, continues to perplex psychological theorists. If human behavior reflects adaptive evolution and the goal of evolution is for individuals to find an unexplored niche in life and use it for their adaptation, then why would people behave self-destructively? Perhaps the need for the "fittest to survive" is involved but it is hard to know. Whatever the underlying mechanisms, a fact of human behavior is that people behave in ways to hurt themselves.

Years ago (Prigatano et al., 1986), I presented a cartoon that demonstrates how laypeople may conceive of psychotherapy. In this cartoon, Dr. Sigmund Void tells a patient to cheer up and assume a positive attitude toward life. The public often sees psychotherapy as a very expensive form of holding an individual's hand during a difficult time. They see it as an attempt to cheer patients and reject the need to pay $125 to $175 an hour for such hand holding. This description, of course, does not capture psychotherapy in any form. Nevertheless, some psychotherapists, one way or another, embody this approach to treatment.

In supportive psychotherapy, therapists listen carefully to individuals and support or reinforce positive aspects of their adaptive behavior without delving into all areas of conflict. This approach may be important in the overall management of persons who cannot, for one reason or another, deal with a given problem at a particular time. For example, a young woman in group psychotherapy became quite upset and stated to her fellow patients that psychotherapy was a sham and a complete waste of their time. She said that her life, as well as their lives, had been ruined by their brain injuries. No matter what was said in psychotherapy, this situation would not resolve. Their lives had been damaged permanently and the sooner they faced that fact, the better they would be.

Her statements provided an unusual opportunity to discuss openly with the patients what psychotherapy is and is not. I thanked the patient for her comments and then reinvoked the bear-trap analogy. Perhaps for the first time, this group of patients began to understand that psychotherapy was not geared toward cheering them up. Rather psychotherapy was geared toward helping them understand and cope with reality.

The part of the analogy about slowly turning the lights up is perhaps more powerful than it might first seem. The point of this analogy is that people are *slowly* helped to see. If the lights in a dark room are turned on too quickly, people will squint and have a hard time focusing. Likewise, if therapists immediately or rapidly pursue difficult topics, patients will squint psychologically and be unable to focus on an issue, particularly at a crucial time. The process of turning the lights up slowly is analogous to having patients slowly and progressively understand the realities of their life. Those realities may include coping with the problem of lost normality and the existence of permanent neurological and neuropsychological deficits.

Symbols of Work, Love, and Play After Brain Injury

In an edited text entitled *Man and His Symbols*, C. G. Jung (1964) provided a historic and artistic demonstration of the psychological reality that human beings create symbols to help them deal with a variety of challenging experiences that they cannot fully understand or deal with (see Jung, 1964; p. 21). Persons with neuropsychological and neurological deficits related to an acquired brain injury seldom can fully understand the sequelae of their injuries. They struggle with questions (and answers) related to whether they will ever be "normal again." They may wonder if life is worth living after the serious losses imposed by brain damage (Prigatano, 1995a).

As they struggle to cope with these issues and questions, they often produce a variety of reactions: *"If I only try harder, I can make a complete recovery." "If I can find the right rehabilitation program, I will be back to normal in no time." "Just remember to be 'positive,' negative thinking cannot be allowed." "If I could just get a job (or a girlfriend or a certain car), life will return to normal again." "I just need to get out of this hospital and back home where I can really recover."*

Other partial responses could be added to this list. Ultimately, however, reality hits the patient (and family). *"I can't remember what was said in class!" "People speak too fast for me to follow what they say." "I don't understand the concept (or idea) even when it is explained to me." "I can't keep up with the workload in school anymore." "I did say something that offended the customer, but I'm not sure what." "I can't dance like I used to." "I don't feel feminine any longer." "I lost my boyfriend. He said I was too 'childish.' "* This list could continue for several pages.

Eventually, the patient and family recognize that their lives have been changed permanently by the patient's brain injury. I refer to this process as coming to grips with the problem of lost normality (Prigatano, 1995a). In the presence of their sadness, anger, depression, and anxiety, individuals must begin to rebuild their lives. Focusing on activities that relate to three human and living symbols can be quite helpful in this process.

The symbols are work, love, and play (Prigatano, 1989). These symbols help provide meaning for many people in Western cultures and beyond.

Work

The symbol of work is the experience of being productive, and a sense of productivity is important for the psychological well-being of a person. It is the experience of being competent, of being needed, of being useful. Why do we crave this experience? Initially, it seems to foster a sense of security and hence well-being. As Eric Erickson pointed out (see Hall and Lindzey, 1978), as we age and develop psychologically, productivity can assume different meanings. In his seventh stage of psychosocial development, Erickson talks about generativity versus stagnation. In this stage, individuals produce something to pass on to others who may benefit from what they had previously done or learned. The purpose is to improve another's quality of life. Such generativity allows a person to avoid psychological stagnation, and the virtue of caring for other people develops during this time.

During most stages of psychosocial development, work is important. When brain-injured persons ask whether they can or cannot do a certain job, it is helpful to provide them a "model" of the components of work (Fig. 9-1). Success at work can be conceptualized as having four basic ingredients, which can be symbolized by the sides of a square. To work successfully, people must first be cooperative. They must be willing to work with others and to postpone some of their own actions or personal gratifications to complete a job. This capacity defines cooperative effort. Second, people must be reliable, that is, they must do what they say they will do. Reliability includes arriving at work on time. It means following through with assigned responsibilities in a serious fashion. Cooperation and reliability are the first two building blocks of the capacity to work.

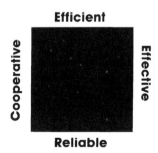

Figure 9-1. A model for work presented to brain dysfunctional patients. Reprinted with permission from Prigatano, G. P. and Klonoff, P. S. (1988). Psychotherapy and neuropsychological assessment after brain injury. *Journal of Head Trauma Rehabilitation* 3: 45–56. Copyright © 1988 Aspen Publishers, Inc.

Third, people must be effective in whatever work effort they choose. That is, they must be able to do the job. Being effective, however, is not enough. People must also be efficient, that is, they must be able to complete a job at a rate that others agree is "normal" or at least cost effective. If they cannot do a job efficiently, their positions rarely last.

When psychotherapists treat adults who have suffered brain injury, they often begin with work and ask patients to reflect on how their neuropsychological and psychiatric problems may or may not interfere with these four ingredients of work or productivity. In this context, their neuropsychological and psychiatric deficits clearly dictate how psychotherapy proceeds. A few case vignettes may clarify this point.

A young man suffered a traumatic brain injury (TBI) 1 year before he was evaluated. His injuries included damage to the frontal and temporal lobes. In addition to memory disturbances, the patient had a tendency toward paranoid ideation. Before his injury, he had a similar problem but to a lesser degree. Afterward, however, he was unable to maintain jobs and was frequently convinced that people were undercutting him in various ways. He believed that people snickered at him, talked behind his back, and told lies about him. His paranoia also emerged at home. He became extremely hostile toward his mother and stepfather and felt that he was not wanted there (in truth, they attempted to provide a reasonable home for him).

As the therapeutic alliance developed, it became necessary to guide this patient to make work choices aligned with his psychiatric and neuropsychological impairments. His problem of paranoia was clearly a neuropsychiatric problem and was described to him in a matter of fact fashion. Eventually, the patient understood that working with multiple people seemed to fuel his paranoia. Both he and the psychotherapist agreed that it would be more practical for him to work at a job that required minimum contact with other people. He then began to change his work options (for example, he stopped working as a waiter in a restaurant). He agreed to work on a task that involved preparing documents. Serendipitously, he found a night job that involved working with only one or two people each shift. With this restricted contact with people, his paranoid ideation actually decreased. The patient, however, also was on antipsychotic medications, which contributed to his improved clinical picture. Yet, even when placed on the antipsychotic medications after his brain injury, his paranoia clearly influenced his work capacity negatively until the environment was changed.

As he experienced some success at work, we reviewed roles at which he could be effective and efficient. He had, at times, unrealistic aspirations that did not match his residual memory difficulties. When he recognized this mismatch, he found it valuable to stay at a particular job, even though it paid less money than he had originally hoped to make. As he became effective and efficient at the job, he was offered a permanent position. His initial capacity to be reliable and cooperative, in part, was based on persuading him to accept a type of work that was compatible with his neuropsychological and personality difficulties.

Another case involved a 21-year-old man who suffered a severe brain injury after falling from a bridge. This patient reported that he wanted to be either a "helicopter pilot or a short order cook." Instead of challenging him and stating that his aspirations were impossible, the model of work depicted in Figure 9-1 was reviewed with him. His therapist agreed that he was cooperative and reliable. However, they discussed the questions of effectiveness and efficiency at length. The roles of both helicopter pilot and short order cook require fairly fast reaction times and speeds of performance. The patient had bilateral injury to the frontal lobes and basal ganglia: he talked, walked, and thought slowly. The patient began to recognize that his job choices were unrealistic and not in his best self-interest. He eventually accepted another type of work without major conflict. This case study demonstrates how the neuropsychological picture dictates how patients are approached and can be helped to see what course is in their best self-interest.

Love

In addition to the symbol of work, the symbol of love is of major importance to human beings. The symbol of love also is the most difficult to define. It is the experience that another's existence and quality of life are as important as one's own. It is, in essence, a transcendental state and enables psychological relatedness. A person who loves another and who is loved in return is not alone psychologically. Love also permits the experience of being valued by another. This experience, in turn, allows individuals to value themselves more honestly and to value others in return.

The symbol of love is intimately connected with the experience of *passion* (see Sternberg, 1986). As Rod Stewart's song tells us "everyone needs passion." People who have lost their passion for life are truly alone and isolated. This sense of passion helps tremendously with the creative force behind so many discoveries—personally as well as collectively.

Although passion is the necessary force behind love, love does not equal passion. Love involves at least two other ingredients (Fig. 9-2). Sternberg (1986) has suggested a triangular theory of love, in which love begins by having some passion or drive to move toward another. From that passion emerges the possibility of intimacy. When passion and intimacy are present, the capacity for commitment may develop.

Intimacy is also difficult to define. It often refers to an individual's capacity to reveal the most private aspects of self to another and to have the courage to listen to what the other says in return. Intimacy is never stagnant. It is as dynamic as passion. Failure to establish true intimacy

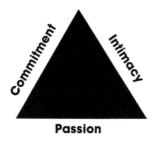

Passion

Figure 9-2. Model regarding love. Adapted with permission from Sternberg, R. J. (1986). A triangular theory of love. *Psychol. Rev.* 93: 119–135. Copyright © 1986 Aspen Publishers, Inc.

shatters love and is, perhaps, the single biggest cause of divorce in our society.

If passion and intimacy remain vibrant and alive, commitment becomes possible and realistic. Commitment can be defined as a pledge freely given, which is realistic and based on the mutual self-interest of the two parties "in love." Passion and intimacy sustain commitment; commitment sustains passion and intimacy.

This triangular theory of love suggests that various forms of "love" relationships can exist. If persons have a lot of passion but little capacity for intimacy or commitment, they typically relate by "one-night stands." Scant passion and intimacy coupled with considerable commitment create situations in which people have been married for 50 years but sleep in separate bedrooms. The most satisfying love relationship is one that balances these three elements—that is, passion, intimacy, and commitment are present in equal amounts.

One might think that work and love alone would provide a psychological sense of meaning in a person's life (see Prigatano, 1989). Although these symbols greatly contribute to a sense of meaning or purpose in life, as Master Yoda says in the movie *Star Wars*, "there is another."

Play

This other force is the symbol of play. Play does not mean recreation. It means the freedom to do what one wants to do in fantasy. By exploring via play and fantasy what individuals want, feel, and desire, a deeper sense of self begins to emerge and reveal itself. Thus, people who can be playful and who recognize both their "light" and "dark" sides seem to be most at home with themselves and others.

Unlike work and love, play can be difficult to depict in a simple geometric form. It is captured in facial expressions, tones of voice, body postures, and utterances that reflect intense, satisfying feelings. The picture presented in Figure 9-3 illustrates a person in "play." In this picture, the fishing guide is happy to see his client catch a fish. His business will obviously increase for this picture appeared in *Sunset Magazine.* The woman who caught the fish, however, shows another emotion. She is not only happy, her face reveals a different, deeper emotion. She is close to being in ecstasy. The experience of play touches the deepest level of the psyche, or soul.

In the play *Zorba, the Greek* (Prigatano, 1994), Zorba reminds us that "in work I am your man, but in play, I am my own—I mean, free." The capacity to develop this sense of freedom to be who one is and to do so within the context of play is crucial for the development of individuality.

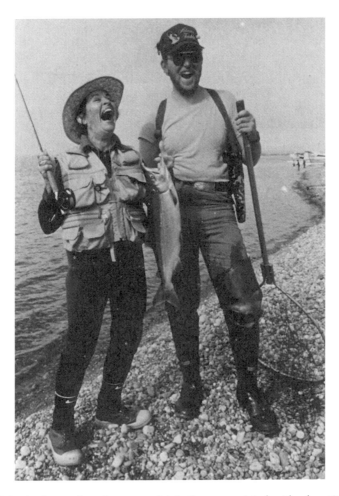

Figure 9-3. A picture denoting powerful feelings associated with play. Copyright 1988 by R. Valentine Atkinson. With permission.

Play is especially difficult for most people—and this statement is true of people both with and without brain injury. Yet, once the capacity for work and love is established, the capacity for play becomes extremely important because play pays closer attention to the inner world. In some ways, work reflects our capacity to deal with the outer world and play our capacity to deal with the inner world; love integrates these two polarities. Individuals must develop each of these components to live a complete or full life. It is the purpose of psychotherapy to foster such an existence.

Thus, the ability to work, love, and play helps individuals to cope with suffering and to establish meaning despite the inevitable losses at each stage in life. Patients with brain dysfunction therefore need to be helped to relate to living symbols to cope with the problem of lost normality after brain injury.

Individuality, Lesion Location, and Psychotherapy After Brain Injury

The process by which people begin to deal with their losses, anxieties, and depression psychologically requires courage and commitment to begin to face the truth in their lives. Although the symbols of work, love, and play often help persons to rediscover meaning and purpose in life, relating to these symbols might be viewed as the intermediate and end-stages of a given journey.

Typically, the process of beginning the journey of psychotherapy (i.e., turning the lights on in a room full of bear traps) begins with what has been termed the "hero's journey" (Campbell, 1968; Prigatano, 1991; Prigatano, 1995a). A given individual has to take the first step of leaving the security of home. Home is a symbol of what is comfortable, secure, and known. It is a person's most natural and earliest sense of identity. The problem, however, is that home often reflects our parents' identity, not our own.

Thus, we must leave the security of home (i.e., a psychological position in time and space) and move out to face an apparently sinister force that exists in the "outer" world. In fairy tales, this force might be a dragon, a giant, an evil queen, a sorcerer, or a bad knight. Beginning the journey requires courage and a commitment to deal with a threatening challenge. Often, the threat first appears to be external to the self. This perspective may be a projection; that is, the threat often is within us but can only be approached indirectly by externalizing the problem. When individuals come face to face with the threatening force, they must be both brave and cunning to neutralize the threat. Heroes always seem to outsmart the enemy, and they do so against a background of courage. In all such journeys, heroes return home "often by another way" (see the song of James Taylor) and re-embrace family and friends in their homeland but now with more maturity. This is a never-ending cycle of psychological growth and maturity (Prigatano and Ben-Yishay, 1999).

This motif is repeated in many forms (including fairy tales; Prigatano, 1991; Brun, et al., 1993). Two recent examples come from popular movies dealing with outer space (a projected image of our need to explore inner space?) In *Star Trek*, Captain Kirk, with the help of Engineer Scottie and Science Officer Spock, places a heat-seeking missile device on a torpedo to find a "cloaked bird of prey"—a Klingon ship that is firing upon them but that they cannot see and which will surely destroy their starship *Enterprise*. Although they could not see the enemy, they found an ingenious way to protect themselves and, in so doing, delivered a fatal blow.

A second example comes from perhaps the most well-known space adventure movie—*Star Wars*. Luke faces Darth Vader (a play on words for the dark father) and is locked in mortal battle using his laser sword. As they fight, Luke finally delivers a decisive blow and decapitates his (unknown) father. As the head rolls to the ground, in the famous Darth Vader helmet, it begins to transform and the face of Luke Skywalker is seen in the helmet of Darth Vader. Why? Because the face of the father is another version of the face of the son. Both have positive and negative forces within them. Awareness of these forces is the beginning of the self-knowledge that is the basis for psychological growth, and Jung recognized the importance of symbols for revealing such mysteries about human beings. As the various movies, stories, and fairy tales reveal, individuals have their own paths that they must follow. Each confronts different, frightening images, but the hero's journey is repeated over and over again. The process of the hero's journey is the process of ultimately developing what Jung called individuation.

Jung (1957) beautifully described the process of individuation as accomplishing two major goals. First, it permits the integration of both positive and negative forces within the self. This integration can greatly aid the process of creativity and accomplishment in life. Second, individuation permits "objective interpersonal relationships." When persons fail to individuate, multiple marriages or difficulties in sustaining relationships often result. Only when individuals know who they are can they relate objectively to another human being. This theme is often reflected in movies as well.

In the movie *Moonstruck*, an elderly lady discovers that her husband has been having an affair. Later, she meets a middle-aged man, who suggests that they return to her home when her husband is absent. She refuses, stating unequivocally that she knows who she is but she is convinced that this man does not know who he is. Erickson (Hall and Lindzey, 1978) makes the same point when he states that only when individuals have established a sense of identity can they be faithful to their spouse, profession, or other activities. Identity and fidelity go together:

no identity, no fidelity. Individuals cannot be faithful if they do not know who they are. Creative people often have a fluid sense of identity, and some have been notoriously unfaithful sexually. The observation is not meant to condone their behavior but to understand it from a psychological perspective.

How do these observations relate to the various types of patients seen after brain injury? Who individuals are before their brain injury as well as who they are after their brain injury (including their neuropsychological deficits) determines the process that they will follow to cope with their unique set of problems. Psychotherapists who understand this basic process in psychotherapy and who can also appreciate the predictable neuropsychological problems of various types of brain-injured patients can greatly assist patients along their hero's journey.

Case Examples

At various places throughout this text, I have referred to a patient I have known for almost 8 years. This young woman suffered a TBI when a large boulder broke loose from the side of a mountain and crashed onto her vehicle. Before the injury, the woman was energetic and athletic and lived a somewhat bohemian life. Although she could have easily attended any university and sought professional training, she elected not to. In her home environment, she had questioned authority and particularly had rebelled against organized religion. Her major goals in life were to have fun and to be athletically fit. After her brain injury, she was no longer athletically fit and fun was very hard to reach.

Initially, she passively engaged in a neuropsychological rehabilitation program but became increasingly resistant as time passed. She insisted that all she wanted was physical therapy. She clearly had no interest in working on cognitive and personality difficulties in rehabilitation. As noted earlier, she was allowed to withdraw from the rehabilitation program with no reprisals.

The clinical director attempted to provide her an opportunity to obtain the therapies that she wanted and at whatever locations that she desired (she often stated that she did not like Phoenix and wanted to have her therapy someplace else). In the course of working with her, she revealed that she had considerable fear of her mother and had felt that way for many years. This fear was her dragon that had to be approached. She began to approach her fear in different ways but eventually recognized, like Dorothy in the *Wizard of Oz*, that she needed to grow up and face who she was and that she needed to live with her mother for a while as a consequence of her injury. She moved in with her mother and eventually was able to accept a lower level of work compared to her preinjury functioning. Her injuries were severe, but her hero's journey consisted of facing her fear. In that context, she was able to move to a more normal lifestyle after significant neuropsychological and neurological problems.

A second patient was a victim of a drive-by shooting. She was angry about being victimized and later had complications related to her injury (e.g., the onset of a seizure disorder). She often struggled with why this tragedy had happened to her. During rehabilitation, she drew a picture demonstrating her frustrations, confusion, isolation, and anger (i.e., Figure 2-3, Chapter 2). As Dora Kalff indicated, once she had externalized her inner problem, she was better able to handle it.

Initially, she refused to show the picture to any of the therapists because she was especially angry at one of them whom she considered insensitive. Eventually, however, she described what the picture meant to her and from this process was able to rekindle an interest in returning to school. She also faced her fear and eventually began to relate to the symbols of work and love in a manner that was productive for her.

The third case is a young man who suffered cerebral anoxia. His neuropsychological impairment was substantial and included profound memory impairment. He had little insight into his disabilities and insisted on returning to his previous studies at a major university. When he did so, he developed a variety of somatic complaints, panic attacks, and severe headaches.

With time, he returned to Phoenix and began to face what frightened him the most, namely, describing himself as an individual who had a brain injury. Once he was able to face this fear and to identify himself as a student with a disability, he was able to relate to the symbols of work and love. He was able to complete his bachelor's degree at a less demanding university and to obtain additional help as a student with disabilities. With time, he met a young woman and a romantic relationship unfolded.

Each of these three patients still struggles with the symbol of play. That struggle is understandable. They are all in their late twenties or early thirties. The capacity to enter fantasy, however, does not stop at any particular point, and several years may elapse before they can use fantasy to foster adult integration and psychological development. Their process of psychotherapy, however, has been positive because they were able to relate to these symbols and to face their initial fears.

Strengths and Limitations of Psychotherapy After Brain Injury

Psychotherapy after brain injury is associated with definite strengths and limitations (Prigatano, 1995b). Although I will not repeat many of these points made elsewhere, I want to highlight some of the observations most relevant to this chapter.

Although the overall goal of psychotherapy is to establish or reestablish a sense of purpose or meaning in a patient's life, many "subgoals" must be addressed before this major goal can be achieved. One of the strengths of psychotherapy is the ability to assist patients in learning to control verbally some aspect of their behavior to facilitate the adjustment process. Such verbal control allows patients to begin to observe their behavioral reactions as well as the reactions of others. They can begin to recognize how poorly identified feeling states can greatly contribute to their maladaptive responses. Also, through the interpersonal relationship that they establish with their therapists, they are able to control or reduce some of their impulsivity and to become more cooperative in activities that enhance their adaptation.

A clear strength of psychotherapy is its ability to establish emotional contact with another human being and to allow that therapeutic alliance to help guide the patients' behavior. Sometimes individuals act not because they understand why they should or should not, but because someone else has asked them to do or not do something. Relationships can have a powerful influence on persons' behaving in a manner that promotes positive choices. Prigatano and Ben-Yishay (1999) have discussed Goldstein's statement that health requires some choices. That is, to live a healthy life, people must make choices and these choices inevitably mean giving up certain things and embracing others. Psychotherapy with brain dysfunctional patients can facilitate this process.

There are, however, definite limitations to psychotherapy. If patients have severe cognitive disturbances, they may have a difficult time establishing verbal control of behavior or entering into a useful dialogue with a psychotherapist. Also, patients' attitudes about themselves and life problems are not easily modified despite the best psychotherapeutic efforts. Individuals may not be able to change long-term ingrained attitudes easily.

Finally, numerous factors outside the course of the psychotherapeutic experience can negatively influence a person's adjustment, and psychotherapy cannot address these issues (e.g., loss of a job, illness, economic pressures).

Some patients who have suffered brain injury absolutely do not need psychotherapy (Prigatano, 1991). These persons tend to have a philosophy of life that helps them to endure suffering. They often view life from a philosophical perspective that gives them a sense of calm even when faced with frightening events. For example, a patient who had suffered a brain injury in the United States was originally from Vietnam. He had been an attorney as well as a pilot during the Vietnam war. Raised in South Vietnam, he had been trained to view life from a different perspective than that of the typical Westerner. In the context of group psychotherapy, he revealed a story that had helped him place the effects of his brain injury in perspective. His story is related in detail in Prigatano (1991) and discussed in Chapter 14. At this point, we need only note that people often do not fully appreciate the meaning of an event until later in their lives. This attitude helps patients place their brain injury into a perspective that many persons cannot achieve.

When something bad happens to people, they automatically assume it is the worse thing that could possibly happen to them. In fact, the event may be a "wake-up call" to change their life. In other instances, it may give them extraordinary opportunities to learn something about themselves or the nature of life that they never would have learned otherwise. This line of reasoning is not intended to talk someone out of feeling their depression or sense of loss. The intent is for them to realize, realistically, that they cannot understand the meaning of an event in their life until they have lived longer. Persons who can internalize this perspective often have the capacity to continue to be productive and to maintain interpersonal relationships even after they have experienced a significant loss.

Psychotherapy may not be helpful at certain times after brain injury. For example, during the acute phases of brain injury, many patients are so severely cognitively impaired that they cannot benefit from formal psychotherapy. Yet, they might benefit from interventions aimed at helping them with difficult situations. Prigatano and Ben-Yishay (1999) describe such situations.

Finally, even when psychotherapy is attempted with patients who seem to be suitable candidates, psychotherapy is sometimes ineffective. Two case examples highlight this all-too-common phenomenon. A 35-year-old woman suffered a severe brain injury in a motor vehicle accident. She had a true amnestic disorder and significant cognitive impairments. She came from a very fundamentalist religious background and felt that God would cure her of any neurological or neuropsychological disabilities. Obviously, therapists would not challenge this view. Rather, they would try to help the patient recognize that she might not recover as much as she expected, regardless of her religious convictions. The goal, therefore, is to help patients learn to cope with their disability as much as possible.

In this case, numerous psychotherapy sessions were spent discussing the extent of her impairment and practical steps that she might take to cope with the disabilities. This patient did not seem to recognize the extent of her disability. In fact, my initial impression was that she was in a state of denial. Despite repeated attempts to break through this so-called denial, she made no progress. The sessions only seemed to upset her and to make her more angry and depressed. Despite intensive neuropsychological rehabilitation, she achieved no practical changes. Eventually, she became more isolated, depressed and, eventually, paranoid. Her case demonstrates a psychotherapeutic failure, presumably because of her severe cognitive deficits and rather rigid approach to life's problems. The quote from Taylor (1971) that introduces this chapter also captures this well-known phenomenon.

In another case, a 16-year-old girl sustained a severe brain injury in a motor vehicle accident. She was extremely childish and impulsive and had very little insight into her behavior. She had almost no verbal control of her behavior. Efforts at behavior modification, interpersonal-oriented psychotherapy, and even psychoanalytically oriented psychotherapy produced no positive effects. Her behavior remained impulsive and childlike, probably reflecting the severity of her cognitive deficits. The money spent on psychotherapy was wasted.

As therapists, we must face these realities and not blindly "do psychotherapy" with each patient referred for that purpose. Whatever form of psychotherapeutic intervention is attempted, therapists must have a clear understanding of what they are trying to accomplish with a given patient. If, after a reasonable time, the therapy is not working, the psychotherapist should accept the failure and terminate the therapy. This acceptance is not abandoning the patient. It is being realistic about what one can and cannot do. It is also being ethically responsible by not charging for services that are essentially ineffective.

Practical Considerations of Doing Psychotherapy with a Person Who Has Suffered Brain Injury

1. Go slowly; do not make it too easy to "get into psychotherapy."
2. Explore the patient's capacity for insight and present yourself as a consultant to the patient, not as healer, guru, boss, or parent.
3. Help patients to sharpen their perspective on reality repeatedly.
4. Recognize the complexity of behavior and the role of conscious and non- or unconscious factors that may motivate a given behavior. But, avoid "digging" for childhood conflicts or infantile or repressed memories. See behavior as an ongoing attempt to adapt to the present in the light of past experiences that are consciously or unconsciously represented.
5. Focus on the present but with a sophisticated understanding of how the past may have contributed to patients' behavior. Help patients recognize these relationships by way of the therapeutic dialogue.
6. Help patients to recognize repeatedly that psychotherapy or neuropsychological rehabilitation has time limitations and that both must have a focused problem-solving approach (thus including a beginning, middle, and end). The intent is to help patients become independent of the therapist.
7. Deal with patients' misperceptions, angry outbursts, inappropriate behavior, anxiety, and depression slowly, honestly, and empathetically. Psychotherapy is a slow, persistent dialogue to help patients improve their behavior (and thinking capacity) to achieve greater adaptation. It requires hard work from both parties.
8. Heed Jung's admonishment—if persons think a certain way, they may feel considerably better. "If they think along the lines of na-

ture, they think properly." The degree to which psychotherapists understand human nature from both scientific and nonscientific perspectives, the more effective they tend to be as psychotherapists (thus the role of science and symbolism in brain injury rehabilitation—see Chapter 14).

9. Share the emotional responsibility of working with brain dysfunctional patients in psychotherapy as well as in neuropsychological rehabilitation. Sharing helps to preserve psychotherapists' energy and creativity.

10. Help patients establish a sense of meaning in the presence of (not despite) brain injury. Ultimately, this approach is the best way of dealing with the problem of lost normality. Further guidelines have been outlined in the chapter on psychotherapy after brain injury in a book by Prigatano and colleagues (1986).

Recurring Issues in the Psychotherapy of Family Members

Florian and Katz (1991) have thoughtfully reviewed the impact of TBI on family members—both parents and spouse. They have also discussed the impact on the children of persons with TBI. The reader is referred to their work to clarify many of the issues relevant to working with family members. The question, however, of how to help family members from a psychotherapeutic perspective arises. Because families are as different as patients, there is no simple formula.

As stated earlier, the central goal of psychotherapy is to teach patients to learn to behave in their own best interest, not selfish interest. This goal can also be applied to family members, whether they are parents, spouse, or children. The process, of course, is delicate. How do therapists teach family members to behave in their own best self-interest if it appears to deprive patients of what they need? The issue is how to help patients get their needs met while simultaneously helping family members get their needs met. Some examples may be helpful.

A middle-aged man suffered a severe hypoxic brain injury. Immediately after the onset of his neurological problems, his wife insisted that she take him home to care for him there. Clearly, however, he needed 24-hour supervision, most likely in an extended care facility. The wife would not entertain this option. Eventually, the neurologist who oversaw this patient's medical needs referred the spouse for psychotherapeutic consultation.

Her first words were "don't you dare attempt to change my mind about my keeping my husband at home!" Instead of challenging her decision regarding her husband's care, the psychotherapist asked the wife to explain her position, what she was experiencing, and how she felt her husband's needs could best be met. After several weeks of discussing her view of her husband's needs, the questions eventually emerged: What are your needs and how are they being met? This question immediately resulted in the spouse crying intensely. After she was able to clarify her position about her husband's needs, she could get in touch with what she herself needed.

Several months of psychotherapy ensued. The initial focus of the psychotherapy was to provide practical suggestions to help her achieve some respite from her husband's care. For example, facilities that might care for him during a weekend were suggested so that she might rest and prepare to manage him during the week. Suggestions about how to deal with family members who were actively involved in her husband's care during the week also were offered.

As the woman began to clarify her own needs, she revealed a long history of difficulties with adjustment. After months of working with her, she admitted that she had previously had problems with drug and alcohol abuse and that she had become intoxicated immediately upon hearing of her husband's brain injury and had remained so for several weeks thereafter. At one point, she angrily asked the psychotherapist why he had never asked her about her drinking history. His response was, "I felt you would tell me what you wanted me to know when you were ready." By not forcing her to talk about anything and simply understanding her experience, she ultimately revealed a number of adjustment difficulties, only some of which were related to her husband's brain injury.

At this point, therapists must make a decision. Will they focus on helping a family member to deal with the patient's problems, or will they deal with the family member from the perspective that the patient's difficulties represent one of many conflicts that people experience in their lives? In some cases, it is best to avoid the family member's preinjury history and to focus only on factors that affect the patient's management. This route is especially relevant during the early stages of rehabilitation. However, when a patient is one, two, three, four or five years postinjury, the family member must deal with this altered relationship. In that context, it may be necessary to explore other areas of adaptation as well as areas of conflict.

In the case of this patient's wife, she had numerous dreams that reflected ongoing struggles with her mother and with her very complicated feelings toward her husband. In one dream, she had the foreboding that a wolf was outside of her home, staring at the window. She became frightened to look outside but when she eventually did, she saw the wolf. She later attempted to draw her dream image (Fig. 9-4). It took some time for her to recognize that all the images in the dream were reflections of part of herself and that one part was dangerous and angry. With time, she could begin to discuss her negative feelings and how her husband's disabilities repulsed her. This scenario is extremely difficult for any human being to face.

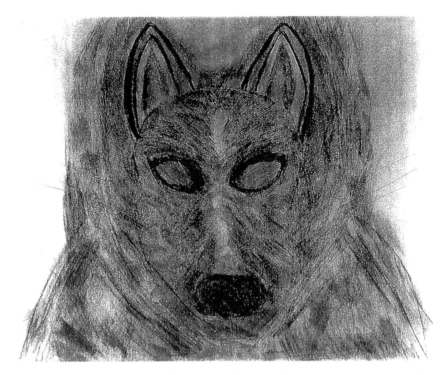

Figure 9-4. The drawing of a dream image by the wife of a patient seen in psychotherapy.

In the same dream, one of her arms was like a wolf's claw. When she turned the arm over, she saw serious wounds or sores on its undersurface. This image was symbolic of what she was experiencing. She, too, in a sense, was wounded from the brain injury and was suffering because of it. Helping her face the complexity of her experiences and feelings toward her husband was crucial for her ultimate ability to adapt to the situation. Eventually, she recognized that she needed to get her own needs met as well as those of her husband. As a result, she placed him in an appropriate long-term nursing facility that could meet his needs.

Dealing with the angry reactions of spouses and parents toward rehabilitation staff is a common issue in neuropsychological rehabilitation. Two cases highlight this point. Several years ago, a woman had suffered a severe brain injury in a car-train accident. Her husband was extremely accepting of his wife's limitations and difficulties and never expressed his own needs. He approached the situation as difficult but manageable. When asked about his own needs, he politely stated that they were of no major concern. He was able to manage his children and his wife, given his religious background and his own method of coping with life. Psychotherapy was not attempted with this spouse.

When the brain-injured patient was seen in psychotherapy, the husband was often present because his wife had severe memory difficulties. It was extremely important that the husband understand some of her difficulties so that he could deal with her emotional reactions outside of psychotherapy. Eventually, the wife's psychotherapist accepted a new position elsewhere. At that point, the outraged husband called the psychotherapist, exclaiming "How dare you leave me to take care of my wife by myself?"

In this instance as in similar ones, a consistent picture seems to emerge. If the family's needs are denied, a negative reaction eventually will occur. The exact form of the reaction is difficult to define or predict, but it is inevitable. The families' "denial" may be extremely resistant to change as the quote from Romano (1974) at the beginning of this chapter illustrates. The denial seems to center on how difficult it is to accept that someone who is loved is no longer the same.

For example, a wealthy oilman constantly insulted his brain-injured son's psychotherapist during regularly scheduled relatives' meetings (see Prigatano, et al., 1986). Eventually, the therapist confronted this man during the relatives' group by stating that he had spent several weeks trying to work with his son and no longer appreciated being berated for his ineptness during these sessions. This father admitted that he had been so upset by his son's brain injury that he literally had to take it out on everyone who was involved with his son's care. With time, he commented that the therapist had, in fact, helped him even more than his son. In other words, the father had been helped to understand the extent of his son's disabilities, which helped him to cope with the situation.

When persons experience brain injury, there is a tremendous ripple effect on those around them, including both family members and the rehabilitation staff who care for them. The next chapter focuses on the staff's reactions to these patients and their own reactions to one another.

Practical Considerations in Doing Psychotherapy with a Family Member of a Person Who Has Suffered Brain Injury

1. Appreciate that the family's situation is difficult. They hurt for the patient. They are frightened and want to ensure that the patient's needs are met. They are hurt for themselves but do not know how or what to do about their pain.
2. Enter the family member's phenomenological field as well as that of the brain-injured patient. Establish some basis for a working alliance.
3. Hear the family members out—take their critiques about the limitations of rehabilitative care seriously.
4. Let them help you understand your "denial" just as you need to help them understand theirs.

5. Help family members get their needs met in a fair and honest way. Achieving this goal may mean changing their relationship to the brain-injured patient. Do not be frightened to work toward this change—it is a part of reality.

6. Recognize that the family's anger is real and must be managed. It will not go away on its own.

7. Do not rush toward psychotherapy if family members are coping adequately with the situation. Establish a good working relationship with them. The family will come to the therapist when they need to talk about what is bothering them.

8. Group work with family members is important, but ultimately it is an individual process with which they must wrestle. Thus, individual psychotherapy may be needed for more than one family member.

9. Symbols of work, love, and play can be helpful to both family members and patients. There is no antidote for human suffering— only useful attempts to establish a sense of meaning in life in the presence of suffering.

10. Have both family members and patient participate as part of the rehabilitation team. As a responsible professional, however, recognize that they do not direct the team efforts. Such decisions must be based collectively on the input of multiple therapists, the attending physician, and the clinical director of rehabilitation.

Two Final Analogies for Psychotherapy After Brain Injury

Two final analogies may be useful in understanding the process of psychotherapy and how it differs for brain dysfunctional individuals. Psychotherapy is much like delivering babies. If one understands the natural process of gestation, the complications that can occur during delivery, and the steps needed to facilitate the delivery process, one is a good physician. The delivery is not rushed nor are forceps used unless necessary. The physician must recognize that critical points during the delivery process can either arrest development or facilitate growth.

Likewise, the effective psychotherapist understands that it is normal for the psyche to develop in different ways in different people. Like the physician who delivers a baby, psychotherapists need to stand by patients as they struggle through various stages of development to facilitate the natural process.

Perhaps the biggest difference, however, in doing psychotherapy with persons who have a brain injury is that the therapist must be a "psychological attorney." That is, patients *occasionally* need specific advice about what course of action is most likely in their best interest as they attempt to cope with the effects of their brain injury (Prigatano and Ben-Yishay, 1999). Traditionally, when patients have few cognitive deficits, psychotherapists impose little of their own values on patients. This is the classic model of psychotherapy as seen from Freudian, Jungian, and Rogerian perspectives. Patients with brain injury, however, have different needs. Therapists must give patients practical advice to help them avoid problems and to adapt as best as possible. Just as attorneys offer specific advice when their clients confront a threatening situation, clinical neuropsychologists involved in psychotherapy with brain-injured patients must do the same thing. A good attorney will help guide clients, while letting them make their own decisions. The same is true in psychotherapy with brain-injured persons. Furthermore, excellent attorneys will recognize when they need to sway their clients in one direction or another to ensure that clients make decisions in their best interest, even if the clients cannot grasp the need. This process is delicate and invokes many ethical issues. Yet, repeatedly, the situation arises: Clinical neuropsychologists who do psychotherapy with brain-injured patients often need to act as a psychological attorney.

Summary and Conclusions

Practical psychotherapy, as Jung referred to it years ago, is extremely important for individuals as they face crisis and change in their life. Dealing with the problem of lost normality after brain injury can be a formidable task. Clinical neuropsychologists who can apply various psychotherapeutic interventions in a sensible manner may greatly help some brain dysfunctional patients with this problem. While the process is by definition highly individualized, helping patients reestablish a sense of meaning in life after brain injury is the cornerstone of such psychotherapeutic interventions. Helping them relate to symbols of work, love, and play ultimately is most adaptive in our culture. It requires, however, courage and guidance to achieve this outcome.

References

Birch, H. (1964). *Brain Damage in Children: The Biological and Social Aspects.* Williams & Wilkins, New York.

Brun, B., Pedersen, E. W., and Runberg, M. (1993). *Symbols of the Soul: Therapy and Guidance Through Fairy Tales.* Jessica Kingsley, Philadelphia.

Campbell, J. (1968). *The Hero with a Thousand Faces.* Princeton University, Princeton, NJ.

Chaplin, C. (1964/1992). *Charles Chaplin: My Autobiography.* Penguin, New York.

Florian, V., and Katz, S. (1991). The other victims of traumatic brain injury: Consequences for family members. *Neuropsychology* 5(4): 267–279.

Hall, C. S., and Lindzey, G. (1978). *Theories of Personality* (3rd ed). John Wiley & Sons, New York.

Hebb, D. (1974). What psychology is about. *Am. Psychol.* 29: 71–79.

Jaffe, A. (1984). *The Myth of Meaning in the Work of C. G. Jung.* Daimon Verlag, Zurich.

Jung, C. G. (1957). *The Practice of Psychotherapy Essays on Psychology of the Transference and Other Subjects.* Princeton University, Princeton, NJ.

Jung, C. G. (1964). *Man and His Symbols.* Aldus, London.

Kalff, D. M. (1980). *Sandplay: A Psychotherapeutic Approach to the Psyche.* Sigo, Boston.

Mohr, D. (1995). Negative outcomes in psychotherapy: a critical review. *Clinical Psychology Science and Practice* 2(1): 1–27.

Prigatano, G. P. (1989). Work, love, and play after brain injury. *Bull. Menninger Clin* 53(5): 414–431.

Prigatano, G. P. (1991). Disordered mind, wounded soul: the emerging role of psychotherapy in rehabilitation after brain injury. *Journal of Head Trauma Rehabilitation* 6(4): 1–10.

Prigatano, G. P. (1994). Individuality, lesion location and psychotherapy after brain injury. In A-L. Christensen and B. Uzzell (eds), *Brain Injury and Neuropsychological Rehabilitation: International Perspective* (pp. 173–199). Lawrence Erlbaum, Hillsdale, NJ.

Prigatano, G. P. (1995a). 1994 Sheldon Berrol, MD, Senior Lectureship: The problem of lost normality after brain injury. *Journal of Head Trauma Rehabilitation* 10(3): 87–95.

Prigatano, G. P. (1995b). Strengths and limitations of psychotherapy after brain injury. *Advances in Medical Psychotherapy* 8: 23–34.

Prigatano, G. P., and Ben-Yishay, Y. (1999). Psychotherapy and psychotherapeutic interventions in brain injury rehabilitation. In M. Rosenthal (ed), *Rehabilitation of the Adult and Child with Traumatic Brain Injury* (3rd ed). F. A. Davis, Philadelphia.

Prigatano, G. P., and Klonoff, P. S. (1988). Psychotherapy and neuropsychological assessment after brain injury. *Journal of Head Trauma Rehabilitation* 3: 45–56.

Prigatano, G. P. et al. (1986). *Neuropsychological Rehabilitation After Brain Injury.* Johns Hopkins University, Baltimore.

Prigatano, G. P., and Summers, J. D. (1997). Depression in traumatic brain injury patients. In M. M. Robertson and C. L. E. Katona (eds), *Depression and Physical Illness* (pp. 341–358). John Wiley & Sons, New York.

Prigatano, G. P., and Weinstein, E. A. (1996). Edwin A. Weinstein's contributions to neuropsychological rehabilitation. *Neuropsychological Rehabilitation* 6(4): 305–326.

Prigatano, G. P., Wong, J. L., Williams, C., and Plenge, K. (1997). Prescribed versus actual length of stay and inpatient neurorehabilitation outcome for brain dysfunctional patients. *Arch. Phys. Med. Rehabil.* 78: 621–629.

Romano, M. D. (1974). Family response to traumatic head injury. *Scand. J. Rehabil. Med.* 6: 1–4.

Schafer, R. (1967). *Projective Testing and Psychoanalysis: Selected Papers.* International Universities, New York.

Sternberg, R. (1986). A triangular theory of love. *Psychological Review* 93: 119–135.

Taylor, E. M. (1971). *Psychological Appraisal of Children with Cerebral Deficits.* Harvard University, Cambridge, Mass.

Watzlawick, P. (1983). *The Situation Is Hopeless, but Not Serious: The Pursuit of Unhappiness.* W. W. Norton, New York.

10

Working with Interdisciplinary Rehabilitation Teams

> In a recent *Archives* article Dr. John Melville called to our attention the distinction between multidisciplinary and interdisciplinary activity that may be summarized as follows: Both involved efforts by people from several disciplines and both require that these people have at least passing familiarity with the knowledge and methods of the other disciplines. But interdisciplinary differs from multidisciplinary in that the end product of the effort—the outcome, can only be accomplished by a truly interactive effort in combination from the disciplines involved. In Melville's words, "the product is more than the sum of its parts."
>
> W. Fordyce, "ACRM Presidential Address on Interdisciplinary Peers," 1981, p. 51

Principle 8 of this text states: "Working with brain dysfunctional patients produces affective reactions in both the patient's family and the rehabilitation staff. Appropriate management of these reactions can greatly facilitate the rehabilitation and adaptive process." In Chapter 4, the impact of various forms of brain injury on family members was briefly discussed. In Chapter 8, a model of neuropsychological rehabilitation that explicitly discussed the importance of working with family members was outlined. Chapter 9 further considered possible psychotherapeutic interventions with family members.

The importance of working with rehabilitation staff, especially interdisciplinary teams, has been discussed elsewhere (Prigatano et al., 1986; Prigatano, 1989; Gans, 1983). Seldom, however, are the dynamics and distress that interdisciplinary rehabilitation teams experience discussed explicitly. Such knowledge does not automatically lead to effective group leadership. Yet, a discussion of these issues may help leaders of interdisciplinary rehabilitation teams, as well as team members, work more effectively together.

An earlier version of this chapter was presented as the 17th John S. Young Lecture delivered on April 9, 1993, at the Craig Hospital, Denver, Colorado. The title of that lecture was "Dynamics and distress in interdisciplinary rehabilitation teams." The author especially thanks Dr. Don Gerber at Craig Hospital for the invitation to give this lecture.

Why Have Interdisciplinary Teams?

In his 1980 presidential address to the American Congress of Rehabilitation Medicine, Wilbert Fordyce (1981) reflected on the problems and the potential power of interdisciplinary teams in the field of rehabilitation. He compared interdisciplinary and multidisciplinary approaches and cited John Melvin's work stating that interdisciplinary teams were superior to multidisciplinary teams because they produced better outcomes in rehabilitation (see quote introducing this chapter). Although this conclusion appears to be accurate, it is supported by no scientific data.

Multiple therapies may be needed to treat traumatically brain-injured patients adequately, but how does the interdisciplinary team actually produce a good outcome? The answer may lie in the feature that distinguishes interdisciplinary teams from multidisciplinary teams. True interdisciplinary teams function in an orchestrated manner. Orchestration means that someone directs the activities of team members so that they are controlled, coordinated, and interdependent on one another to produce a specific outcome.

Orchestration is not easy for at least three reasons. First, when higher cerebral deficits are present, it is often difficult to conceptualize exactly what is wrong with the patient's functioning (see Principle 4; also Prigatano, 1989). Thus, knowing what to do from a rehabilitation perspective is not always clear. Second, as is discussed in more detail later, team or group members both want and yet resist leadership. Thus, the capacity to orchestrate depends on the talents and attitudes of both the therapists and clinical director. Third, a good orchestra leader must understand timing and balance to produce a symphony instead of noise. Sometimes, activities performed in the name of rehabilitation often resemble noise.

Interdisciplinary teams are important and needed. They appear to be more useful than multidisciplinary teams, but again systematic data supporting this notion are unavailable.

Interdisciplinary Teams and Group Dynamics

By definition, interdisciplinary teams are small groups. Thus, like other groups, they obey the laws of group dynamics and structure. What are some of these laws?

First, a group forms to meet the needs of its members and will dissolve when it fails to do so. Sherwood Washburn's (1960) article on "Tools and Human Evolution" (in Isaac and Leakey, 1979) noted five distinctive attributes of human evolutionary development: (1) locomotion of the two hind limbs (bipedalism) with the forelimbs free for nonlocomotor functions; (2) dependence on skillfully made tools and equipment for adaptations and survival; (3) enlargement and reorganization of the brain relative to the brains of other higher primates; (4) development of speech and language, and (5) development of social patterns involving cultural controls on aggression and sexual actions and involving the division of labor.

Present neurorehabilitation therapies can readily be identified along this continuum of evolutionary development. Problems related to bipedalism are addressed by physical therapy. Problems related to the skillful use of tools for adaptation are addressed by occupational therapy. Assessment of brain function and attempts at conceptualizing ways of reorganizing brain function are addressed by neuropsychology. Disorders of speech and language are addressed by speech and language therapy. Cultural control of sex and aggression is addressed by a number of disciplines but often includes psychiatry, neurology, clinical psychology, and social work. Both pharmacological and nonpharmacological interventions may be attempted to reinstitute "cultural" control of behavior.

Most relevant to the present discussion, however, is the division of labor. When applied to neurorehabilitation, it appears that interdisciplinary teams have evolved primarily to enable a division of labor. Interdisciplinary teams also evolved to protect rehabilitation groups as a whole. That protection includes providing an administrative and financial structure by which team members can function and provide their services. In the context of this group, a mechanism is provided that allows each therapist to apply his or her specific skills to help a patient to restore function and adapt to impaired functioning after a brain disorder. If the group cannot accomplish these goals adequately, it will dissolve. Thus, a rehabilitation group can dissolve because of inadequate financial and professional support; it can also dissolve because it has failed to achieve its specific goals of an orchestrated effort. The development of the case manager model in neurorehabilitation, as well as in other forms of rehabilitation, in part reflects the failure of interdisciplinary teams to achieve their own goals.

In attempting to maintain themselves and to form their own identity as a group, interdisciplinary teams, as well as other small groups, often develop what can be described as a "we" versus "them" focus. This focus reflects the second law of group dynamics. Groups identify their particular constituency and attempt to support that constituency along some dimension. Individuals who are not members of the group and who may threaten the group's achievement of its goals are considered "them." In interdisciplinary neurorehabilitation teams, persons comprising "them" can become patients themselves, the patients' family, hospital administrators, or insurance carriers. This dynamic can produce significant tensions between the interdisciplinary team and these four groups. The degree to which the interdisciplinary team has insight into these dynamics and attempts to build bonds with each of the external forces often ultimately determines its survival and the rehabilitation outcome for patients. This task, however, is difficult and requires sophistication on the part of group members about the dynamics of interpersonal interaction, small group interaction, and, in some instances, individual member's own intrapsychic dynamics and conflicts.

The famous "Stanford University prison experiment" conducted by Philip G. Zimbardo and colleagues (1973; Haney et al., 1973) gives some valuable clues about the "we" versus "them" phenomenon. Zimbardo produced a "mock prison with a homogeneous group of people who could be considered 'normal-average' on the basis of clinical interviews and personality tests" (p. 38). The experiment had to be stopped prematurely because the college student participants became so abusive to one another that the situation was nothing short of dangerous. Normally functioning college students appeared to overidentify with their role as guards or prisoners and began to act out these roles in a frightening manner. Rumors started, anger emerged, paranoid ideation was common, and unduly harsh and punitive behavior was often exhibited.

Once a group begins to feel "powerless, arbitrarily controlled, dependent, frustrated (and) hopeless . . ." (p. 39), a great deal of intolerant behavior for the "other" group can be expected to emerge. Sincere complaints of feeling sick, for example, may be perceived as manipulative by the other group. Perhaps not as dramatically as observed in Zimbardo's experiment, patients' behavior is still often viewed as manipulative when it may be a response to feeling powerless, arbitrarily controlled, dependent, and frustrated. Brain dysfunctional patients state that their two most common experiences are frustration and confusion (see Chapter 2 and Prigatano, 1992). No wonder significant stresses can develop between patients and staff. Although therapists have definite professional roles to play, their failure to appreciate patients' phenomenological experience can result in the mismanagement or mistreatment of patients, their families, or both (see Principle 1). Two clinical examples highlight this potential.

A young man with an amnestic disorder repeatedly failed to use his memory notebook to compensate for his memory failures. The rehabilitation team understandably tired of reminding him to use his notebook and perhaps became more frustrated than usual with his apparent indifference to their advice.

On a planned outing, it was this patient's responsibility to bring hamburger for barbecue. His therapist, typically supportive and caring, secretly purchased the hamburger because she anticipated that he would forget to do so. On the morning of the planned event, she asked the patient if he had remembered to get the hamburger. The patient had forgotten to do so, immediately panicked, and wanted to go to a store to buy the hamburger. Despite his emotional reaction, the therapist told him that he failed to write the assigned task in his notebook and he would have to face the consequences of his behavior.

The patient remained upset and agitated for the next several hours. When he arrived at the picnic, the therapist finally told him that the hamburger had been purchased because it had been anticipated that he would forget to fulfill his responsibilities. Although the therapist's intent was to teach the patient a lesson, he rightfully felt betrayed. The incident had a powerful negative effect on their working alliance.

This caring therapist had done a frankly uncaring (punitive) act, in part, from her frustration about failing to teach the brain dysfunctional patient the need to use compensatory devices. Such behavior can emerge in the most supportive interdisciplinary teams. The rehabilitation team's ability—both individually and collectively—to recognize that their actions can be punitive as well as caring is extremely important in their maturation.

A second example highlights the we-versus-them phenomenon. On another outing, a group of patients was taken several miles from the rehabilitation center by bus. On the return trip, the therapists responsible for planning the event noticed that they had not refueled the vehicle. An astute patient also observed that the gas tank was reading close to empty. From the patient's perspective, the therapists had repeatedly badgered her for failing to follow through with responsibilities. She therefore immediately pointed out the therapists' shortcomings. Rather than admitting that they had made a mistake, the therapists insisted that they had enough gas for the return trip. In truth, they arrived home with minimal gas in the bus.

This event occurred on Friday. On the following Monday morning, the therapists involved immediately cornered the clinical director as he entered the rehabilitation center. They insisted that he listen to their point of view before he accepted the patients' assertions.

During the ensuing milieu session, the therapists clearly tried to protect their authority rather than admit to their mistake. Their dynamics were discussed at a later staff meeting, where the facts revealed that the therapists had failed to plan for the outing. However, they were concerned that if they admitted their oversight they would lose their credibility with the patients.

The clinical director insisted the opposite was the case. If the therapists could not admit the truth, they would be unable to maintain a working alliance with their patients. Despite their discomfit, the therapists admitted their mistake during the next milieu meeting. To their surprise, the patients were not especially retaliatory. Rather, they were relieved that the therapists could also admit their frailties. Thus, the experienced interdisciplinary team and clinical director must constantly be vigilant for these types of problems and foster honest dialogue among themselves as well as with the patients.

A third law influencing group behavior reflects the group's simultaneous desire both to have and not to have a leader. Groups perform best if they have a sense of direction. It is therefore natural for a leader to rise and take control of the group's activity. The group, however, is composed of individuals, each with his or her own aspirations, feelings, values, and so on. The group is often willing to follow the direction of a leader if that leader is sensitive to their individual needs, helps provide experiences that aid their individual growth and development, and demonstrates that his or her leadership protects the individual members. If a leader fails to meet these needs, other group members will vie for the leadership role and the observing group members will become sensitive to slight shifts in power and control. If these dynamics are not managed properly, the group's activity can be disrupted significantly. The clinical leader's ability to help achieve the overall group's needs as well as to help members meet their individual needs is, perhaps, the most demanding yet essential task confronting a group leader.

The fourth group law is that each group often seeks a scapegoat for its own failures and limitations. One member's perceptions and values are often identified as conflicting with those of the rest of the group. This situation tends to develop when the group's activities are frustrated by reality. That is, when the group is unable to achieve their specific economic, political, or professional goals, they blame somebody other than themselves. This tendency to find a scapegoat can be intense. It is also recurring, a process that never seems to be satisfied fully. It is almost as if the "gods demand a sacrifice" when humans face their daily failures. A clinical director must be able to sense these dynamics and work with team members as they emerge. Specific members sometimes work poorly with the group and must modify their behavior to meet the group's needs. At other times, a divergent perspective is crucial to balance the team. This is a powerful and challenging phenomenon that a sophisticated team must understand and address regularly.

A final corollary embedded in these observations is that a group can be punitive toward other groups as well as toward individual members of its own group if the group's needs are thwarted. Such behavior occurs throughout daily activities. It occurs in local, state, and world politics. It occurs within families and it occurs within professional organizations. Before discussing how these factors can be managed when combining divergent professionals into a group to help patients with brain dysfunction accomplish their goals, we consider some of the major stressors confronted by such interdisciplinary teams.

Stress and Distress in Postacute Brain-Injured Rehabilitation Programs

Health care professionals are at high risk for burnout (Maslach, 1982). Why does caring for other individuals cause such emotional distress? Elsewhere I have discussed therapists' need for patients to be cured or healed in order for therapists to feel a sense of personal well-being (Prigatano, 1989). This may be one of the major unconscious motivations involved in health care delivery and may explain some of the irrational behavior that individual team members may show toward patients and families. However, there are other important sources of stress, particularly for those who work with brain dysfunctional patients (Table 10-1).

Franzen and Myers (1973) observed the social behavior of rhesus monkeys after bilateral ablation of prefrontal or anterior temporal cortex (see Chapter 4). The monkeys displayed several deficits in social behavior. For purposes of this discussion, however, one finding is particularly important: Nonoperated monkeys often withdrew from the monkeys with a brain injury. Franzen and Myers further noted:

> Coinciding with and likely precipitated by the primary behavioral changes induced in the individual monkeys by the specific cerebral lesions were changes in the structuring of the social groups. A long-term reduction in group solidarity became apparent after the prefrontal and anterior temporal lesions. Following these ablations, the number of normal animals remaining to sustain normal social interactions in any given group was reduced. In addition, pronounced emotional disturbances followed the reintroduction of the lesioned animals due to their decreased and inappropriate social signaling (p. 153).

This study highlights that mere interaction with brain dysfunctional patients can distress normal individuals, who tend to withdraw from injured individuals because of their socially inappropriate behavior. This stress is constant for interdisciplinary teams working with postacute brain dysfunctional patients and is a dimension that must be understood and worked with.

Table 10-1. Stressors experienced by interdisciplinary teams in postacute brain injury rehabilitation

---

Inappropriate social reactions of patients with brain injury
Patient's and family's resistance to treatment/rehabilitation
Insurance "hassles"
Administration "hassles"
Lack of scientifically based evidence supporting rehabilitation

---

A second source of distress is patients' resistance and, occasionally, the family's resistance to rehabilitation activities. This problem has been discussed elsewhere (Prigatano et al., 1986; Prigatano, 1989; Ben-Yishay and Prigatano, 1990), but it is worth mentioning that resistance comprises at least two components. One component emanates from disturbances of self-awareness (see Prigatano and Schacter, 1991). Patients do not fully understand how their injuries have affected them and consequently do not perceive a need for treatment. A major goal (and stress) on the rehabilitative team is to find ways to engage patients in rehabilitation despite their socially inappropriate behavior and their resistance to treatment.

Besides these neurologically based difficulties, personality or nonneurological variables can contribute to patients' resistance. Before their injury, patients might have had manipulative, distrustful, or other negative personality characteristics whose presence still prevents them from following the guidance of therapists after their injury.

Furthermore, some family members may be so exhausted by the changes in their brain-injured relative that they doubt that rehabilitation can provide any useful assistance. They may resist rehabilitative efforts either passively or actively, especially when the cost of treatment is high and insurance coverage is low.

The health care delivery system also can be a source of stress for rehabilitation therapists. A growing literature documents that quality of life is not just measured by significant life changes, as the early work by Holmes and Rahe (1967) indicated. Rather, hassles and minor events that affect our daily functioning make a considerable contribution to an individual's sense of well-being. Chamberlain and colleagues (e.g., Zika and Chamberlain, 1987; Chamberlain and Zika, 1990) noted that chronic daily stressors (or hassles, as they call them) have a direct effect on a person's sense of well-being. They also found that individuals' sense of mental health is often related to whether they derive a sense of meaning from their work (Zika and Chamberlain, 1992).

What hassles typically confront a treatment team? A major hassle is the requirement of insurance companies for excessive documentation about progress in rehabilitation. A more important stressor is the growing tendency for third-party payers to determine appropriate lengths of stay and treatments. This tendency, of course, is managed care at its worst: payers dictating treatment based on a bottom-line mentality rather than the patients' needs. Gabbard (1990) described the predictable negative impact of this scenario on milieu-based treatment programs. This problem, however, partially reflects interdisciplinary teams' failure to demonstrate their efficacy and to provide outcome studies to support the need for their interventions. A recent research project has addressed this question as it applies to inpatient neurorehabilitation (Prigatano, et al., 1997).

Another major stress is related to dealing with administrative personnel in the delivery of services. Although any form of health care service needs to make an appropriate profit, hospital administrators may have an unrealistic perspective concerning legitimate fees for services and rates of return for investments in providing rehabilitative services. Dealing with administrators who do not fully understand that rehabilitation services cannot be equated to "EEGs per unit of time" or "echocardiograms per unit of time" is an ongoing battle in many settings.

Because providing billable services is emphasized, therapists must obtain a certain number of "billable hours" each day, week, and month to feel secure in their jobs and for hospital administrators to feel comfortable with their financial investment in a program. Frank discussions about legitimate rates of economic growth that can be expected from rehabilitation are necessary. The therapeutic impact of neurorehabilitation may be limited, but its contributions are still valuable and important. Appropriate economic goals must be established with this basic clinical fact in mind.

The final stressor concerns professional responsibilities. Interdisciplinary neurorehabilitation teams have not done their scientific homework. Few controlled studies have examined the efficacy of various forms of neurorehabilitation for patients with brain dysfunction (see Prigatano et al., 1997). Elsewhere, I have discussed the importance of neurorehabilitation teams identifying their outcome goals for a given patient group, of clarifying entry criteria for a given program, and of studying the efficacy of neurorehabilitation activities with some type of controlled method of observation (Prigatano et al., 1984; Prigatano et al., 1986; Prigatano et al., 1994; Prigatano et al., 1997). There are many arguments why people involved in rehabilitation do not investigate the efficacy of their interventions. None of these arguments, however, are professionally or ethically responsible. Until this problem is rectified, therapists will experience this stress in many forms and, frankly, deserve to do so.

Methods of Managing Interdisciplinary Teams

The management of an interdisciplinary team is a formidable task. The clinical director must attend to the needs of the team, patient, family, third-party payers, and administration. The clinical director of such teams must be alert to the role of group dynamics and to the stresses experienced by interdisciplinary teams. Often managing team members is more stressful than managing brain dysfunctional patients and their families.

Why, then, form and attempt to manage interdisciplinary teams? The answer is because interdisciplinary teams have the potential to provide comprehensive care to brain-injured patients. This method of treatment

Table 10-2. Advantages and disadvantages of interdisciplinary teams

Positive	Negative
Different sources of information about the patient create a more comprehensive patient profile	Adds needless information and can disrupt priorities
Different patients get along with different therapists	Certain patients and staff do not get along with each other (can reflect an indirect assault on a fellow staff member)
Staff can learn from each other	Staff can be territorial about "their" job duties and responsibilities
Burden of care is shared	Increases burden of care
Group benefits from effective leadership	Group may both want and reject a leader. Also, the team is only as strong as its weakest member

attends to the whole person and consequently has the chance to make a great impact. This model also permits a meaningful way to assess the total impact of neurorehabilitation as opposed to assessing the impact of each discipline. In short, if conducted properly, interdisciplinary teams provide a meaningful, although at times stressful, work setting.

Attempting to manage interdisciplinary teams and my own reactions to them, I find that reflecting on the pros and cons of such teams is important (Table 10-2) for maintaining perspective. Interdisciplinary teams offer different sources of information that can provide a comprehensive profile of patients. With interdisciplinary teams, different therapists can work with a patient so that if a given therapist does not "click" with a given patient or family member at a given time in treatment, others may fill that role. This flexibility can help establish a working alliance when resistance to treatment surfaces early in the rehabilitation process. Interdisciplinary team members can teach one another about patients' difficulties. When approached properly, this aspect permits the burden of care to be distributed among team members. It is hoped that both interdisciplinary teams and the patients and families will benefit from a group's leadership.

There is always a downside, of course. Sometimes team members provide needless or erroneous information, which can create confusion about a patient's problems and the issues most in need of attention. Staff can also react negatively to given patients and their reaction can disrupt the patients' overall care. Staff can also project their feelings about other staff members onto patients and hence react negatively to them. Therefore, interstaff conflict can sometimes be played out by a patient-staff conflict. Staff members can also become territorial rather than shar-

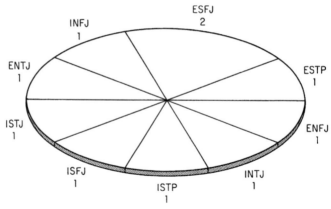

Figure 10-1. Myers-Briggs personality profiles obtained in a heterogenous group of brain dysfunctional patients involved in a milieu-oriented neuropsychological rehabilitation program.

ing the responsibilities of caring for patients. Finally, interdisciplinary teams increase the burden of care and produce a more costly venture for both administration and clinical director. Nevertheless, when team members are selected and managed properly, a balanced perspective can emerge. Writing practice critiques like this one also helps clinical directors gain perspective that may be lost in the daily routine.

Clinical directors also must consider the actual differences in each team member's personality style and psychodynamics. Trying to accommodate and use these differences to clarify rather than confuse treatment approaches is helpful. For example, Figures 10-1 and 10-2 represent typical personality types of various team members and their patients in a neurorehabilitation setting. Based on the Myers-Briggs Type Indicator (Myers and McCaulley, 1989), various patient types are treated in a neuropsychologically oriented milieu-based program. Some patients tend to be introverted, others are extroverted; some rely on intuition as a major source of information whereas others prefer sensory information; and some use feelings to make decisions and others use thinking.

In contrast, rehabilitation staff who do this type of work seem to cluster along certain dimensions. One group tends to be introverted, intuitive, and feeling (Fig. 10-2). In some ways, these therapists represent the traditional prototype of a psychotherapist who has not worked with brain dysfunctional patients. Other therapists, however, tend to be more extroverted and more sensory in their orientation, even though they tend to focus on feelings when making decisions. In our program, this group tends to be the physical, occupational, and recreational therapists. Therapists with an extrovert-sensory-thinking profile may be viewed by other team members as "cold" toward patients. In fact, one therapist with this profile left our milieu-oriented rehabilitation program, in part, because

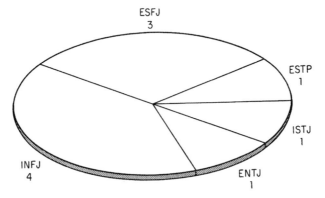

Figure 10-2. Myers-Briggs personality profiles obtained on the rehabilitation staff and supportive personnel of a milieu-oriented neuropsychological rehabilitation program.

she felt unaccepted by her coworkers. Therapists with extrovert-intuitive-thinking profiles are needed to help make policy decisions and to present neuropsychological patient findings to the scientific and lay communities.

Thus, a clinical director must accommodate different personality styles to achieve a balanced team, and the team must recognize that their psychological approach to the world may be quite different from the patients' experience of the world. This argument underlines the importance of entering patients' phenomenological fields when attempting to engage them in rehabilitation.

A third method of managing interdisciplinary teams is to provide a forum for the regular review of patient-staff and staff-staff relations. Such a review can be done within the context of a daily staff meeting and is extremely helpful (Prigatano et al., 1986). Both administrative and patient issues can be reviewed, and interstaff tension can be approached.

Five other tools are useful in managing interdisciplinary teams (Table 10-3). First, for any rehabilitation program, patients must be selected carefully. Selecting patients who have a realistic chance of benefitting from a given program goes a long way to raise the morale of interdisciplinary staff and to allow them to use their talents most effectively. Second, staff, too, must be selected carefully. Not everyone can work on an interdisciplinary team. However, staff members who enjoy interacting with other disciplines and combining efforts and who can look at their own dynamics form an extremely important subgroup of therapists who are able to work effectively in this setting. Third, external consultants can also be helpful in managing a team. Having a consultant psychiatrist listen to the staff's personal reactions to patients and to the difficulties they have with one another has helped clarify issues that can then be

Table 10-3. Methods of managing interdisciplinary teams

Review pros and cons of interdisciplinary teams
Appreciate different personality styles of interdisciplinary team members
Provide a forum for regular review of patient-staff and staff-staff relationships
Select patients carefully
Select staff carefully
Use external consultants
Take periodic respites from work
Incorporate clinical research as a part of the interdisciplinary team's
    responsibilities

---

resolved. Fourth, interdisciplinary team members need a respite from this type of work, which can be provided through a vacation policy and a flexible schedule. Sabbaticals from this form of work are another option. Finally, staff must be involved in clinical research projects that measure the efficacy of their work. Such involvement is extremely important for the team's growth and development. Research provides an opportunity to evaluate the efficacy of therapeutic interventions objectively and also checks therapists' assumptions about the work that might be wrong. By renewing the commitment to analyze the effectiveness of rehabilitation, therapists can maintain an attitude of wonder and learning, which is crucial to maintaining a creative approach to the work.

Change in Interdisciplinary Teams

Even the most well-developed and smooth-running interdisciplinary team will experience changes in membership and leadership. These changes can improve the neuropsychological rehabilitation effort or herald its decline. Neuropsychological programs are dynamic entities (Principle 9). It is often difficult to determine immediately if such changes in membership are positive or negative. Typically, 1 or 2 years elapse before the impact of the changes is revealed.

The outcome measures of such change can be seen in the group's clinical and research productivity. Do the outcome statistics reveal a greater percentage of patients returning and maintaining a productive lifestyle? Are team members innovative about their conceptions of the various patient problems they encounter? Do the team members, individually or collectively, publish their observations in peer-reviewed journals? Do the team members, individually and collectively, show evidence of enhanced professional development as reflected by their capacity to remain creative despite inevitable conflicts? These questions must be answered to determine how to help interdisciplinary rehabilitation teams best and to determine which types of patient problems such teams can best address.

Summary and Conclusions

Interdisciplinary rehabilitation teams are groups and, by their nature, demonstrate many of the positive and negative characteristics associated with group behavior. Patients with brain injuries present formidable challenges to such teams, particularly during the postacute phase of rehabilitation. By understanding some of the typical group dynamics and stressors of interdisciplinary teams, clinical directors may be in a better position to manage the team. This task, however, is not easy. As noted in Principle 8, daily contact and work with brain-damaged patients produce powerful negative reactions in both the patient's family and rehabilitation staff. If the rehabilitation team can manage their reactions to these patients and their interpersonal behaviors toward one another, neuropsychological rehabilitation programs develop in a positive manner. Otherwise, the neuropsychological rehabilitation efforts typically deteriorate after 1 to 2 years (Principle 9).

For rehabilitation team members to remain active and creative in their work, they must learn to manage their personal reactions to patients and their fellow staff members. They also must learn to expand their knowledge about mechanisms of change associated with various forms of brain injury so that neuropsychological rehabilitation can continue to develop on a firm scientific basis. Failure to do so often results in selecting inappropriate patients and maintaining ineffective rehabilitation activities. This course ultimately leads to a lack of credibility for the entire field (Principle 10). Such failures can also destroy the morale and creativity of the rehabilitation staff.

Neurorehabilitation therapists tend to attribute positive outcomes to their therapeutic interventions (Macciocchi and Eaton, 1995). In contrast, they often attribute negative outcomes to factors other than their professional skills. The need for objective evaluation of neurorehabilitation outcomes is crucial both for teams to continue to mature and for establishing scientific credibility.

References

Ben-Yishay, Y., and Prigatano, G. P. (1990). Cognitive remediation. In E. Griffith, M. Rosenthal, M. R. Bond, and J. D. Miller (eds), *Rehabilitation of the Adult and Child with Traumatic Brain Injury* (pp. 393–409). F. W. Davis, Philadelphia.
Chamberlain, K., and Zika, S. (1990). The minor events approach to stress: support for the use of daily hassles. *Br. J. Psychol.* 81: 469–481.

Fordyce, W. E. (1981). ACRM Presidential Address on Interdisciplinary Peers. *Arch. Phys. Med. Rehabil.* 62: 51–53.

Franzen, E. A., and Meyers, R. E. (1973). Neural control of social behavior: prefrontal and anterior temporal cortex. *Neuropsychologia* 11: 141–157.

Gabbard, G. O. (1990). The therapeutic relationship in psychiatric hospital treatment. *Bull. Menninger Clin.* 56(1): 4–19.

Gans, J. S. (1983). Hate in the rehabilitation setting. *Arch. Phys. Med. Rehabil.* 64: 176–179.

Haney, C., Banks, C., and Zimbardo, P. (1973). Interpersonal dynamics in a simulated prison. *International Journal of Criminology and Penology* 1: 69–97.

Holmes, T., and Rahe, R. (1967). The social readjustment rating scale. *J. Psychosomatic Research* 11: 213–218.

Isaac, G., and Leakey, R. E. F. (1979). Introduction. In G. Isaac and R. E. F. Leakey (eds), (pp. 2–8) *Readings from Scientific American. Human Ancestors.* W. H. Freeman, San Francisco.

Macciocchi, S. N., and Eaton B. (1995). Decision and attribution bias in neurorehabilitation. *Arch. Phys. Med. Rehabil.* 76: 521–524.

Maslach, C. (1982). *Burnout—The Cost of Caring.* Prentice Hall, New York.

Myers, I. B., and McCaulley, M. H. (1989). *Manual: A Guide to the Development and Use of the Myers-Briggs Type Indicator.* Consulting Psychologist, Palo Alto, Calif.

Prigatano, G. P. (1989). Bring it up in milieu: toward effective traumatic brain injury rehabilitation interaction. *Rehabilitation Psychology* 34(2): 135–144.

Prigatano, G. P. (1992). What does the brain injured person experience? Implications for rehabilitation. Centennial Lecture in Brain Injury Rehabilitation, American Psychological Association Convention, Washington, D.C.

Prigatano, G. P., Fordyce, D. J., Zeiner, H. K., Roueche, J. R., Pepping, M., and Wood, B. (1984). Neuropsychological rehabilitation after closed head injury in young adults. *J. Neurol. Neurosurg. Psychiatry* 47: 505–513.

Prigatano, G. P., Klonoff, P. S., O'Brien, K. P., Altman, I., Amin, K., Chiapello, D. A., Shepherd, J., Cunningham, M., and Mora, M. (1994). Productivity after neuropsychologically oriented, milieu rehabilitation. *Journal of Head Trauma Rehabilitation* 9(1): 91–102.

Prigatano, G. P., et al. (1986). *Neuropsychological Rehabilitation After Brain Injury.* Johns Hopkins University, Baltimore.

Prigatano, G. P., and Schacter, D. L. (1991). *Awareness of Deficit after Brain Injury: Theoretical and Clinical Issues.* Oxford University Press, New York.

Prigatano, G. P., Wong, J. L., Williams, C., and Plenge, K. (1997). Prescribed versus actual length of stay and inpatient neurorehabilitation outcome for brain dysfunctional patients. *Arch. Phys. Med. Rehabil.* 78: 621–629.

Washburn, S. (1960). Tools and human evolution. In G. Isaac and R. E. F. Leakey (eds), *Readings from Scientific American. Human Ancestors* (pp. 1–21). W. H. Freeman, San Francisco.

Zika, S., and Chamberlain, K. (1987). Relation of hassles and personality to subjective well-being. *J. Pers. Soc. Psychol.* 53(1): 55–162.

Zika, S., and Chamberlain, K. (1992). On the relation between meaning in life and psychological well-being. *Br. J. Psychol.* 83: 133–145.

Zimbardo, P. G., Haney, C., Banks, W. C., and Jaffe, D. (1973). The mind is a formidable jailer: a Pirandellian prison. *New York Times Magazine* April 8, 38–60.

11

The Outcome of Neuropsychological Rehabilitation Programs that Incorporate Cognitive Rehabilitation and Psychotherapeutic Intervention

You can't be a sourpuss and be rehabilitated.
Y. Ben-Yishay, Degendorf, Germany, 1993

Neuropsychological rehabilitation that is holistic in scope and embedded in a milieu day-treatment program often seems to produce the best outcomes for patients with traumatic brain injuries (TBIs), but opinions on this proposition differ (Malec and Basford, 1996). This chapter focuses on the clinical and scientific evidence that supports the clinical usefulness (or efficacy) of such programs of care. To aid this analysis, four interconnected questions must be considered (as outlined in Chapter 4).

1. Do holistic "milieu-oriented" neuropsychological rehabilitation programs improve the psychosocial functioning of persons with brain injury?
2. Do cognitive retraining and rehabilitation improve higher cerebral functioning?
3. Do certain forms of cognitive rehabilitation substantially help individuals with brain dysfunction to compensate for persistent and residual impairments?
4. Do psychotherapeutic interventions help patients adjust to the permanent effects of brain damage in a meaningful and long-lasting manner?

The Efficacy of Holistic Milieu-Oriented Neuropsychological Rehabilitation Programs

Prigatano and colleagues (1984) first studied the efficacy of a holistic milieu-oriented rehabilitation program by using an untreated control group (*not* a historical control group as reported by Malic and Basford, 1996). Eighteen TBI patients were compared to 17 TBI patients who either elected not to enter the treatment program or who lacked the financial resources for the treatment. The groups were compared on neuropsychological tests, personality measures, relatives' ratings of the patients' emotional status, and employment measures. Treated patients had a higher incidence of employment, and their emotional status, as reported by relatives, was considerably better than that of the untreated group. This study provided the first empirical evidence that such programs of care have useful psychosocial consequences. In this and a following study with a larger sample (Prigatano, et al., 1986), these authors emphasized that *both* cognitive and personality factors related to a "successful outcome" (i.e., return to work). Disturbances in self-awareness, complicated disturbances that often reflect both neurological and non-neurological factors, were identified as important for outcome and as areas that needed to receive considerable attention during treatment.

Soon thereafter, Ben-Yishay and colleagues (1985) summarized their experiences and outcome with 100 brain dysfunctional patients treated within a holistic neuropsychological rehabilitation program. They reported that 50% of their TBI patients returned to work, a statistic identical to that reported by Prigatano and colleagues (1984) for patients in a completely different environment (i.e., Oklahoma City versus New York City). These studies represent the first cross-validation of outcomes of neurorehabilitation programs.

Albeit in a limited scientific fashion, these studies documented the potential psychosocial usefulness of a holistic milieu-oriented neuropsychological rehabilitation program for postacute TBI patients. Scherzer (1986) then reported outcomes that Malec and Basford (1996) correctly classified as "contrastingly dismal results (e.g., 69% unemployed at follow-up)" (p. 201). A careful reading of Scherzer (1986), however, clarifies this discrepancy. Scherzer's (1986) program did not appear to devote adequate attention to personality disturbances associated with brain dysfunction. Patients had only 1 hour of individual counseling each week for 30 weeks. Therapeutic community meetings, also held only once each week, dealt with issues of awareness and acceptance and attempted to teach patients emotional control. The group activity also attempted to help patients express their feelings about how they had been affected and to improve their social or interpersonal interactions.

Affective disturbances of TBI patients, however, require much more attention if patients are to improve in terms of their personality function and the associated problems of impaired awareness and lack of acceptance of their permanent neuropsychological disabilities (Prigatano and Ben-Yishay, 1999). Individual and small group therapy activities aimed at these problems often are needed daily (Prigatano, et al., 1986). Therefore, Scherzer's (1986) program appears to have been substantially different than the programs described by Prigatano and colleagues (1984) and Ben-Yishay and colleagues (1985). These differences likely account for their "contrastingly dismal results."

Later, Ezrachi, Ben-Yishay, Kay, Diller, and Rattok (1991) specifically addressed the question of what factors "appeared to predict who will benefit vocationally from a neuropsychological rehabilitation program . . ." (p. 72). The authors noted that from their clinical experience, the patients whose awareness and acceptance of their deficits improved benefited the most from their holistic neuropsychological rehabilitation program. The study included 59 patients with moderate to severe TBIs who underwent rehabilitation at the New York University (NYU) Head Trauma Program. The impact of several sets of variables on treatment outcome was evaluated: demographic characteristics, neuropsychological test findings, functional behavioral ratings of the group process, ratings of the rehabilitation staff concerning the patient's behavior before and after brain injury, and the patients' acceptance of their condition. The staff also rated the degree to which patients received ongoing family support. Repeatedly, patients' capacity to "regulate affect" before and after rehabilitation related to their vocational outcome. Prigatano and colleagues (1984) made a similar point: Patients who were free of psychiatric disturbance before and after brain injury tended to return to a productive lifestyle more frequently than patients who lacked these characteristics.

The capacity for realistic self-appraisal also correlated with vocational outcome (r values ranged from .60 to .67; Ezrachi, et al., 1991). Verbal problem-solving skills and the ability to be involved with others appropriately correlated with vocational outcome at a similar level. Unfortunately, Ezrachi and colleagues (1991) included no control group to demonstrate that untreated TBI patients' poor awareness and acceptance of their disabilities related to unemployment or social isolation. These authors, however, made the following point:

> . . . the concept of awareness as a prerequisite to successful rehabilitation after TBI makes contact with a concept of developing a therapeutic alliance as a prerequisite to successful psychotherapy. Recent research in psychotherapy outcome research points to a confluence of studies that suggest that measures of alliance in the course of treatment are powerful predictors of outcome (p. 83).

Prigatano and colleagues (1994) later confirmed that the working or therapeutic alliance with brain dysfunctional patients and their families related to patients' productivity status after they had completed a neuropsychologically oriented rehabilitation program (Table 11-1). A similar relationship exists between patients' productivity status and the strength of the working relationship with family members ($\chi^2=7.3$; df $= 1, p<.01$).

Table 11-1. Therapists' modal ratings of working alliance with patients related to patients' productivity status

Productivity Status	Therapists' Modal Ratings	
	Excellent/Good	Fair/Poor
Productive	21	8
Nonproductive	2	6

$\chi^2=5.99$; df$=1$; $p<0.05$.

Reprinted with permission from Prigatano, G. P., Klonoff, P. S., O'Brien, K. P., Altman, I., Amin, K., Chiapello, D. A., Shepherd, J., Cunningham, M., and Mora, M. (1994). Productivity after neuropsychologically oriented, millieu rehabilitation. *Journal of Head Trauma Rehabilitation* 9(1): 91–102. Copyright © 1994 Aspen Publishers, Inc.

These studies provide empirical support for the notion that outcome depends on the quality of the therapeutic alliance.

Prigatano and colleagues (1994) also demonstrated that patients who participated in neuropsychologically oriented rehabilitation programs have a high incidence of productivity, replicating their early findings (Prigatano, et al., 1984). Thirty-five brain dysfunctional patients were matched to 36 historical untreated control patients in terms of admitting Glasgow Coma Scale (GCS) score and other variables. Almost 49% of the treated patients returned to full-time employment compared to 36% of the control patients. Furthermore, 14% of the treated patients were working in meaningful voluntary positions. None of the controls reported such work. In the treated group, only one of the 35 (2.9%) patients reported being "unable to work." In contrast, 13 (36.1%) of the untreated control patients reported being "unable to work" (Table 11-2). Apparently, the holistic milieu-oriented neuropsychological rehabilitation program helped change the attitudes of many TBI patients and in so doing helped them to obtain a productive lifestyle.

For patients to regain a productive life after TBI requires far more intervention than a traditional supportive employment model offers (Malic and Basford, 1996). It often requires daily work in dealing with the emotional and motivational disturbances of TBI patients. Often, some form of psychotherapeutic interventions must be included (Prigatano and Ben-Yishay, 1999). When these ingredients are part of a neuropsychological rehabilitation program, the psychosocial outcomes of TBI patients appear to be enhanced.

Two additional studies further support this contention. Christensen and colleagues (1992) reported the psychosocial outcomes of primarily Danish-speaking brain dysfunctional patients treated at the Center for Rehabilitation of Brain Damage at the University of Copenhagen. As these authors recognize, their program borrowed heavily from the programmatic activities developed by Ben-Yishay and coworkers and Pri-

Table 11-2. Frequency analysis of responses to the question: "What best describes what the patient was doing most of the last week?"

	Treated Patients		Control Patients	
	Number out of 35	Percent	Number out of 36	Percent
Working full time	17	48.6	13	36.1
Working part time	5	14.3	4	11.1
Looking for work	2	5.7	2	5.6
Unable to work	1	2.9	13	36.1
Homemaker	—		1	2.8
Retired	—		1	2.8
Other	5	14.3		—
Unknown	—		2	5.6
Volunteer	5	14.3		—

Reprinted with permission from Prigatano, G. P., Klonoff, P. S., O'Brien, K. P., Altman, I., Amin, K., Chiapello, D. A., Shepherd, J., Cunningham, M., and Mora, M. (1994). Productivity after neuropsychologically oriented, millieu rehabilitation. *Journal of Head Trauma Rehabilitation* 9(1): 91–102. Copyright © 1994 Aspen Publishers, Inc.

gatano and associates. Christensen and colleagues (1992) stated that "the general objectives of the program are to achieve independence in the home and the community, and, as far as possible, to return to productive work" (p. 33).

They reported a significant improvement in a number of these dimensions, including the number of hours spent at work activities before and after rehabilitation. Teasdale and Christensen (1994) showed that these gains decreased the use of health care services and were substantially sustained across a 3.5-year follow-up. Moreover, the cost of treatment was recuperated by the reductions in the use of health care services during the 3.5 years of follow-up (Table 11-3, Mehlbye and Larsen, 1994). "The economic analysis shows that an average saving of approximately DKK 190,000 per student was achieved with regard to the costs of public treatment and care (the costs of the stay at the Center not included)" (p. 263). The average cost of the rehabilitation program paid for itself. Assuming many of these patients maintained their increased functional independence and social integration, additional savings would accrue and support the long-term cost-effectiveness of this form of postacute neuropsychological rehabilitation.

Rattok and colleagues (1992) compared three combinations of neuropsychological treatments in terms of various outcome measures and found differential effects. One treatment mix balanced various forms of cognitive remediation, small-group interactions, which emphasized interpersonal adjustment skills and community activities, and personal counseling. The second treatment condition lacked several hours of cognitive remediation and the third lacked small-group interaction thera-

Table 11-3. The costs before, during, and after treatment at the center

Time	Costs/Month/Person (DKK)
Before treatment	11,630
During treatment	5,331
Just after treatment	5,843
1 year after treatment	7,802
3 years after treatment	3,675
Reduced costs in the whole period	−190,400

From Mehlbye, J. and Larsen, A. (1994). Social and economic consequences of brain damage in Denmark: a case study. In A. L. Christensen and B. P. Uzzell (eds), *Brian Injury and Neuropsychological Rehabilitation. International Perspectives* (pp. 257–267). Lawrence Erlbaum, Hillsdale, NJ. With permission from Lawrence Erlbaum.

pies. While their findings are limited because of the absence of an untreated control group, they noted the following:

> ... the gains achieved through participation in the program can be attributed, in the case of most subjects, to improvement in general alertness and ability to maintain focused attention, and to increased efficiency in applying residual abilities (Rattok, et al., 1992, p. 406).

These findings continue to suggest that neuropsychologically oriented rehabilitation programs, which foster a holistic milieu approach, can help some patients use their residual cognitive skills more effectively.

The study of Rattok and colleagues (1992) also suggested that training in interpersonal skills was specifically related to achieving greater regulation of affect—an important adaptive ability. They also noted that such training helped patients improve their self-appraisal.

Although there were no differences on employability measures among the patients who received the different mixtures of therapy, patients who received cognitive rehabilitation performed better on selected cognitive measures. Patients who received more small group or interpersonal exercises performed proportionately better on the measure of self-appraisal as noted above. The authors concluded that psychometric tests scores are useful but may not be strong indications of change after neuropsychological rehabilitation because they are too insensitive to reflect a number of important changes that actually occur.

Collectively, these studies suggest the three following points:

1. A day-treatment, milieu-oriented holistic neuropsychological rehabilitation program, which, by definition, includes cognitive remediation and psychotherapeutic interventions, appears to improve the psychosocial outcome of postacute TBI patients (i.e., increases the likelihood of employment, reduces social isolation, and increases emotional adjustment and control of disruptive affect).

2. Working on different domains of function (cognitive versus inter-personal) appears to be associated with differential changes in some (but not all) patients.
3. Holistic neuropsychological rehabilitation programs can be cost effective for postacute brain dysfunctional patients.

As Malec and Basford (1996) concluded, well-designed clinical trials aimed at evaluating postacute brain injury rehabilitation programs are needed. The initial answer to whether holistic milieu-oriented rehabilitation programs improve the psychosocial functioning of persons with brain injury is yes. This affirmation, however, must be tempered: These therapies must be provided by a competent team that understands the strengths and limitations of such forms of interventions.

Does Cognitive Retraining-Rehabilitation Improve Higher Cerebral Functioning?

Some postacute brain dysfunctional patients seem to improve in several cognitive domains in a clinically meaningful way after cognitive rehabilitation (Rattok, et al., 1992). Yet cognitive rehabilitation aimed at directly remediating an impairment of brain function remains controversial. Ben-Yishay and Diller (1993) concluded that "It would be premature to draw definitive conclusions regarding its validity and use for rehabilitation purposes based on current evidence" (p. 294).

Clinically, postacute TBI patients often fatigue easily and may become increasingly depressed as time passes (Fordyce, et al., 1983). The daily cognitive and group exercises may improve their overall mental energy. This phenomenon, however, is difficult to measure because we have no psychometric for "mental energy" (Prigatano and Henderson, 1997). After the first few days of treatment, many TBI patients who participate in such rehabilitation programs go home and sleep for several hours. With time the patients seem to need less rest and sleep, and they are able to engage the various cognitive and associated rehabilitation activities adequately. Thus, these neurorehabilitation activities may improve patients' overall level of mental energy, even though the variable is difficult to measure.

Another possibility is that interpersonal interactions coupled with the various forms of psychotherapeutic interventions substantially reduce the severity of patients' depression. Depression can affect mental status adversely, particularly memory and concentration (Strubb and Black, 1985). It is often assumed that the capacity of depressed patients is inadequate to sustain the effort needed to perform various psychometric tasks. Perhaps neuropsychologically oriented rehabilitation affects this broad dimension.

Pliskin and colleagues (1996) have written a scholarly and accurate review on the effectiveness of cognitive rehabilitation when used to treat patients with cerebral vascular accidents (CVAs). Considering the evidence on the efficacy of cognitive retraining for remediating language, attention, and perceptual disorders, they note that the overall scientific database is at best nonconclusive and at worst negative, despite reports of positive results. In terms of the efficacy of language therapy, for example, they state the following: "A study by Wertz, et al. (1986) indicated that the effectiveness of treatment cannot be demonstrated when variables that influence recovery are tightly controlled (e.g., age, number and location of CVAs, premorbid psychological condition, premorbid physiological condition, and social support)" (p. 198).

This comment could equally apply to the treatment of various cognitive deficits when the focus is the restoration of impaired function in adult brain dysfunctional patients. Neither the technology nor the methodology exists for treating these basic cognitive impairments in the mature brain. Consequently, Wilson (1997) recently reminded us that contemporary cognitive retraining focuses more on the management of disability than on the treatment of the underlying impairment. As discussed in Chapter 13, however, understanding the variables that influence change after brain injury (both recovery and deterioration) may lead to more effective forms of cognitive retraining in the future, particularly in the developing brain.

Prigatano and colleagues (1996) observed the following about cognitive rehabilitation after TBI:

> Cognitive rehabilitation is not used so much to restore lost higher cerebral functioning, but to use residual functions to maximum capacity. In this regard, one specific goal of cognitive rehabilitation is to help the patient attend to and process information more effectively. This in turn helps patients positively respond to feedback from individual therapists as well as from others in various group settings. This capacity to learn from small group interaction has been reported to be an important predictor for vocational outcome in TBI patients (Ben-Yishay and Prigatano, 1990) (pp. 233–234).

Thus, the answer to the question, does cognitive retraining or rehabilitation directly improve higher cerebral functioning in adults after acquired brain injury, is at present no.

Given this sober conclusion, why should cognitive rehabilitation be considered an important part of neuropsychological rehabilitation as described in Chapter 8? The answer is clear. Cognitive rehabilitation helps patients to use their residual capacities to improve their abilities to problem solve and adapt. This assertion is supported by two clinical scenarios. First, cognitive retraining may help patients understand the nature of their impairment or disability better. This is an extremely valuable contribution (Prigatano, 1987; Klonoff, et al., 1989). Cognitive retraining can help patients choose specific courses of action that help them succeed. For example, via cognitive retraining, patients may choose to learn specific skills like data entry (Glisky and Schachter, 1987). This choice may help them obtain a job. Second, by teaching patients appropriate compensatory skills for their various impairments (Prigatano, et al., 1986), cognitive retraining aids adaptation.

Does Cognitive Rehabilitation Help Patients to Compensate for Persistent and Residual Impairments?

Before a brain dysfunctional patient can seriously consider the need to use compensatory strategies to cope with cognitive impairments to reduce their disabilities, they must recognize that they have an impairment that debilitates their function. As noted, one of the most fascinating aspects of disturbed higher cerebral functions is that consciousness about these impairments is often impaired (see Chapter 12). Thus, helping patients become "more aware" of how their brain injury has actually affected them is emphasized.

Why make patients aware, however? Improved awareness for what purpose? The answer is that improved awareness improves adaptation. Adaptation can be improved by avoiding destructive choices (see Chapter 9 on psychotherapeutic interventions) or by using appropriate compensatory techniques to fulfill commitments in life. But what is the evidence that present compensation techniques work? How can patients be helped to recognize the need to use compensation techniques?

Prigatano and colleagues (1993) studied whether adults with TBIs would spontaneously use compensatory techniques when attempting to perform a simple but demanding paired-association learning task. TBI patients did not use self-initiated compensations as often as non–brain dysfunctional control subjects. When TBI patients did use a self-generated compensation, it did not appear to help improve their performance. In contrast, controls who used compensations performed better than controls who did not use compensations.

At least two important lessons can be learned from this study. First, TBI patients may not spontaneously recognize the need to use compensatory techniques. Second, even if they do use such techniques, they may not benefit from them. Many of the cognitive retraining activities briefly described in Chapter 8 give patients an opportunity to observe their behavior systematically over time and to determine under what conditions compensation may be helpful to them. Such "objective" feedback about their performance when they do not use compensation techniques (as well as interpersonal feedback) often helps patients to become more realistic about the nature of their disabilities and the need to use compensatory strategies. This process seldom depresses patients. Rather, as their perplexity about "what is wrong" seems to be reduced, they begin to recognize their need for compensatory techniques.

Compensatory techniques help patients to reduce their disability (Wilson, 1995). For example, a densely amnestic patient treated within the context of neuropsychological rehabilitation was able to maintain a voluntary job precisely because she used an extensive compensatory technique based on external queuing (Kime, et al., 1996). Patients who achieve greater levels of functional independence use more compensations in their daily activities than patients who do not (Wilson, 1991). The actual level of memory impairment (as measured by psychometric scores) does not relate to the degree of independence.

Patients with focal lesions and more restrictive cognitive deficits may be in a good position to recognize the need to use compensatory techniques. Patients with more diffuse lesions, particularly those involving the heteromodal cortex (see Chapter 12), often have reduced levels of self-awareness about their impairments and disabilities. Patients often appear indifferent to or resist using compensatory techniques, especially after severe TBI. Consequently, the programs directed by Ben-Yishay and colleagues and Prigatano and colleagues have been developed primarily to deal with this problem.

In terms of the usefulness of cognitive rehabilitation to help patients compensate for impairments and thereby reduce disability, the greatest success yet has been in compensating for memory disorders (Baddeley, et al., 1995). The efficacy of compensation in other areas of functioning (i.e., judgment and problem solving) has been much less impressive (von Cramon and Matthes-von Cramon, 1992).

Compensations often fail to restore an individual to a premorbid level of functioning. Rather, after significant brain injury, compensatory techniques help individuals to return to a productive and independent lifestyle albeit in a less demanding environment. At the appropriate time, this intent must be made explicit to patients and family. These techniques can be extremely useful in improving the functional independence of some brain dysfunctional patients. Consequently, they can indirectly reduce the emotional and motivational disturbances frequently found in these patients (Prigatano, 1991).

Thus, the answer to whether certain forms of cognitive rehabilitation help persons with brain dysfunction compensate for persistent and residual impairments is yes. There are, however, important provisos. Not all impairments can be compensated for equally, and the level of functional independence achieved by using such compensatory techniques is often lower than patients' premorbid levels. New, more sophisticated compensatory devices are badly needed, and various computer and associated memory aids are under development (see Kapur, 1995).

Do Psychotherapeutic Interventions Help Patients Adjust to the Permanent Effects of Brain Damage?

After any major change or loss, a person's sense of stability and security can be shaken. When the change or loss is caused by brain damage, patients experience the predictable problems of frustration and confusion (Chapter 2). Sometimes these problems can be managed by the patients themselves, but they often need some form of psychotherapeutic intervention (Prigatano, 1995; Prigatano and Ben-Yishay, 1999).

This process, however, is delicate. Psychotherapy is a highly individual venture, as noted earlier (Prigatano, 1991). Therefore, the application of the traditional scientific method of controlled observation to determine the efficacy of psychotherapy is extremely difficult. As Strupp (1996) has noted,

> The simple incontrovertible truth, it seems to me, is that if you are anxious or depressed or if you are experiencing difficulties with significant people in your life, chances are that you feel better if you talk to someone you can trust (p. 10).

This statement is true of persons both before and after brain damage.

Strupp's comment on the *Consumer Report* (1995) survey regarding the usefulness of psychotherapy is informative. He reviewed his tripartite model of mental health and the implications for measuring outcome after psychotherapy in terms of the findings of that survey. He suggested that mental health status can best be captured by three classes of measurement: adaptive behavior, personal sense of well-being, and personality structure. These three dimensions reflect societies' view, individuals' view of themselves, and professionals' view:

> In brief, each person's mental health may be judged differently, depending on whether society, the individual, or a mental health professional makes the judgment. Concomitantly, a given individual is regarded as being in need of professional help to the extent that he or she deviates from the standards and values governing each of the vantage points (p. 1019).

Because of this reality, psychotherapeutic outcomes are difficult but not impossible to measure.

The usefulness of psychotherapy with persons with brain dysfunction has been measured indirectly. Rehabilitation programs that actively employ psychotherapy or psychotherapeutic interventions can be compared to programs that do not use these techniques. Outcome measures should include levels of productivity and the capacity to maintain mutually satisfying interpersonal relationships (e.g., the capacity to work and to love). Outcomes must be measured across time to determine the immediate, intermediate, and possible long-term effects of such interventions. Measurements at discharge are necessary but not sufficient.

Psychotherapy does not magically transport people into a euphoric state. Rather, it should help patients to make more reasonable choices as judged by the individual and, perhaps, by society. Individuals experience many choices throughout the course of their life. Their behavior and interactions with others should demonstrate that their choices are adaptive: They have been able to deal with broader issues in life, particularly those surrounding the meaning of life in the context of their personal losses. Thus, studies on the efficacy of psychotherapy should consider patients' behavioral functioning as it relates to work and interpersonal relationships over an extended period.

Unfortunately, no such studies have been performed, but three studies provide indirect evidence of the importance of psychotherapy in the postacute rehabilitation of TBI patients. As noted above, Prigatano and colleagues (1984) documented that patients treated within the context of a neuropsychological rehabilitation program that actively used psychotherapy had a higher incidence of employability at discharge. Family members judged these individuals to be considerably less emotionally distressed than did the relatives rating untreated patients. The finding on employment was replicated 10 years later in a different treatment setting using the same methods and philosophy of care (Prigatano, et al., 1994).

Ben-Yishay and colleagues (Rattok, et al., 1992) also made similar observations regarding patients' emotional status. Patients who underwent neuropsychologically oriented rehabilitation that incorporated psychotherapeutic interventions showed improved interpersonal relationships and better control of their emotions. Prigatano and colleagues (1994) also found that the strength of the therapeutic alliance between patient and staff related to employment outcome at discharge. These findings support the contention that psychotherapy can be a practical and useful service for some brain dysfunctional patients. Yet, clear, unambiguous scientific data supporting this position are unavailable.

Psychotherapists must apply the spirit of the code of ethics of the American Psychological Association when making decisions about the appropriateness of psychotherapy for brain-injured patients. A good rationale should exist either for attempting or not attempting psychotherapy with a given brain dysfunctional patient. The intended outcome should be clear as should an understanding about the cost of services. The cost-benefit ratio of implementing such service should be considered. If someone other than the patient is paying for the service, the costs that will be engendered and the intended outcome need to be clearly explained in writing. With this type of professional vigilance, the field will grow. Without it, however, psychotherapy will be viewed with considerable skepticism and its level of coverage will dwindle.

Thus, the answer to whether psychotherapeutic interventions help patients to adjust to the permanent effects of brain damage in a meaningful and long-lasting manner is yes for some brain dysfunctional patients and no for others. Continued research is needed to clarify why this is the case. Ultimately, classification of the types of patients best treated by certain types of therapies will be necessary to determine when psychotherapy will most likely have a positive outcome for a patient. The work of Strupp and his colleagues provides excellent guidelines for such research (Strupp, 1996).

Definitions and Guidelines for Neuropsychological Rehabilitation

For neuropsychological rehabilitation to continue to develop, its usefulness and scientific basis must be evaluated further. The various services provided should be clearly defined as should guidelines for their implementation. Although this text focuses on overall principles of neuropsychological rehabilitation, my hope is that guidelines of care will eventually emerge from these principles.

In Chapter 9 and elsewhere (Prigatano, et al., 1986), I have attempted to define psychotherapy and how it can be applied to brain dysfunctional patients. The question of defining cognitive rehabilitation, however, is somewhat more challenging. Different authors with considerable experience in the field have proffered different definitions as the following sample demonstrates.

1. "Cognitive remediation (Diller and Gordon, 1981a, 1981b; Gordon, 1987) is a form of intervention in which a constellation of procedures are applied by a trained practitioner (usually a neuropsychologist, speech-language pathologist, or occupational therapist) to provide brain-injured individuals with the skills and strategies needed to perform tasks that are difficult or impossible for them, due to the presence of underlying cognitive deficits" (p. 13, Gordon and Hibbard, 1991).

2. "Cognitive retraining can be defined as those activities that improve a brain-injured person's higher cerebral functioning or help the patient to better understand the nature of those difficulties while teaching him or her methods of compensation" (p. 37; Klonoff, et al., 1989).

3. "Cognitive retraining is a systematic attempt to improve their resultant intellectual deficits that interfere with the processing of information at some level. Cognitive rehabilitation is broader in scope

than cognitive retraining since the goal of rehabilitation is functional adaptation in daily life activities" (p. 219; Berrol, 1990).

4. "Cognitive rehabilitation, as used in this text, refers to the therapeutic process of increasing or improving an individual's capacity to process and use incoming information so as to allow increased functioning in everyday life" (p. 3; Solberg and Mateer, 1989).

All of these definitions have merit. In my opinion, however, cognitive rehabilitation should be defined as a teaching activity that helps restore higher cerebral functioning by facilitating processes responsible for partial recovery and by avoiding processes responsible for deterioration after brain injury. Such cognitive rehabilitation or retraining should aim at restoring function against a background of understanding mechanisms of change associated with various brain injuries (Geschwind, 1985). Compensatory techniques can actually help patients avoid deterioration not only in the present but several years after brain injury as well (see Chapter 14).

Neuropsychological rehabilitation, however, still needs clinical guidelines for its work. Although no comprehensive guidelines are currently available, the following discussion should be considered in terms of the data presented in this and preceding chapters.

Toward Clinical Guidelines

Acute Stage

During the first few weeks and possibly for 2 to 3 months after the acute onset of a cerebrovascular accident (CVA) or moderate to severe TBI, rehabilitation should focus on improving patients' physical functioning, reducing their disorientation, and providing an environment conducive to recuperation. A brief neuropsychological examination is often warranted. When patients' speech and language, orientation, visuospatial, memory, affective, and awareness capabilities are identified, effective rehabilitation activities can be planned (Prigatano and Wong, 1999).

Early neurorehabilitation must aim to improve patients' basic physical functioning while teaching them how to control basic bodily activities and helping them to process information more realistically and practically. Considerable effort should be exerted to avoid needlessly tiring or frustrating patients (Brodal, 1973). During this time, making patients comfortable and facilitating the natural processes of recovery should be emphasized.

As Prigatano and Wong (1999) have recently noted, helping patients to predict accurately how they would perform on various tasks without challenging them may be helpful. Also helping patients improve basic affective and cognitive functions should be seriously considered during the inpatient phase.

Intermediate phase

The intermediate phase can be classified as the time during which individuals leave the hospital and begin to receive some form of outpatient treatment. The outpatient treatment should help patients maintain their physical stamina and foster good judgment about the issues of safety and basic self-independence. Physical and occupational therapies continue to be of primary importance for many individuals. However, speech and language therapy and various forms of cognitive therapy should now focus on helping patients to recover as much of their higher cerebral functions as possible. Slowly and progressively demonstrating how compensatory techniques can be useful is extremely important during this phase. Equally important, however, is the actual attempt to restore higher cerebral functions. The intermediate phase can last 3 to 12 months after a brain injury. Specialized programs of neuropsychological rehabilitation devoted to the acute and intermediate phases after diffuse and focal brain injury have not been adequately developed.

Postacute Phase

The postacute phase begins about 12 months after injury and can continue indefinitely. Typically, patients who are 1 to 2 years beyond their TBI who recovered inadequately during the acute and intermediate phases may well need a holistic neuropsychological rehabilitation program embedded in a milieu day-treatment program. The day-treatment program described in Chapter 8 is geared toward this type of patient. The focus is to help patients compensate for their difficulties and to deal with a wide variety of emotional and motivational disturbances that undercut their adjustment.

During this phase, it may be extremely important to help patients understand how their brain injury has created numerous difficulties in their ability to adapt to the vicissitudes of life. The role of psychotherapy, cognitive remediation, protected work trials in a therapeutic milieu, and family education becomes crucial. Establishing meaning in life with full recognition of permanent losses is the focus of the postacute phase. Figure 11-1 illustrates the process and outcome of postacute neuropsychological rehabilitation from my perspective.

As patients become progressively engaged in the rehabilitation task, they learn about their strengths and weaknesses (i.e., improved awareness). This process can lead to choices that improve the patients' mastery of certain skills and thereby give them greater control of their lives. At this point, greater social integration is possible and further social isolation is avoided. This process is difficult and can be aptly described as the "hero's journey." The person now begins to face limitations and endures the suffering associated with brain injury. However, they endure this pain in an adaptive, not a destructive or depressive manner. Thus,

PHILOSOPHICAL PATIENCE IN THE FACE OF SUFFERING

SOCIAL RE-INTEGRATION

CONTROL

MASTERY

AWARENESS

ENGAGEMENT

Figure 11-1. Components of the process and outcome of neuropsychological oriented rehabilitation. Originally adapted with permission from Ben-Yishay, Y. and Prigatano, G. P. (1990). Cognitive remediation. In E. Griffith, M. Rosenthal, M. R. Bond, and J. D. Miller (eds), *Rehabilitation of the Adult and Child with Traumatic Brain Injury*. F. A. Davis, Philadelphia.

the initial quote by Dr. Ben-Yishay reminds us that one "cannot be rehabilitated and be a sourpuss." This statement captures the true spirit of the process and outcome of neuropsychological rehabilitation.

Summary and Conclusions

Holistic milieu-oriented neuropsychological rehabilitation for postacute brain dysfunctional patients can improve their psychosocial outcomes. Such improvements are reflected in patients' higher incidence of employability and their reduced level of emotional distress. These programs appear to be cost effective. Studies supporting this view, however, have not been randomized, prospective investigations. Thus, their findings must be interpreted as suggestive (not definitive) evidence. Cognitive retraining of underlying impairments continues to be a controversial area of clinical intervention. Yet the techniques employed can help establish a better working alliance with patients. They can also help patients to become progressively more realistic about (aware of) their strengths and limitations. When this occurs, patients may be more willing to use compensatory techniques to aid their adjustment.

Psychotherapeutic interventions appear useful in this regard, but again systematic data are unavailable. Existing data provide indirect evidence that appropriately implemented psychotherapy can help some brain dysfunctional patients. The field, however, needs further guidelines to establish when and how neuropsychological rehabilitation activities will be most helpful to brain dysfunctional patients.

References

Baddeley, A. D., Wilson, B. A., and Watts, F. N. (1995). *Handbook of Memory Disorders*. John Wiley & Sons, Chichester, England.

Ben-Yishay, Y., and Diller, L. (1993). Cognitive remediation in traumatic brain injury: update and issues. *Arch. Phys. Med. Rehabil.* 74: 204–213.

Ben-Yishay, Y., and Prigatano, G. P. (1990). Cognitive remediation. In E. Griffin, M. Rosenthal, M. R. Bond, J. D. Miller (eds), *Rehabilitation of the Adult and Child with Traumatic Brain Injury* (pp. 393–409). F. A. Davis, Philadelphia.

Ben-Yishay, Y., Rattok, J., Lakin, P., Piasetsky, E. D., Ross, B., Silver, S., Zide, E., and Ezrachi, O. (1985). Neuropsychological rehabilitation: quest for a holistic approach. *Semin. Neurol.* 5: 252–258.

Berrol, S. (1990). Issues in cognitive rehabilitation. *Arch. Neurol.* 47, 219.

Brodal, A. (1973). Self-observations and neuro-anatomical considerations after a stroke. *Brain* 96: 675–694.

Christensen, A.-L, Pinner, E. M., Pedersen, M. P., Teasdale, T. W., and Trexler, L. E. (1992). Psychosocial outcome following individualized neuropsychological rehabilitation of brain damage. *Acta Neurol. Scand.* 85: 32–38.

Diller, L., and Gordon, W. A. (1981a). Interventions for cognitive deficits in brain injured adults. *J. Consult. Clin. Psychol.* 49: 822–834.

Diller, L., and Gordon, W. A. (1981b). Rehabilitation and clinical neuropsychology. In S. Filskov and T. Boll (eds), *Handbook of Clinical Neuropsychology* (Vol. 1, pp. 702–733). John Wiley & Sons, New York.

Ezrachi, O., Ben-Yishay, Y., Kay, T., Diller, L., and Rattok J. (1991). Predicting employment in traumatic brain injury following neuropsychological rehabilitation. *Journal of Head Trauma Rehabilitation* 6(3): 71–84.

Fordyce, D. J., Roueche, J. R., and Prigatano, G. P. (1983). Enhanced emotional reactions in chronic head trauma patients. *J. Neurol. Neurosurg. Psychiatry* 46: 620–624.

Geschwind, N. (1985). Mechanisms of change after brain lesions. In F. Nottebohm (ed), *Hope for a New Neurology* (pp. 1–12). Annals of the New York Academy of Sciences, New York.

Glisky, E. L., and Schacter, D. L. (1987). Acquisition of domain-specific knowledge in organic amnesia: training for computer-related work. *Neuropsychologia* 25: 893–906.

Gordon, W. A. (1987). Methodological issues in cognitive remediation. In M. Meir, A. L. Benton, and L. Diller (eds), *Neuropsychological Rehabilitation* (pp. 111–131). Churchill Livingston, London.

Gordon, W. A., and Hibbard, M. R. (1991). The theory and practice of cognitive remediation. In J. S. Kreutzer and P. H. Wehman (eds), *Cognitive Rehabilitation for Persons with Traumatic Brain Injury. A Functional Approach* (pp. 13–22). Paul H. Brookes, Baltimore.

Kapur, N. (1995). Memory aids in the rehabilitation of memory disordered patients. In A. D. Baddeley, B. A. Wilson, and F. N. Watts (eds), *Handbook of Memory Disorders* (pp. 533–556). John Wiley, Chichester, England.

Kime, S. K., Lamb, D. G., and Wilson, B. A. (1996). Use of a comprehensive programme of external cueing to enhance procedural memory in a patient with dense amnesia. *Brain Injury* 10(1): 17–25.

Klonoff, P. S., O'Brien, K. P., Prigatano, G. P., Chiapello, D. A., and Cunningham, M. (1989). Cognitive retraining after traumatic brain injury and its role in facilitating awareness. *Journal of Head Trauma Rehabilitation* 4(3): 37–45.

Malec, J. F., and Basford, J. R. (1996). Postacute brain injury rehabilitation. *Arch. Phys. Med. Rehabil.* 77: 198–207.

Mehlbye J., and Larsen A. (1994). Social and economic consequences of brain damage in Denmark: a case study. In A. L. Christensen and B. P. Uzzell (eds), *Brain Injury and Neuropsychological Rehabilitation. International Perspectives* (pp. 257–267). Lawrence Erlbaum, Hillsdale, NJ.

Pliskin, N. H., Cunningham, J. M., Wall, J. R., and Cassisi, J. E. (1996). Cognitive rehabilitation for cerebrovascular accidents and Alzheimer's disease. In P. W. Corrigan and S. C. Yudofsky (eds), *Cognitive Rehabilitation for Neuropsychiatric Disorders* (pp. 193–222). American Psychiatric Press, Washington, DC.

Prigatano, G. P. (1987). Recovery and cognitive retraining after craniocerebral trauma. *Journal of Learning Disability* 20(10): 603–613.

Prigatano, G. P. (1991). Disordered mind, wounded soul: the emerging role of psychotherapy in rehabilitation after brain injury. *Journal of Head Trauma Rehabilitation* 6(4): 1–10.

Prigatano, G. P. (1995). 1994 Sheldon Berrol, MD, Senior Lectureship: The problem of lost normality after brain injury. *Journal of Head Trauma Rehabilitation* 10(3): 87–95.

Prigatano, G. P., Amin, K., and Jaramillo, K. (1993). Memory performance and use of a compensation after traumatic brain injury. *Neuropsychological Rehabilitation*, 3(1): 53–62.

Prigatano, G. P., and Ben-Yishay, Y. (1999). Psychotherapy and psychotherapeutic interventions in brain injury rehabilitation. In M. Rosenthal (ed), *Rehabilitation of the Adult and Child with Traumatic Brain Injury* (3rd ed). F. A. Davis, Philadelphia.

Prigatano, G. P., Fordyce, D. J., Zeiner, H. K., Roueche, J. R., Pepping, M., and Wood, B. (1984). Neuropsychological rehabilitation after closed head injury in young adults. *J. Neurol. Neurosurg. Psychiatry* 47: 505–513.

Prigatano, G. P., Glisky, E. L., and Klonoff, P. S. (1996). Cognitive rehabilitation after traumatic brain injury. In P. W. Corrigan and S. C. Yudolfsky (eds), *Cognitive Rehabilitation for Neuropsychiatric Disorders* (pp. 223–242). American Psychiatric Press, Washington, DC.

Prigatano, G. P., and Henderson, S. (1997). Cognitive outcome after subarachnoid hemorrhage. In J. B. Bederson (ed), *Subarachnoid Hemorrhage: Pathophysiology and Management* (pp. 27–40). American Association of Neurological Surgeons, Park Ridge, Ill.

Prigatano, G. P., Klonoff, P. S., O'Brien, K. P., Altman, I., Amin, K., Chiapello, D. A., Shepherd, J., Cunningham, M., and Mora, M. (1994). Productivity after neuropsychologically oriented, milieu rehabilitation. *Journal of Head Trauma Rehabilitation* 9(1): 91–102.

Prigatano, G. P., Fordyce, D. L., Zeiner, H. K., Roueche, J. K., Pepping, M., and Wood, B. C. (1986). *Neuropsychological Rehabilitation After Brain Injury.* Johns Hopkins University, Baltimore.

Prigatano, G. P. and Wong, J. L. (1997). Speed of finger tapping and goal attainment after unilateral cerebral vascular accident. *Arch. Phys. Med. Rehabil.* 78: 847–852.

Prigatano, G. P. and Wong, J. L. (1999). Cognitive and affective improvement in brain dysfunctional patients who achieve inpatient rehabilitation goals. *Arch. Phys. Med. Rehabil* (in press).

Rattok, J., Ben-Yishay, Y., Ezrachi, O., Lakin, P., Piasetsky, E., Ross, B., Silver, S., Vakil, E., Zide, E., and Diller, L. (1992). Outcome of different treatment mixes in a multidimensional neuropsychological rehabilitation program. *Neuropsychology* 6(4): 395–415.

Scherzer, B. P. (1986). Rehabilitation following severe head trauma: results of a three-year program. *Arch. Phys. Med. Rehabil.* 67, 366–374.

Sohlberg, M. M. and Mateer, C. A. (1989). *Introduction to Cognitive Rehabilitation: Theory and Practice* (pp. 3–13). Guilford, New York.

Strubb, R. L. and Black, F. W. (1985). *The Mental Status Examination in Neurology* (2nd ed). F. A. Davis, Philadelphia.

Strupp, H. H. (1996). The tripartite model and the Consumer Reports study. *Am. Psychol.* 51(10): 1017–1024.

Teasdale, T. W. and Christensen, A.-L. (1994). Psychosocial outcome in Denmark. In A.-L. Christensen and B. P. Uzzell (eds), *Brain Injury and Neuropsychological Rehabilitation: International Perspectives* (pp. 235–244). Lawrence Erlbaum, Hillsdale, NJ.

von Cramon, D. Y. and Matthes-von Cramon, G. (1992). Reflections on the treatment of brain-injured patients suffering from problem-solving disorders. *Neuropsychological Rehabilitation* 2(3): 207–229.

Wertz, R. T., Weiss, D. G., Aten, J. L., Brookshire, R. H., Garcia-Buñuel, L., Holland, A. L., Kurtzke, J. F., LaPointe, L. L., Milianti, F. J., Brannegan, R., et al. (1986). Comparison of clinic, home, and deferred language treatment for aphasia: a Veterans Administration Cooperative Study. *Arch. Neurol.* 43(7): 653–658.

Wilson, B. A. (1991). Long-term prognosis of patients with severe memory disorders. *Neuropsychological Rehabilitation* 1: 117–134.

Wilson, B. A. (1995). Management and remediation of memory problems in brain-injured adults. In A. D. Baddeley, B. A. Wilson, and F. N. Watts (eds), *Handbook of Memory Disorders* (pp. 451–479). John Wiley, Chichester, England.

Wilson, B. A. (1997). Cognitive rehabilitation: how it is and how it might be. *Journal of International Neuropsychological Society* 3: 487–496.

III

THEORETICAL AND
EMPIRICAL ISSUES

12

Disorders of Self-Awareness After Brain Injury

> "We are coming now rather into the region of guesswork," said
> Dr. Mortimer. "Say, rather, into the region where we balance
> probabilities and choose the most likely. It is the scientific use of
> the imagination, but we have always some material basis on
> which to start our speculation."
>
> Sherlock Holmes, *The Hound of the Baskervilles*, written by
> Sir Arthur Conan Doyle, 1902, p. 30

Disorders of self-awareness are common after brain injury but poorly understood and managed (Principle 11). Is the patient's apparent lack of insight a result of brain dysfunction or a psychological defense (i.e., denial) against recognizing impairments and disabilities? The answer to this question has important implications for managing patients and for understanding the mechanisms responsible for human consciousness (Principle 11).

In the clinical arena, one of the most dramatic forms of impaired awareness is anosognosia for hemiplegia. Patients literally cannot move the entire left side of their bodies and yet report no impairment! Sandifer's (1946) verbatim account of one such patient exemplifies the power of this disorder. Although patients momentarily may be forced to admit that their position is illogical, their words reveal that they do not experience what their examining physician's logic forces them to admit.

Such anosognosia may improve rapidly within a few days or weeks of an acute brain injury. Yet, in many patients, subtle disorders of consciousness seem to persist weeks, months, or even years after their brain injury. For some, the disorder may be permanent. Because the physician, psychologist, and rehabilitation therapist may not follow a given patient from the emergency room through acute care to rehabilitation and beyond, their view of acquired disturbances in human consciousness or awareness may be limited, if not distorted. This partial exposure is analogous to seeing only the first few or last minutes of a movie and being asked to give a complete account of the film.

When patients are followed from the time of injury to well thereafter, a different picture of impaired awareness emerges and suggests a new classification for these disorders. This chapter attempts to formalize such a classification juxtaposed against a brief historical review of disorders of self-awareness. Historical facts are integrated with more contemporary insights: Disorders of self-awareness appear to assume different forms, depending on the brain regions damaged, and to change with time, much like aphasic syndromes.

The proposed classification system is brief and incomplete but offers initial guidelines for understanding disorders of self-awareness. Such disorders may be considered either "complete" or "partial" manifestations of impaired self-awareness that are related to specific neurological and neuropsychological disturbances. Patients who retain partial awareness may use nondefensive, premorbid methods to cope after a brain injury, or they may rely on defensive mechanisms such as denial or projection. Both defensive and nondefensive methods of coping with partial syndromes are also classified. Understanding the latter class of behavior may be especially important during attempts to engage and manage patients in neurorehabilitation.

Historical Perspective of Impaired Self-Awareness

Although the work of von Monakow in 1885 is often cited as the earliest historical description of anosognosia, Bisiach and Geminiani (1991) remind us that disturbances of self-awareness have been recorded since antiquity.

> In one of the letters addressed to his friend Lucilius (*Liber V, Epistula IX*), L. A. Seneca dealt with beliefs related to the self. Although primarily interested in moral implications of such beliefs, he related the following anecdote.
> "You know that Harpastes, my wife's fatuous companion, has remained in my home as an inherited burden. . . . This foolish woman has suddenly lost her sight. Incredible as it might appear, what I am going to tell you is true: She does not know she is blind. Therefore, again and again she asks her guardian to take her elsewhere. She claims that my home is dark."

Further on, Seneca remarked that there are instances in which "it is difficult to recover from illness just because we are unaware of it" (p. 17).

These remarks document that disorders of self-awareness associated with brain injury likely existed long before the formal study of neurology and neuropsychology began. The early scientific work related to this problem, however, was conducted by Herbert Munk (1881; cited by Blakemore, 1977). Munk experimentally placed lesions in the association cortex of dogs and produced a phenomenon that he referred to as "mind blindness." These animals often approached objects in the manner that revealed that they were seen, but their familiarity remained unknown (i.e., they might not bump into an object when walking near it but failed to recognize the object as their master). With time, the term mind blindness was replaced by the term agnosia. Bauer and Rubens (1985) credited Sigmund Freud for introducing this term in 1891.

Research on agnosia quickly focused on visual object agnosia. As Rubens (1979) noted, in 1889 Lissauer proposed that visual object agnosia be separated into two types: *apperceptive* and *associative*, depending on whether lower or higher levels of sensory processing were disturbed. Apperceptive visual object agnosia exists in patients who "cannot draw misidentified items or match them to sample" (Rubens, pp. 236–237). In contrast, patients with associative visual agnosia can draw objects but have considerable difficulty with identifying their meaning. Rubens and Benson (1971) reported a patient who could draw several items adequately but still failed to identify them. Interestingly, many patients who exhibit associative visual object agnosia have bilateral lesions that affect not only cortical areas but limbic regions as well.

In 1885, von Monakow described a patient's failure to recognize cortical blindness. The patient, however, also seemed to have confabulatory tendencies, and diffuse brain injury was considered a high probability. Therefore, the lack of insight could not be distinguished from a general dementia. In 1898 Gabriel Anton, however, described a patient with focal brain dysfunction who lacked awareness of his cortical blindness. This important clinical observation suggested that the lack of insight was independent of generalized intellectual impairment. Consequently, it could not be interpreted as an epiphenomenon of an impaired cognitive state.

At about the same time, Charcot (1882) demonstrated that paralysis could be caused by psychological rather than neurological disturbances. Using hypnosis, Charcot could break a patient's "hysterical paralyses" at least for brief periods. Freud observed some of Charcot's patients and became convinced that mechanisms of repression and denial could be responsible for many syndromes that appeared to have neurological substrates.

The next important contributions were made by Felix Babinski and Arnold Pick. In 1914 Babinski introduced the term anosognosia as it applied to a lack of awareness of hemiplegia. Arnold Pick, however, is credited for actually describing the phenomenon of anosognosia years earlier but he did not introduce the term anosognosia (Prigatano and Schacter, 1991).

Since these early observations, numerous articles in the field of neurology have provided additional clues about important factors involved in disorders of self-awareness. For example, Henry Head (1920), a leading antilocalization theorist of higher cerebral functioning, noted that lesions in one cerebral hemisphere can affect the patient's emotional responses to the "so called" affected side. He described a patient who was unable to go to a place of worship because he could not tolerate how the religious hymns affected his "affected side" (p. 560). Roeser and Daly (1974) reported the interesting case of a 49-year-old woman with a right thalamic tumor who expressed paresthesias and "perversions of sensations" on the left side of her body:

> About 1 month after the onset of the sensory disturbances, she had noted altered perception of music but had no difficulty in perceiving speech. Initially, she had thought that her high-fidelity phonograph was defective since music sounded "fuzzy and blurred." She mentioned this to her husband who commented that there was no disturbance in the music coming from the phonograph (p. 556).

In Roeser's and Daly's case, as in the cases described by Head, the patients' initial response was to describe the problem as external to themselves rather than recognizing their problem processing information. This tendency is a hallmark of impaired self-awareness after brain injury. Patients attribute problems to external rather than internal causes. The human brain seems to attempt to make sense out of a disordered experience or perception by any available method. In some instances, these methods can be viewed as nondefensive methods of coping; in other instances, they can be viewed as defensive methods of coping, as described later.

Weinstein and Kahn (1955) also made an important observation that greatly influenced the study of impaired self-awareness after brain injury. In their scholarly review, they noted that denial phenomena can exist with many medical conditions when the brain has not been damaged directly. They argued that while brain damage would produce certain neuropsychological impairments, it would not produce the mechanism of denial. In fact, they argued that denial was independent of patients' symptoms and simply reflected the symbolic way in which individuals attempt to cope with their impaired condition.

Unfortunately, this perspective discouraged many clinical neuropsychologists and neurologists from seriously considering impaired awareness as a true neuropsychological disturbance. However, various case studies in the literature eventually made it clear that individuals who knew a considerable amount about both the nervous system and psychiatry could exhibit anosognosia if they sustained a brain injury.

Anosognosia, Denial, and Altered Awareness in People Who Should Have Known Better

Among the most striking pieces of evidence that impaired self-awareness after brain injury is a neuropsychological disturbance are the writings of experienced individuals who have experienced various forms of anosognosia after brain injury. As noted earlier, Brodal (1973) wrote an extraordinary article on his observations of himself after an infarction in the right internal capsule. He described his clinical picture as others had as consisting of a "pure motor hemiplegia." By that he meant hemiplegia "without somatosensory impairment, visual field defects, aphasia, or apractagonosia" (p. 676).

Brodal discussed his difficulties with mental energy, problems with handwriting, difficulties with communication, and so on (Chapter 6). He also observed that the most helpful activity during physical therapy was passive range of motion of his affected arm. Subjectively, the sensory information produced by this passive range of motion seemed to help him "reexperience" normal movement of the affected limb. This activity helped him not only by initiating a motor act but by helping him understand his own baseline (normal) experience. He noted that attempting to move the arm required a great deal of mental energy and frequently resulted in considerable fatigue. He had lost the experience of a normal movement or position for that limb, and the passive range of motion helped him to reexperience what was normal. His case demonstrates that impairments in self-awareness can be associated with even very focal brain lesions.

Discussing his own case, he commented as follows:

> During a lifelong occupation with the anatomy of the central nervous system, especially its fiber connections, the author [referring to himself] has been increasingly struck by the tremendous complexity in the organization of the brain. Two aspects, apparently contradictory, are particularly conspicuous. There is an extremely high degree of specificity and at the same time a far-going diffuseness in the patterns of organization (p. 687).

This important observation is relevant to the phenomenon of impaired awareness as discussed later. It also is relevant to understanding mechanisms of recovery, which are discussed in Chapter 13.

The psychiatrist Wallace LaBaw is another noted example. In his article "Denial: Inside Out: Subjective Experience with Anosognosia and Closed Head Injury," LaBaw (1969) described how he dismissed feedback from nurses that his records of patients whom he saw after his own head injury were inadequate. As discussed in Chapter 2, he indicated that it was one thing to overcome the head injury and another to overcome his "denial."

LaBaw's description is compatible with what is frequently reported as "denial of disability" (Prigatano and Klonoff, 1997). Individuals have some knowledge of impaired functioning but fail to see that the impairment restricts them in any way. Such patients often perceive that the best "therapy" is to return to their previous lifestyle. Patients recognize that *some* problem exists but think that others are overstating the extent of the problem or its implications. Clinical psychologists and psychiatrists should read and reread LaBaw's article to form a clear understanding of denial in the presence of brain damage and how it can differ from denial in non–brain dysfunctional individuals.

The last case is that of William J. German. With colleagues, German (1964), at the time Chairman of Neurosurgery at Yale University, wrote a remarkable paper entitled *"Remarks on a Subdural Hematoma and Aphasia,"* describing what it was like to be aware of some changes in higher cerebral functioning but not others:

> In April 1964 he [referring to himself] attended the meeting of the Harvey Cushing Society, in Los Angeles. Following these meetings he visited Disneyland with his family. There, at the request of his two younger children, he accompanied them on a ride on the Bobsled. Those who have had this experience will probably recall a certain hairpin curve in which the angular acceleration reaches a very considerable number of radians per second per second. About two-thirds of the way through this left curve the patient felt a dull thud which seemed to be inside his right frontal cranium. An immediate response was the thought: "Wouldn't it be silly if I got a subdural hematoma from this?" That evening he had a little difficulty locating one portion of his railroad tickets and was aware of mild dullness of mood. During this succeeding week there were occasional frontal headaches, usually on the right, sufficiently annoying to raise the query that a long gone migraine might be returning. There was then little of note until about the third week, when in dim light, a small flash of brightness was noted in the extreme periphery of the left visual field, on turning the head quickly to the left. After that time, it was possible to reproduce this phenomenon consistently. The fourth and fifth weeks were notable for progressive difficulty in sequential thought and speech, and for a diminution of right hand dominance. There was even a trend toward left preference and occasional uncertainty in right-left differentiation.
>
> Normal ability to retain temporarily the usual seven digit telephone numbers was lost, requiring one or two rechecks while dialing. Even semiautomatic, internal speech seemed to lose its natural continuity.
>
> As he approached the end of the fifth week there was evident inattention to the right side; leaving a slipper on the right foot when getting into bed; neglecting to bring the right foot into bed; even an impression that the right side of his car took up too much room on the road and needed particular care in steering (pp. 344–345).

Even a trained neurosurgeon attributed difficulties with hemi-inattention and problems of neglect to external rather than to internal causes. It was his car that took up too much room on the road and needed extra care in steering, rather than he himself who was having the problems.

German is another striking example of altered self-awareness after a brain insult.

These three individuals, an internationally known neuroanatomist, a psychiatrist, and a neurosurgeon, all experienced alterations in self-awareness after and associated with their brain injury. These individuals were all well-trained and undoubtedly familiar with the phenomenon of anosognosia before their brain injury. Yet when their brain was injured, they could not apply previously learned technical knowledge to their own case. With true disturbances of brain functioning, people are deprived not only of memories but of the experience of impaired functioning. If it is true that consciousness is the highest of all integrated brain functions, then any brain injury will alter persons' ability to perceive themselves objectively. Untangling these and related phenomena now confronts us.

Observations Relevant to Impaired Self-Awareness

Many observations must be attended to in order to untangle the facts as they relate to impaired self-awareness after brain injury. The following historical observations are important:

1. Patients can have a hemiplegia and not be aware of it (Pick, 1908; Babinski, 1914).
2. The striking phenomenon of anosognosia of hemiplegia often improves with time (Prigatano, 1988).
3. Anosognosia for hemiplegia is more common after right hemisphere sessions than after left hemisphere lesions (Weinstein and Kahn, 1955).
4. Anosognosia can exist for other neurologic deficits, such as cortical blindness (von Monakow, 1885).
5. In some cases, the lesions are focal and a general decline in intellectual function is not present (Anton, 1898).
6. When an impairment of brain function causes a sensory or motor deficit, persons often attribute the problem to external causes rather than to some problem within themselves or what they experience (e.g., Head, 1920; Roeser and Daly, 1974; German, et al., 1964; LaBaw, 1969).
7. The latter phenomenon occurs even in people highly knowledgeable about brain function and psychiatric defense mechanisms (e.g., German, et al., 1964; LaBaw, 1969).
8. Even relatively small subcortical lesions can deprive people of the experience of what is normal for any given function or activity (e.g., Brodal, 1973).
9. No straightforward neurological or neuropsychological markers

automatically predict the sequelae of impaired self-awareness or denial (Weinstein and Kahn, 1955).

10. Denial of disability can exist in persons with no brain damage and can be difficult to distinguish from impaired self-awareness after brain injury (Weinstein and Kahn, 1955).

The preceding 10 observations have been known since the late 1800s to the mid-1900s. Additional observations were made in the latter half of the twentieth century:

11. Cultural factors can influence self-reports of disabilities or impairments after brain injury (Gainotti, 1975; Prigatano and Leathem, 1993; Prigatano, et al., 1997).
12. Anosognosia can occur with left hemisphere lesions (Lebrun, 1987).
13. Anosognosia in patients with cerebrovascular lesions is unrelated to the presence or absence of depression (Starkstein, et al., 1992).

These observations must be kept in mind during attempts to classify disorders of self-awareness. A more detailed analysis of these last three observations is warranted.

Recent Studies on Anosognosia for Hemiplegia

Starkstein and colleagues (1992) studied anosognosia in patients with acute cerebrovascular lesions. They noted that 28% of their subjects originally demonstrated some form of anosognosia for hemiplegia. Anosognosia was assessed by a questionnaire (i.e., the clinician asked patients specific questions about their illness). Between 40% and 75% of their patients who had had a cerebrovascular accident (CVA) showed hemispatial neglect. Earlier, Cutting (1978) had estimated that 52% of his anosognostic patient showed hemispatial neglect as did 24% with "anosognostic phenomena."

Starkstein and colleagues (1992) and Cutting (1978) also noted that CVA patients with disorders of self-awareness showed affective changes. Both reported that about 10% of patients with severe or moderate anosognosia exhibited major signs of depression. Depression and anxiety, however, did not distinguish CVA patients with anosognosia for hemiplegia from those without it.

Other mood changes can be associated with classic anosognosia. Cutting (1978) reported that 51% of his anosognostic patients were apathetic. Starkstein and colleagues (1992) found that anosognostic CVA patients had significantly more difficulties recognizing facial emotion and performed significantly worse on a test of receptive aprosody than patients without anosognosia. In both studies, measures of overall cognitive functioning failed to distinguish between patients with and without anosognosia. Both also reported that patients with right or left hemisphere strokes could demonstrate anosognosia for hemiplegia.

As has been observed historically, a right hemisphere CVA is more frequently associated with this phenomenon than a left hemisphere CVA. Cutting (1978) reported that 58% of his left hemiparetic patients (right hemisphere–damaged individuals) showed clear anosognosia. Of the right-hemiplegic patients (left hemisphere–damaged patients) who were testable (i.e., not severely aphasic), 14% also showed anosognosia. In the study by Starkstein and colleagues (1992), 80% of the severely anosognostic patients had right-hemisphere lesions documented by computed tomography (CT). The remaining 20% of severely anosognostic patients had bilateral lesions. Some of the patients with moderate anosognosia, however, had left hemisphere lesions (Table 12–1).

As Table 12–1 illustrates, right hemisphere and bilateral lesions are associated with anosognosia more often than left hemisphere lesions, as reflected by their presence on CT scans. As described below, however, both behavioral data (Prigatano and Wong, 1997) and positron emission tomography (PET) studies (Perani et al., 1993) suggest that bilateral cerebral dysfunction, which cannot be detected by CT, can follow unilateral

Table 12-1. Results of neurological examination in 80 stroke patients

	No Anosognosia No. (%)	Mild Anosognosia No. (%)	Moderate Anosognosia No. (%)	Severe Anosognosia No. (%)
*Hemineglect**				
Left	2 (4)	6 (75)	5 (56)	4 (40)
Right	0 (0)	0 (0)	0 (0)	0 (0)
Visual field deficits†				
Left hemianopsia	6 (11)	3 (38)	4 (44)	4 (40)
Right hemianopsia	1 (2)	0 (0)	0 (0)	0 (0)
Cortical blindness	0 (0)	0 (0)	0 (0)	1 (10)
Side of neurological signs‡				
Left	24 (45)	0 (0)	3 (33)	0 (0)
Right	24 (45)	7 (88)	6 (67)	8 (80)
Bilateral	5 (10)	1 (12)	0 (0)	2 (20)

*χ^2=17.4, df=3, p=0.0006; †χ^2=22.5, df=3, p=0.0001; ‡χ^2=13.0, df=6, p<0.05

From Starkstein et al. (1992). With permission from Scientific Publishing, American Heart Association.

CVAs. The potential for bilateral cerebral dysfunction, irrespective of whether bilateral lesions are imaged, becomes important in understanding syndromes associated with disorders of self-awareness.

Starkstein and colleagues (1992) also described a relationship between generalized brain dysfunction and anosognosia. They found a significant association between measures of atrophy and anosognosia. Their regression analysis to predict anosognosia showed that "two variables accounted for 57% of the variance: the frontal horn ratio ($R=0.69$, $R^2=0.49$, $F=21.0$, $p<0.01$) and lesion location (right temporoparietal or thalamic) ($R=0.76$, $R^2=0.57$, $F=4.03$, $p<0.05$)" (p. 1451). Frontal horn ratio was defined as the "area of the frontal horn contralateral to the lesion at the level of the foramen of Monro, divided by the area of the whole brain at the same level, multiplied by 1,000" (p. 1448). We return to the importance of these observations during the discussion of classifying disorders of self-awareness.

Anosognosia for Aphasia

It is difficult to assess disorders of self-awareness in aphasic patients for obvious reasons. The patients' verbal report regarding their functioning is used to judge the presence or absence of anosognosia. Anosognosia, however, can exist in aphasic patients who have left-hemisphere lesions (Lebrun, 1987). The classic example is jargon aphasia. Patients' language output may be fluent, but they produce paraphasic and neologistic verbal responses. In other words, their language output is nonsensical to the listener. Patients with Wernicke's aphasia can also exhibit jargon aphasia.

Years ago, I had an opportunity to examine a young adult male within the first few weeks of his traumatic brain injury (TBI). He exhibited a classic fluent aphasia, making numerous paraphasic errors in his free speech. Several months after his injury, his aphasic disturbance had substantially improved but was not completely eliminated. I asked him if he remembered his notable difficulties in communicating with me soon after his injury. He looked at me perplexed. He felt he had always been able to speak normally but remembered not understanding why others had looked at him strangely when he spoke. He was still unaware of his aphasic output. This important phenomenon has been documented by Lebrun (1987) and others (Rubens and Garrett, 1991).

The theoretical importance of these observations is that lesions in regions other than the right hemisphere can cause disturbances in self-awareness. Patients can be unaware of a deficit in one area while simultaneously aware of a deficit in another area. This paradox does not necessarily suggest the presence of psychological denial. Rather, specificity may exist in terms of the types of impaired awareness that follow brain injury.

Anosognosia for Hemiplegia and Hemianopia

Bisiach and colleagues (1986) found that 30% of 97 right-handed, right-brain–damaged patients showed anosognosia for motor impairments after a CVA. Some persons exhibited anosognosia for motor impairments but not for their visual defect and vice versa—evidence that two forms of anosognosia can be disassociated in the same patient.

Bisiach and colleagues (1986) make the following points:

1. "... anosognosia for left hemiplegia is not simply a manifestation of inattention ..." (p. 478).
2. "... anosognosia for hemiplegia fails to show any association to unilateral neglect" (p. 480).
3. "... four of the 10 patients with severe anosognosia for hemianopia had minimal (if at all) anosognosia for hemiplegia" (p. 480).
4. "... unawareness of a failure of a particular function betrays a disorder at the highest levels of organization of *that* function. This implies that *monitoring of the internal working is not secured in the nervous system by a general, superordinate organ, but is decentralized and apportioned to the different functional blocks to which it refers*" (p. 480).

Anosognosia When Traditional Neurological Deficits Are Absent

The classic study of anosognosia has centered around specific neurological syndromes or deficits: anosognosia for hemiplegia (Babinski, 1914), anosognosia for cortical blindness (Anton, 1889), anosognosia for hemianopia (Bisiach and Gemeniani, 1991), and anosognosia for aphasia (Rubens and Garrett, 1991). In the latter stages of progressive dementia, anosognosia for the dementing condition can also occur (McGlynn and Kaszniak, 1991). These cases, however, do not reflect important disturbances in self-awareness associated with specific neuropsychological impairments present in the absence of frank neurological syndromes.

For example, a patient with a right frontal oligodendroglioma showed a relatively normal neuropsychological test performance. Yet, his wife noted that he tended to overestimate his ability to remember his daily schedule. She also noted that he tended to overestimate his ability to handle arguments with people he knew well. The perspective of the patient's wife was that her husband's personality had changed dramatically, but he did not seem to recognize the changes (Prigatano and O'Brien, 1991).

In contrast, a patient with the same type of brain tumor but in the right parieto-occipital region showed a different pattern of disturbed awareness. This patient's wife reported that his personality was the same, but he had difficulties performing mechanical and visuospatial problem-solving tasks that had not previously been troublesome for him. She also noted a curious behavior. Immediately after surgery, her husband complained that she must be turning his clothes inside out because he was finding it difficult to dress in the morning. Apparently, the patient had a dressing apraxia but did not perceive himself as having the problem. Rather, he attributed the problem to an external cause—his wife playing a trick on him.

Disorders of self-awareness repeatedly manifest by persons failing to recognize their inability to function. Perhaps, as Bisiach suggests, disorders of consciousness reflect an impairment of the highest level of organization of a given function. These last two cases seem to support this interpretation. These two cases also reinforce that disturbances of self-awareness can be quite specific and unaccompanied by a generalized disturbance in self-awareness. This possibility must be kept in mind when evaluating and managing patients.

Attempts to rehabilitate postacute TBI patients with bilateral and diffuse cerebral dysfunction of the frontal and parietal areas have provided another important source of information for understanding this complex set of disorders. These patients' insight about their socially inappropriate behaviors or the impact that their neuropsychological deficits would have on their ability to function in the real world often seems reduced (Prigatano, et al., 1984). Such patients frequently have low average intelligence quotients (IQ) with moderate to severe memory impairments. They are also often young, somewhat impulsive males with limited social judgment. These patients raise the question of whether their impaired self-awareness is a true reflection of brain damage, their premorbid psychological makeup, or the tendency of young males to perceive no limitations in terms of themselves.

Impaired Self-Awareness Across Cultures in Patients with Moderate to Severe TBI

Prigatano and colleagues (1990) asked 64 TBI patients to rate their functional competency on a 30-item questionnaire referred to as the Patient's Competency Rating Scale (PCRS). This scale was developed to supplement information obtained during diagnostic interviews and formal neuropsychological testing. TBI patients were predicted to underestimate their behavioral limitations, social interactions, and emotional control compared to their relative's ratings of these patients' abilities. This hypothesis was clearly supported and replicated 5 years later with an independent sample of 31 TBI patients (Prigatano, 1996). Moreover, a "neuropsychological control group" tended to see themselves as less competent than their relatives reported (Fig. 12-1), a pattern exactly opposite that of the TBI patients.

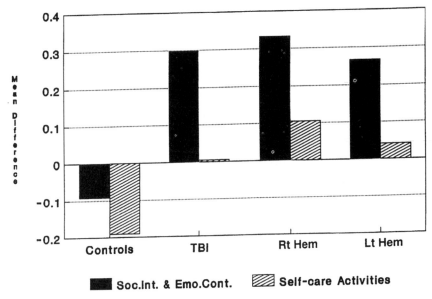

Figure 12-1. Mean difference scores for different patient groups on selected PCRS items reflecting social interaction and emotional control or self-care activities. Each item is scored on a scale from 1 to 5 (higher score represents higher level of behavioral competency). The patients' ratings (i.e., scores) were subtracted from relatives' ratings and the mean difference across items obtained. It can be seen that traumatically brain-injured patients report a higher level of competence than their relatives do regarding them on items dealing with social interaction and emotional control. Among other findings, the neuropsychological control group shows the opposite pattern. From Prigatano, G. P. (1996). Behavioral limitations TBI patients tend to underestimate: A replication and extension to patients with lateralized cerebral dysfunction. *The Clinical Neuropsychologist* 10(2):191–201. With permission from Swets & Zeitlinger.

Using other methods, similar findings have been reported (Fleming, et al., 1996). Thus, TBI patients who are not demented and who have low-average IQ scores repeatedly tend to overestimate their ability to interact in a socially appropriate manner and to control their emotional reactions.

Although this tendency to underestimate impairment or disabilities in social interactions or emotional control could appear to be a direct effect of brain damage, patients' personalities could also influence their self-reports about their neurological or neuropsychological disturbances (Weinstein and Kahn, 1955). In fact, Northern Italian demented patients from a Roman Catholic background exhibit less denial of illness than Swiss demented patients of a Calvinistic Protestant heritage (Giannotti, 1975). This finding suggests that personality and cultural variables can influence TBI patients' perceptions about their disability and therefore how they would answer specific questions about their disability posed by neurologists or neuropsychologists.

Two cross-cultural studies were conducted to explore whether brain dysfunction or personality variables affected self-reports of TBI patients. Prigatano and Leathem (1993) attempted to cross-validate the earlier findings by studying New Zealand TBI patients. The New Zealand TBI patients were composed of two subgroups: one of English ancestry and the other of Maori ancestry. Both groups were predicted to underestimate their behavioral competencies in social and emotional interactions because of their brain damage. New Zealand TBI patients of English ancestry showed the same response patterns as American TBI patients; the Maori patients did not. The Maori TBI patients, however, also had a higher incidence of left hemisphere dysfunction than the English ancestry group (Prigatano and Leathem, 1993). The presence of this confounding variable limits the cross-validity of the study.

A second study was conducted with Japanese TBI patients to clarify the degree to which brain damage influences self-reports of disability (Prigatano, et al., 1997). A Japanese translation of the PCRS was administered to both TBI and CVA patients. Very impaired Japanese patients (mean IQ scores in the low 70s) reported levels of competency on the PCRS that would be impossible given the severity of their neuropsychological impairments.

Interestingly, the relatives' ratings of these patients on the PCRS correlated with the patients' performance on the *BNI Screen for Higher Cerebral Functioning* (Table 12-2). In contrast, the self-reports of the Japanese TBI patients' about their competency and their actual performance on the screening test showed no relationship. These findings have also been reported in other cultures (Table 12-2). The same pattern was observed, for example, with Maori and non-Maori TBI patients in the New Zealand study. These relationships are true of TBI patients but not of normal control subjects. The findings (Table 12-2) suggest that TBIs negatively affect self-perceptions of functional limitations across the cultures studied.

The Japanese cross-cultural study, however, illustrates a more important lesson. Contrary to the prediction, some Japanese TBI patients did *not* overestimate their ability to control emotions or to behave appropriately in social settings. Rather, they overestimated their ability to perform self-care activities. In the Japanese culture, modesty is a virtue and the ability to care for oneself is important socially. These findings, therefore, raise an interesting possibility.

Perhaps severe TBIs, which are known to produce bilateral frontal and anterior temporal lesions in the context of diffuse brain damage, negatively affect the ability to be aware of any socially relevant impairment in a given culture. That is, these lesions might affect context-dependent judgments. This interpretation would help explain why the findings have not been fully cross-validated across the cultures studied thus far.

Table 12-2. Correlations of BNI Screen for Higher Cerebral Functions and PCRS total scores in three studies

Population studied	Correlation Coefficient	Number in Group
Prigatano and Leathem (1993)		
Non-Maori, English ancestry TBI patients	+.26	18
Non-Maori, English ancestry TBI relatives	+.46*	17
Maori ancestry TBI patients	−.04	14
Maori ancestry TBI relatives	+.50*	17
Prigatano (1996)		
U.S. TBI patients (some received neuropsychological rehabilitation)	+.43*	31
U.S. TBI relatives	+.51*	31
U.S. neuropsychological controls (patients)	.64†	20
U.S. neuropsychological controls (relatives)	.66†	20
Prigatano, Ogano, and Amakusa (1997)		
Japanese TBI patients	−.09	21
Japanese TBI relatives	+.68*	21

PCRS = Patient's Competency Rating Scale; TBI = traumatic brain injury.
*p = .05; †p = .01.

Speed of Finger Tapping and Impaired Self-Awareness in TBI Patients

A post hoc analysis of the Japanese study revealed another important finding. The speed of finger tapping on the Halstead Finger Oscillation Test (Reitan, 1955) by Japanese TBI patients who consistently overestimated their abilities for self-care and appropriate social interactions tended to be slow (mean speed of 35 taps or less, Table 12-3). This finding was true when the patients' ratings were compared to their relatives' ratings and to the physical therapist's ratings of the patients' functional capacities.

The implications of this finding broaden when three other studies are considered. Prigatano and Altman (1990) noted that the speed of finger tapping of American TBI patients who consistently overestimated their behavioral limitations (i.e., Group 1) was slow bilaterally, but the effect was only significant for the patients' left hand (Table 12-4). On numerous other psychometric measures, the patients who overestimated their functional capacity (Group 1) did not differ from groups who did not overestimate their neuropsychological impairments. The groups differed only in terms of the speed of finger tapping.

Table 12-3. Post hoc analysis of possible relationship between speed of finger tapping and PCRS ratings in Japanese patients with severe TBI

	Mean	SD	F Ratio	p
Patient vs. relative social-emotional subscale				
Speed of FT ≤ 35 (n = 8)	6.88	(11.36)		
Speed of FT > 35 (n = 11)	−2.00	(8.25)	3.9180	.0642
Self-care subscale				
Speed of FT ≤ 35 (n = 8)	5.13	(8.04)		
Speed of FT > 35 (n = 11)	−1.00	(3.92)	4.8673	.0414
Patient vs. physical therapist social-emotional subscale				
Speed of FT ≤ 35 (n = 6)	15.33	(10.44)		
Speed of FT > 35 (n = 3)	−.667	(7.51)	5.4468	.0523
Self-care subscale				
Speed of FT ≤ 35 (n = 6)	11.17	(8.13)		
Speed of FT > 35 (n = 3)	−4.33	(1.53)	10.0253	.0158

PCRS = Patient Competency Rating Scale, TBI = traumatic brain injury, SD = standard deviation, and FT = finger tapping.

From Prigatano, et al., 1997. With permission from Lippincott-Raven.

The speed of finger tapping in both the dominant and nondominant hands of TBI patients also correlates with the amount of time that it takes them to respond to commands in a meaningful way (Dikmen, et al., 1995). The correlation between these variables was about 0.50. This finding suggests that the speed of finger tapping is related to the severity of the initial injury. After mild to moderate TBIs, the speed of finger tapping also recovers less than grip strength (Haaland, et al., 1994). Although this evidence is indirect, speed of finger tapping could be extremely sensitive to brain injury and therefore recover less well than grip strength. If speed of finger tapping reflects the severity of brain injury, it could also serve as an indirect marker of impaired self-awareness.

The question then arises: Does impaired self-awareness correlate with severity of brain injury? Two recent studies suggest that it does. Sherer and colleagues (1998) found a correlation of +0.39 ($p < .05$) between admitting Glasgow Coma Scale (GCS) scores and later judgments of awareness. Less severely injured TBI patients were more aware several months after injury. With Spanish TBI patients, Prigatano and colleagues (1998) reported a correlation of −0.39 ($p < .05$) between admitting GCS scores and a measure of impaired awareness. The more severely injured TBI patients showed more impaired awareness several months after injury. The magnitude of the correlation between the two studies was identical.

Table 12-4. Neuropsychological test scores by groups

Test	Group I	Group II	Group III	F	df	p
WAIS-R (mean scale scores)						
Information	7.5	8.4	7.2	.96	2,53	.39
Similarities	9.4	8.8	8.6	.43	2,28	.65
Block design	9.1	9.5	8.9	.17	2,59	.23
Digit symbol	6.6	8.0	7.9	1.52	2,59	.23
WMS and WMS-R (mean raw scores)						
Visual reproduction						
card A	5.4	5.8	5.9	.96	2,53	.39
card C	6.3	7.2	7.1	.83	2,53	.44
Total hard paired-associates	5.3	6.3	5.1	1.42	2,60	.25
Halstead manual finger tapping (mean taps/10 sec)						
Right hand	35.7	44.4	39.3	1.92	2,52	.15
Left hand	31.4	41.9	42.4	5.90	2,52	.005
WCST						
Categories achieved	4.7	5.3	5.7	1.37	2,48	.26
Cards used	107.2	91.1	100.0	.95	2,48	.35

WAIS-R = Wechsler Adult Intelligence Scale-Revised, WMS-R = Wechsler Memory Scale-Revised; WCST = Wisconsin Card Sorting Test
From Prigatano and Altman, 1990. With permission from W. B. Saunders.

A Model of Impaired Self-Awareness

As the quote introducing this chapter suggests, we have reached an area of speculation—but the speculation is based on empirical and clinical observations. Disorders of self-awareness are perplexing for several reasons. First, they manifest in a wide variety of forms. Furthermore, in some patients the apparent lack of insight appears to be "organically" based and in others it appears to reflect some effort at psychological coping. How can this conflicting array of observations be resolved?

The place to begin is to recognize that different forms of impaired awareness emanate from damage to different brain regions. Second, like all neurological syndromes, impairments of awareness can change over time. The severity of the syndrome is based on the extent of the disturbed brain area involved. As dysfunctional brain regions partially recover, the syndrome changes from a "complete" anosognosia to a "partial" anosognosia.

No simple descriptive terms have emerged to describe these phenomena adequately. When language disorders follow brain damage, the term aphasia has been used to refer to the initial loss of language function. To reflect a partial recovery of language function even though the deficit remains, the term aphasia is replaced by the term dysphasia. Yet, neither of these terms adequately reflects that a disturbance is complete or partial. Hence, they are unsatisfactory. For the time being, it might be best then to refer to complete or partial syndromes of impaired self-awareness.

Next, we must recognize that a syndrome depends on which region of heteromodal cortex has been damaged. Although discussed elsewhere (Prigatano, 1991), the basis of this existing model is summarized below.

Mesulam has reconceptualized the organization of the cerebral hemispheres (Fig. 12-2). Traditional neurology has focused on the primary sensorimotor cortex (blue areas). S1 and M1, regions surrounding the central sulcus, are extremely important to the perception of factual information and the ability to perform basic sensorimotor functions, respectively. A1, Heschl's gyrus, is crucial for the perception of auditory inputs. V1 and V2 refer to the occipital notch and the calcarine fissure, areas crucial for visual perception. All of these areas are important for processing information about the exterior world, that is, the world outside of the "skin."

The regions known as the limbic system, which Mesulam has renamed the *paralimbic belt* or *paralimbic region* (green areas), process information about the world "under the skin." In other words, these regions are extremely important to the perception of the internal bodily milieu—aspects such as body temperature or certain crude emotional states.

The rest of the brain has traditionally been referred to as association cortex. Mesulam (1985) further divides this area into *unimodal* (yellow areas) and *heteromodal* (pink areas) regions. The unimodal cortex primarily responds to stimuli in one modality but at a complex level. For example, areas in the inferior temporal cortex often respond to changes

Figure 12-2. Mesulam's distribution of functional zones in relation to Brodmann's map of the human brain. The boundaries are not intended to be precise. Much of this information is based on experimental evidence obtained from laboratory animals and needs to be confirmed in the human brain. AA = auditory association cortex; AG = angular gyrus; A1 = primary auditory cortex; CG = cingulate cortex; INS = insula; IPL = inferior parietal lobule; IT = inferior temporal gyrus; MA = motor association cortex; MPO = medial parietooccipital area; MT = middle temporal gyrus; M1 = primary motor area; OF = orbitofrontal region; PC = prefrontal cortex; PH = parahippocampal region; PO = parolfactory area; PS = peristriate cortex; RS = retrosplenial area; SA = somatosensory association cortex; SG = supramarginal gyrus; SPL = superior parietal lobule; ST = superior temporal gyrus; S1 = primary somatosensory area; TP = temporopolar cortex; VA = visual association cortex; V1 = primary visual cortex. From Mesulam, M. M. (1985). *Principles of Behavioral Neurology.* F. A. Davis, Philadelphia. With permission from F. A. Davis.

in the angle of a visual stimulus. Heteromodal regions are the last to develop both phylogenetically and ontogenetically. These regions involve large areas of the prefrontal and frontal cortex, the inferior parietal lobule, the supramarginal and angular gyri, and portions of the temporal lobe.

As noted elsewhere (Prigatano, 1991), different forms of impaired awareness seem to emerge from damage to different areas of heteromodal cortex. Injuries to the inferior parietal lobule often produce unawareness of disorders of hemiplegia. Disturbances to the angular gyrus are often associated with aphasic syndromes in which individuals are unaware of their impaired language output. Damage to the frontal and prefrontal areas often elicits disturbances in social behavior, judgment, planning, and the capacity for empathy of which patients are unaware.

Different syndromes of impaired awareness can therefore be broadly conceptualized, depending on which region of the heteromodal cortex is damaged (Table 12-5). Within the context of this model, individuals could have *frontal heteromodal* disorders of impaired self-awareness, *parietal heteromodal* disorders of impaired self-awareness, *temporal heteromodal* disorders of self-awareness, and *occipital heteromodal* disorders of self-awareness. Theoretically, the presence of bilateral cerebral dysfunction in these heteromodal regions would result in a complete syndrome. Otherwise, a partial syndrome would manifest.

This model could account for the rapid changes in anosognosia for hemiplegia that are observed clinically. Soon after a unilateral stroke, bilateral cerebral dysfunction may often be present even though only unilateral damage is visualized on CT (Prigatano and Wong, 1997). As the so-called unaffected hemisphere begins to regain its functional capacity, the frank phenomenon of complete anosognosia begins to disappear, although residual and important disturbances in self-awareness may remain. The neural circuitry underlying various types of changes in awareness is unknown; however, the model suggests that bilateral cerebral dysfunction would be associated with complete syndromes and unilateral dysfunction with partial syndromes.

The heteromodal cortex integrates information processed by the primary sensorimotor cortex about the external world with the information processed by the limbic regions about the inner world. The model

Figure 12-3. The purple area represents the findings reported by Reiman and colleagues (1996): bilateral hypometabolic activity of the parietal and temporal lobes. Superimposed are the positron emission tomography (turquoise) findings from the 77-year-old woman suspected of dementia of the Alzheimer type who also shows an impairment of self-awareness. This patient's hypometabolic activity primarily involves bilateral temporal and inferior parietal regions and a large area of the posterior cingulate.

Table 12-5 Disorders of impaired self-awareness (direct effects of brain damage)

Disorder	Manifestation	Probable Brain Dysfunctional Regions
Frontal heteromodal		
Complete syndrome	No awareness of impaired self–awareness as a social being. No awareness of socially inappropriate comments. No awareness of one's reduced capacity to plan or anticipate. No awareness of one's reduced capacity for empathy in interpersonal situations.	Bilateral prefrontal and frontal cortices. Diffuse involvement of both anterior cerebral hemispheres. Frontal and cingulate connections particularly disturbed.
Partial syndrome	Limited awareness of inappropriate social behavior, including comments, actions, etc. Limited awareness of one's reduced capacity to plan or anticipate; limited awareness of a change in one's capacity for empathy in interpersonal relationships.	Unilateral cerebral cortex; frontal and cingulate connections impaired in functional integrity.
Parietal heteromodal		
Complete syndrome	No awareness of impaired sensorimotor function. No awareness of hemiplegia. No awareness of hemi-inattention. No awareness of reduced balance or capacity to navigate freely and safely in space.	Bilateral parietal cortex. Inferior parietal and posterior cingulate regions impaired in functional integrity.
Partial syndrome	Limited awareness of motor impairment with no appreciation of the impact it has on safety or the capacity to ambulate independently.	Unilateral cerebral cortex. Inferior parietal and cingulate connection impaired in functional integrity.

(continued)

Table 12-5—Continued

Disorder	Manifestation	Probable Brain Dysfunctional Regions
Partial syndrome	Limited awareness of reduced attentional capacities with no appreciation of implications for functional independence.	

Temporal heteromodal

Complete syndrome	No awareness of a memory impairment being "abnormal" for age or situation. No awareness that visual or auditory perceptions are distorted. Problems with visual and auditory perception explained on the basis of exterior causes (a faulty stereo; dim lights, etc.) Can result in misinterpretation of complex visual and auditory inputs given from others and lead to paranoid thinking.	Bilateral cerebral cortex, particularly the superior temporal and mesial temporal cortex. Temporal limbic connections are disturbed, particularly involving the amygdala and hippocampal regions.
Partial syndromes	Limited awareness of above.	Unilateral cerebral cortex involving superior and mesial temporal region. Temporal limbic connections, particularly involving the amygdala and hippocampus.

Occipital heteromodal

Complete syndrome	No awareness of cortical blindness or hemianopsia.	Bilateral occipital limbic disruptions.
Partial syndrome	Awareness of some disturbance in vision, although difficult to describe. May not recognize implications for safety.	Unilateral occipital limbic disruptions.

therefore suggests that the heteromodal cortex is the basis from which self-awareness ultimately emerges. Consequently, any true anosognosia would involve disruptions of cognitive and affective components of neuropsychological functioning, accounting for the definite changes in both affect and cognition reported in anosognostic patients (Starkstein, 1992; Cutting, 1978).

This clinical fact is often neglected by the disciplines of cognitive neuropsychology and cognitive sciences. It is vital that practicing clinical neuropsychologists bring affective changes associated with disturbances of awareness to the attention of their more theoretical colleagues. Again, however, the disturbance is not psychiatric. Rather, by its very nature, awareness reflects an integration of both thinking and feeling. This contention is difficult to demonstrate empirically, but case examples provide indirect evidence that impaired self-awareness involves more than a pure cognitive dysfunction.

Further Evidence that Impaired Self-Awareness Is Not a Purely Cognitive Function

Individuals with a genetic predisposition for Alzheimer's disease show hypometabolic activity in regions of the hetermodal cortex (Reiman, et al., 1996). This observation is compatible with well-known clinical and empirical literature. For example, patients with Alzheimer's disease often show bilateral atrophy in the parietal regions. As the disease progresses, both temporal lobes are involved. The degree of atrophy is often asymmetrical but it is still bilateral. Furthermore, the posterior cingulate can be surprisingly hypometabolic in patients with a predisposition for Alzheimer's disease.

Against this background, a fortuitous case came to my attention. A 77-year-old woman began to show a memory decline that alarmed her observant daughter. Consequently, the daughter requested that her mother undergo a neuropsychological evaluation. The initial evaluation showed considerable memory impairment relative to the patient's intelligence. Even more startling, the patient seemed totally unconcerned or unaware of the implications of her memory impairment. She stated, for example, that she was 77 years old, widowed, and had little to do each day. The memory failures that she noticed she attributed to her age and environmental circumstances. In contrast, her daughter clearly documented that the memory impairments were substantial and far beyond what would be expected from this intelligent woman.

A PET study was finally obtained to determine the nature of this woman's brain dysfunction (Fig. 12-3). The major area of hypometabolic activity was in the temporal regions. The model would suggest that this patient has a single major syndrome—memory impairment. However, her posterior cingulate area also exhibited hypometabolic activity. Again, the model would suggest that she would have no experience of the memory disorder and hence no affective distress.

As this patient begins to deteriorate and to show signs of impaired social judgment, the model would predict that the hypometabolic activity in the prefrontal regions would increase. If the disturbance, however, is purely cognitive, the posterior dorsolateral surface would be the primary area of dysfunction. And if her disturbance of awareness reflects deterioration of the integration of cognition and feeling, enhanced hypometabolic activity should also be observed in the anterior cingulate region as well. The patient is now being followed up to test the predictive power of the model.

Implications for Neuropsychological Rehabilitation

Principle 11 states that neuropsychological rehabilitation can help clarify the nature of disturbances of self-awareness and thereby lead to better management and rehabilitative care for patients. How is this actually accomplished?

When patients have a complete syndrome of impaired self-awareness, it is futile to try to argue with them. Rather, patients should be examined to determine the extent and the nature of their complete syndrome of impaired awareness. Patients should be kept in a safe environment, one that helps them to establish a relationship with their caregivers (i.e., their therapists, physicians, psychologists, and so on). They need slow and patient guidance, not lectures.

Inevitably, these patients will experience a number of failures that they do not understand. Apathy will give way to frustration. The therapist can then establish a therapeutic alliance by working toward reducing patients' frustration by appropriate management of the environment. The relationship can be used to guide patients to make safe decisions. During this time, patients exhibit little, if any, resistance.

Resistance emerges when their syndrome recovers from complete to partial. With partial syndromes, again, the first step is to evaluate the extent and nature of the impaired self-awareness. If a therapeutic alliance has been established, the relationship can now be built upon. The therapist continues to guide patients slowly toward recognition of how their higher cerebral functions have been affected. This process occurs within the context of cognitive rehabilitation, speech and language therapy, physical therapy, and occupational therapy. Making patients feel safe and comfortable remains a major focus. The patients continue to experience frustration, however, and are often perplexed and confused. Patients sense that something is wrong but may behave in a manner that seems to imply that nothing is really wrong. At this point, many patients will attempt to represent their partial knowledge symbolically (Fig. 12-4).

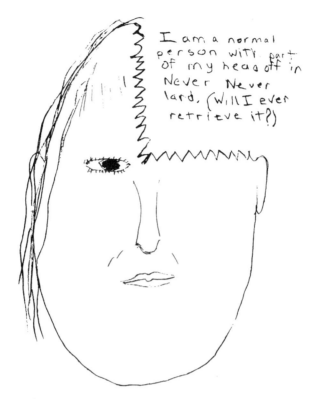

I am a normal person with part of my head off in Never Never land. (Will I ever retrieve it?)

Figure 12-4. Drawing by a brain dysfunctional patient with presumed "partial awareness" of impaired higher cerebral functions that symbolized her feelings about her brain injury. This classic picture was used on the cover of our textbook *Awareness of Deficit After Brain Injury: Clinical and Theoretical Issues.* First published in Prigatano, G.P. and Klonoff, P. S. (1988). Psychotherapy and neuropsychological assessment after brain injury. *Journal of Head Trauma Rehabilitation* 3: (1) 45–60. Copyright © Aspen Publishers, Inc.

At this point, it becomes *very* important for the clinician to try and answer the question: What type of method of coping is the patient using? Some methods simply reflect premorbid coping strategies that are non-defensive in nature. That is, the person is relying on previous ways of thinking and behaving to get his or her needs met in an adaptive fashion. The person, for example, may say he wants to return to his university teaching duties despite visuospatial and memory problems. Patients believe (i.e., do not experience) that such problems will not substantially stop them from being successful. Moreover, they have learned from past experience that their job responsibilities afforded them a sense of prestige, pleasure, and avoidance of normal domestic problems. This is not the use of psychological denial to cope. It is not a defense mechanism as described in the psychiatric literature (American Psychiatric Association, 1994).

This nondefensive method of coping with partial syndromes of impaired awareness can be contrasted to defensive methods of coping with a partial impairment of awareness. A defense mechanism, by definition, is "an automatic psychological process that protects the individual against anxiety and from awareness of internal or external stressor or dangers" (American Psychiatric Association, 1994; p. 765). It is a refusal "to acknowledge some painful aspect of external reality or subjective experience" (American Psychiatric Association, 1994; p. 753).

Brain dysfunctional patients who insist that they are not damaged, who blame others for their shortcomings, and who often resist any clinically sensible approach to rehabilitation often reveal some aspect of defensive coping skills. These defensive coping skills are not limited to denial, but can virtually draw upon any of the known psychological defense mechanisms. For example, the patient may become paranoid and project onto his caregivers internal worries that he experiences (e.g., they are thinking that I am gay! they want to hurt me because I am not a "yes man"; they want to keep me in rehabilitation just to make money).

Defensive methods of coping have to be approached with all of the respect seen in the competent practice of psychiatry and clinical psychology. As defense mechanisms of coping, they can only be addressed slowly and often indirectly (at first). Otherwise, the well-intentioned therapist can precipitate a clinical crisis for the patient as well as the rehabilitation team.

Thus, one can conceptualize both defensive and nondefensive methods of coping that are observed in the rehabilitation setting when patients have partial awareness syndromes (Table 12-6).

Coping strategies thus depend on how well patients can tolerate negative information about themselves, and the unpleasant realities of life. Consequently, coping strategies reflect premorbid personality characteristics. Disturbances in self-awareness reflect the region of the brain that has been damaged or rendered dysfunctional.

Summary and Conclusions

Disorders of self-awareness are beginning to be better understood. As we gain a more sophisticated understanding of how various regions of the brain integrate thinking and feeling, we can appreciate how different lesions actually produce disturbances of self-awareness. Consideration of premorbid methods of coping helps determine to what degree these methods reflect nondefensive or defensive approaches to coping with partial information.

Previously, I attempted to distinguish impaired self-awareness from denial of disability (Prigatano and Klonoff, 1997), but that classification system now appears too simple. The behavioral descriptions of impaired self-awareness reflected a clear disruption of the integration of

Table 12-6. Methods of coping with partial syndromes of impaired awareness
(indirect effects of brain injury)

Methods	Example
Nondefensive	
Use of existing beliefs and values to cope with partial knowledge.	Patient with posttraumatic amnesia explains that she is in the hospital to have a baby. The only reason she would ever be in the hospital would be to have a baby.
Use of preexisting behavioral strategies to solve problems.	Patient insists on returning to work to regain feeling of being effective and to recover from brain injury. Previously, work used to diffuse anxiety-provoking situations.
Defensive	
Denial of existing problem that is partially recognized	"I can't allow you or anyone else to discourage me from going back to work. I am perfectly normal and I will show you."
Projection of existing problem partially recognized	"*You* are making me worse by keeping me in the hospital or this rehabilitation program."
Intellectualization (as a defense) only partially recognized	"Of course I have a memory impairment but I have learned to compensate for it and can therefore return to my previous university."

thinking and feeling. However, the scale reflecting denial of disability did not adequately represent how the distinctions made in this text, that is, methods of coping, could be defensive or nondefensive. And it is inappropriate to use denial to describe nondefensive reactions. It is hoped that this classification can be developed further; the form of different syndromes amplified; the change in these syndromes documented over time; and the most salient ingredients that distinguish the four syndromes of impaired self-awareness highlighted in this chapter clarified.

Understanding and measuring disorders of impaired awareness after TBI can lead to important empirical observations. Recently, for example, Sherer and colleagues (1998) demonstrated that two methods of measuring impaired awareness after TBI predicted employment outcome better than measures of severity of TBI, time since injury, preinjury employment status, preinjury use of alcohol, or the level of cognitive functioning. Understanding complex disturbances of self-awareness and how they may change over time is important for neuropsychological rehabilitation. The next chapter considers both recovery and deterioration phenomena as they impact the field of neuropsychological rehabilitation.

References

American Psychiatric Association (1994). *DSM-IV: Diagnostic and Statistical Manual of Mental Disorders*. Washington, DC: American Psychiatric Association.

Anton, G. (1898). Ueber Herderkrankungen des Gehirnes, welche von Patienten selbst nicht wahrgenommen werden. *Wien. Klin. Wchnschr.* 11: 227–229.

Babinski, J. (1914). Contribution à l'etude des troubles mentaux dans l'hémiplégie organique cérébrale (Anosognosie). *Revue Neurologique* 27: 845–847.

Bauer, R. M., and Rubens, A. B. (1985). Agnosia. In K. M. Heilman and E. Valenstein (eds). *Clinical Neuropsychology* (2nd ed, pp. 187–229). Oxford University Press, New York.

Bisiach, E., Vallar, G., Perani, D., Papagno, and Berti, A. (1986). Unawareness of disease following lesions of the right hemisphere: Anosognosia for hemiplegia and anosognosia for hemianopia. *Neuropsychologia* 24(4): 471–482.

Bisiach, E., and Geminiani, G. (1991). Anosognosia related to hemiplegia and hemianopia. In G. P. Prigatano and R. L. Schacter (eds), *Awareness of Deficit After Brain Injury. Clinical and Theoretical Issues* (pp. 17–39). Oxford University Press, New York.

Blakemore, C. (1977). *Mechanics to the Mind*. Cambridge University Press, London.

Brodal, A. (1973). Self-observations and neuro-anatomical considerations after a stroke. *Brain* 96: 675–694.

Charcot, J. M. (1882). Sur les divers états nerveux déterminés par l'hynotisation chez les hystériques. *Comptes-Rendus hebdomadaires des séances de l'Académie des Sciences* XCIV: 403–405.

Cutting, J. (1978). Study of anosognosia. *J. Neurol. Neurosurg. Psychiatry* 41: 548–555.

Dikmen, S., Machamer, J. E., Winn, H. R., and Temkin, N. R. (1995). Neuropsychological outcome at 1-year post head injury. *Neuropsychology* 9: 80–90.

Doyle, A. C. (1986). *Sherlock Holmes: The Complete Novels and Stories* (Vol. 2, pp. 1–146). Bantam, New York.

Fleming, J. M., Strong, J., and Ashton, R. (1996). Self-awareness of deficits in adults with traumatic brain injury: how best to measure? *Brain Inj.* 10: 1–15.

Gainotti, G. (1975). Confabulation of denial in senile dementia: an experimental study. *Psychiatric Clinics* 8: 99–108.

German, W. J., Flanigan, S., and Davey, L. M. (1964). Remarks on subdural hematoma and aphasia. *Clin. Neurosurg.* 12: 344–350.

Haaland, K. Y., Temkin, N., Randahl, G., and Dikmen, S. (1994) Recovery of simple motor skills after head injury. *J. Clin. Exp. Neuropsychol.* 16: 448–456.

Head, H. (1920). *Studies in Neurology* (pp. 560–561). Oxford University Press, London.

LaBaw, W. L. (1969). Denial inside out: subjective experience with anosognosia in closed head injury. *Psychiatry* 32(1): 174–191.

Lebrun, Y. (1987). Anosognosia in aphasics. *Cortex* 23: 251–263.

McGlynn, S. M. and Kaszniak, A. L. (1991). Unawareness of deficits in dementia and schizophrenia. In G. P. Prigatano and D. L. Schacter (eds), *Awareness of Deficit After Brain Injury. Clinical and Theoretical Issues.* Oxford University Press, New York.

Mesulam, M. M. (1985). *Principles of Behavioral Neurology.* F. A. Davis, Philadelphia.

Perani, D., Vallar, G., Paulesu, E., Alberoni, M., and Fazio, F. (1993). Left and right hemisphere contribution to recovery from neglect after right hemisphere damage—an[^{18}F] FDG PET study of two cases. *Neuropsychologia* 31: 115–125.

Pick, A. (1908). Ueber Störungen der Orientierung am eigenen Körper. Arbeiten aus der psychiatrischen. *Klin. Prag.* 1 (Berlin, Karger).

Prigatano, G. P. (1988). Anosognosia, delusions, and altered self-awareness after brain injury: a historical perspective. *BNI Quarterly* 4(3): 40–48.

Prigatano, G. P. (1991). Disturbances of self-awareness of deficit after traumatic brain injury. In: Prigatano, G. P., Schachter, D. L. (eds) *Awareness of Deficit After Brain Injury: Clinical and Theoretical Implications.* New York, Oxford University Press.

Prigatano, G. P. (1996). Behavioral limitations TBI patients tend to underestimate: a replication and extension to patients with lateralized cerebral dysfunction. *Clinical Neuropsychologist* 10(2): 191–201.

Prigatano, G. P., and Altman, I. M. (1990). Impaired awareness of behavioral limitations after traumatic brain injury. *Arch. Phys. Med. Rehabil.* 71: 1058–1063.

Prigatano, G. P., Altman, I. M., and O'Brien, K. P. (1990). Behavioral limitations that traumatic-brain-injured patients tend to underestimate. *Clinical Neuropsychologist* 4(2): 163–176.

Prigatano, G. P., Bruna, O., Mataro, M., Muñoz, J. M., Fernandez, S., and Junque, C. (1998). Initial disturbances of consciousness and resultant impaired awareness in Spanish traumatic brain injured patients. *Journal of Head Trauma Rehabilitation* 13(5): 29–38.

Prigatano, G. P., Fordyce, D. J., Zeiner, H. K., Roueche, J. R., Pepping, M., and Wood, B. (1984). Neuropsychological rehabilitation after closed head injury in young adults. *J. Neurol. Neurosurg. Psychiatry.* 47: 505–513.

Prigatano, G. P., and Klonoff, P. S. (1997). A clinician's rating scale for evaluating impaired self-awareness and denial of disability after brain injury. *Clinical Neuropsychologist* 11(1): 1–12.

Prigatano, G. P., and Leathem, J. M. (1993). Awareness of behavioral limitations after traumatic brain injury: a cross-cultural study of New Zealand Maoris and non-Maoris. *Clinical Neuropsychologist* 7(2): 123–135.

Prigatano, G. P., and O'Brien, K. P. (1991). Awareness of deficit in patients with frontal and parietal lesions: two case reports. *BNI Quarterly* 7(1): 17–23.

Prigatano, G. P., Ogano, M., and Amakusa, B. (1997). A cross-cultural study on impaired self-awareness in Japanese patients with brain dysfunction. *Neuropsychiatry, Neuropsychology, and Behavioral Neurology* 10(1): 135–143.

Prigatano, G. P., and Schacter, D. L. (1991). *Awareness of Deficit After Brain Injury: Clinical and Theoretical Issues.* Oxford University Press, New York.

Prigatano, G. P., and Weinstein, E. A. (1996). Edwin A. Weinstein's contributions to neuropsychological rehabilitation. *Neuropsychological Rehabilitation* 6(4): 305–326.

Prigatano, G. P., and Wong, J. (1997). Speed of finger tapping and goal attainment after unilateral cerebral vascular accident. *Arch. Phys. Med. Rehabil.* 78: 847–852.

Reiman, E. M., Caselli, R. J., Yun, L. S., Chen, K., Bandy, D., Minoshima, S., Thibodeau, S. N., and Osborne, D. (1996). Preclinical evidence of Alzheimer's disease in persons homozygous for the E4 allele for apolipoprotein E. *N. Engl. J. Med.* 334: 752–758.

Reitan, R. M. (1955). *Manual for Administration of Neuropsychological Test Batteries for Adults and Children.* Neuropsychology Laboratory, Indiana University Medical Center, Indianapolis.

Roeser, R. J., and Daly, D. D., (1974). Auditory cortex disconnection associated with thalamic tumor: a case report. *Neurology* 24: 555–559.

Rubens, A. B. (1979). Agnosia. In K. M. Heilman and E. Valenstein (eds), *Clinical Neuropsychology* (1st ed, pp. 233–267). Oxford University Press, New York.

Rubens, A. B., and Benson, D. F. (1971). Associative visual agnosia. *Arch. Neurol.* 24: 304–316.

Rubens, A. B., and Garrett, M. F. (1991). Anosognosia of linguistic deficits in patients with neurological deficits. In G. P. Prigatano and D. L. Schacter (eds), *Awareness of Deficit After Brain Injury. Clinical and Theoretical Issues.* Oxford University Press, New York.

Sandifer, P. H. (1946). Anosognosia and disorders of body scheme. *Brain* 69: 122–137.

Sherer, M., Bergloff, P., Levin, E., High, W. M., Jr., Oden, K. E., and Nick, T. G. (1998). Impaired awareness and employment outcome after traumatic brain injury. *Journal of Head Trauma Rehabilitation* 13(5): 52–61.

Sherer, M., Boake, C., Levin, E., Silver, B. V., Ringholz, G., and High, W. (1998). Characteristics of impaired awareness after traumatic brain injury. *Journal of International Neuropsychological Society* 4, 380–387.

Starkstein, S. E., Fedoroff, J. P., Price, T. R., Leiguarda, R., and Robinson, R. G. (1992). Anosognosia in patients with cerebrovascular lesions: a study of causative factors. *Stroke* 23(10): 1446–1453.

von Monakow, C. (1885). Experimentelle und pathologisch-anatomische Untersuchungen über die Beziehungen der sogentannen Sehsphäre zu den infracorticalen Opticuscentren und zum N. opticus. *Archiv. für Psychiatrie* 16: 151–199.

Weinstein, E. A., and Kahn, R. L. (1955). *Denial of Illness. Symbolic and Physiological Aspects.* Charles C. Thomas, Springfield, Ill.

13

Recovery and Deterioration
After Brain Injury

> One can probably never speak of a *fixed* neurological lesion.
> N. Geschwind, "Mechanisms of change
> after brain lesions," 1985, p. 8

Observations of patients within a few weeks to several years after a brain insult support the concept of a continued pattern of dynamic change in brain dysfunctional persons. This pattern seems to be true of a variety of neuropathological lesions and disease states. Although recovery is seldom, if ever, complete after significant neuronal loss, the brain is a dynamic organ constantly undergoing change for the better or worse. Thus, Geschwind's (1985) observation that "One can probably never speak of a *fixed* neurological lesion" is important to heed.

Follow-up evaluations of patients who have undergone neuropsychological rehabilitation have taught some important lessons. Some patients exhibit objective signs of continued partial improvement several months and even years after injury and participation in formal rehabilitation. In other instances, patients clearly deteriorate. Both the improvement and the deterioration can be observed in both direct and indirect symptoms, and these phenomena should be studied experimentally and clinically.

This chapter reviews some of these observations and attempts to place them in a perspective based on contemporary concepts of brain plasticity and behavior (Kolb, 1995) and theories of recovery (Stein, 1999). Competent patient management and planning of innovative rehabilitation programs depend on understanding the mechanisms underlying these changes (i.e., Principle 12).

What Is Recovery of Function?

Before specific case examples that highlight different patterns of change associated with various brain insults are discussed, some attempt to de-

Portions of this chapter were presented at a workshop entitled "Recovery and deterioration after brain injury: Implications for neuropsychological rehabilitation." 16th Annual Academy of Neuropsychology Meeting, New Orleans, La, October 30–November 1996.

fine the phrase "recovery of function" is necessary. Laurence and Stein (1978) provided the following definition: "Recovery of function can be generally defined as a return to a normal or near normal level of performance following the initially disruptive effect of injury to the nervous system" (p. 370). These authors, however, commented that even when patients' level of performance appears to approach their premorbid levels, "normal" and "recovered" functions may still have numerous "qualitative" differences. These differences are often noticeable in clinical practice. Recently, Stein (1996) concluded that there is no consensus about the meaning of the terms recovery or function. Strictly speaking, complete recovery means a return to an organism's premorbid state.

Luria (1966) suggested that in biology, function can be defined in two ways. It can refer to "the activity performed by a given organ or tissue" (p. 27), or it can be defined as ". . . an organism's complex adaptive ability" (p. 24). The latter definition implies the existence of a functional system or systems. Luria (1966) further defined functional systems as ". . . complex dynamic 'constellations' of connections, situated at different levels of the nervous system, that, in the performance of an adaptive task, may be changed while the task itself remains unchanged" (p. 24).

From a mathematical perspective, function has a simpler definition: "A function f is a correspondence or relationship that pairs each member of a given set with *exactly* one member of another set" (Lynch and Olmstead, 1998; p. 16). Thus, in mathematical terms, a function is defined via a function rule that can be expressed by an equation. For example, speed of finger tapping (X) has been defined as a function of age (Y) given in the following equation: $Y = -0.03X + 6.92$ (see Shimoyama, et al., 1990).

It should be noted that theoretically a set can refer to numbers (as noted above) or it can refer to names, geometric configurations, neural networks, and so on. The function describes the laws of a relationship. When these laws are expressed in mathematical terms, the laws are called a function rule.

Based on this definition, recovery of function would mean the reestablishment of previous function rules that existed before a brain insult. Input x would result in output y given function rule f. Consider, for example, a possible function rule that might govern rote verbal learning in a young, bright, normal adult *before* brain injury.

Predictable patterns of learning (or a learning curve) on the Rey Auditory Verbal Learning Test (RAVLT) have been documented by Geffen and her colleagues (Geffen, et al., 1990; Forrester and Geffen, 1991). Extrapolating from these data as well as from clinical practice, one often observes the following phenomena. After being exposed to a list of 15 words for the first time and being asked to remember that list, bright, normal adults (aged 19 to 21) often recall 5 to 7 words. After a second repetition, 8 to 10 words are typically recalled. After a third repetition, 11 to 12 words are generally remembered. By the fourth repetition, 13 to 14 words are recalled. By the fifth repetition, all 15 words are typically recalled, even though group norms with individuals of average intelligence may be somewhat lower.

Theoretically, the learning curve could be described as a mathematical function rule. F words/recalled = $5 + 2t$, where t = trial number. Therefore, the expected values for a bright young adult would be as follows:

$$\text{Trial } 1 = 5 + 2(1) = 7$$

$$\text{Trial } 2 = 5 + 2(2) = 9$$

$$\text{Trial } 3 = 5 + 2(3) = 11$$

$$\text{Trial } 4 = 5 + 2(4) = 13$$

$$\text{Trial } 5 = 5 + 2(5) = 15$$

The variability of performance on any given trial could reflect a variety of biological or psychological factors that could alter performance but not necessarily the underlying function rule, which specifies the relationship. For example, fatigue, anxiety, or depression might cause performance to deviate from its predicted level. As bright, normal individuals regain their typical homeostatic function (i.e., adequate sleep, reduced anxiety or depression), the function rule seems to be fully operative.

Age is known to influence the level of performance on neuropsychological tests (see Chapter 3), but the pattern of learning (i.e., learning curve) often remains predictable across age on the RAVLT (Geffen et al., 1990; Forrester and Geffen, 1991). Age, however, may influence the function rule by altering the constant. For example, for a person at age 12, the function rule may be F words/recalled = $3 + 2t$, where t equals the trial number. This function would produce the following performance.

$$\text{Trial } 1 = 3 + 2(1) = 5$$

$$\text{Trial } 2 = 3 + 2(2) = 7$$

$$\text{Trial } 3 = 3 + 2(3) = 9$$

$$\text{Trial } 4 = 3 + 2(4) = 11$$

$$\text{Trial } 5 = 3 + 2(5) = 13$$

For older adolescents, the function rule may be F words/recalled = $4 + 2t$, where t = trial number:

$$\text{Trial } 1 = 4 + 2(1) = 6$$

$$\text{Trial } 2 = 4 + 2(2) = 8$$

$$\text{Trial 3} = 4 + 2(3) = 10$$
$$\text{Trial 4} = 4 + 2(4) = 12$$
$$\text{Trial 5} = 4 + 2(5) = 14$$

Brain damage could temporarily affect the function rule and render it inoperable for a time, or it could permanently alter the function rule in a minor or major way. For example, an 11-year-old boy (D. W.) suffered a moderate traumatic brain injury (TBI) and 10 days later took the RAVLT (Table 13-1). His pattern of scores did not follow the function rule (expected values). Two months after injury, however, this boy's scores began to approach expected values. Theoretically, therefore, the function rule would appear to be operative again. The progressive increment on trials 1 through 4 empirically matches the normal learning curve for adolescents his age. Apparently, 4 months after injury, this boy had re-approximated the preexisting function rule related to rote verbal learning.

In contrast, a 13-year-old boy who suffered a severe TBI failed to show this normal learning curve at either 4 or 12 months after injury (Table 13-2). In his case, apparently, the function rule was permanently and severely damaged. Monitoring this boy's performance over time suggests that the function rule governing rote verbal learning (as measured by the RAVLT) did not return to normal.

Table 13-1. Performance of an 11-year-old boy on the RAVLT 10 days and 2 months after sustaining a moderate brain injury

Obtained Score	Expected Score (range)*
10 Days after injury	
Trial 1 = 3	5–7
Trial 2 = 5	7–10
Trial 3 = 10	8–11
Trial 4 = 8	10–13
Trial 5 = 9	10–13
2 Months after injury	
Trial 1 = 8	5–7
Trial 2 = 9	7–10
Trial 3 = 10	8–11
Trial 4 = 14	10–13
Trial 5 = 15	10–13

*Expected values obtained from the normative data of Geffen, et al. (1990). RAVLT = Rey Auditory Verbal Learning Test.

Table 13-2. Performance of a 13-year-old boy on the RAVLT 4
and 12 months after sustaining a severe brain injury

Scores 4 Months after Injury	Scores 12 Months after Injury	Expected Score (range)
Trial 1 = 3	Trial 1 = 5	5–7
Trial 2 = 5	Trial 2 = 5	8–11
Trial 3 = 3	Trial 3 = 7	9–13
Trial 4 = 3	Trial 4 = 7	9–13
Trial 5 = 5	Trial 5 = 5	10–14

RAVLT = Rey Auditory Verbal Learning Test.

What function rules govern the recovery of different higher cerebral functions? Can they be derived by comparing brain dysfunctional patients to appropriate matched controls? Could empirically derived approximations of these function rules be used to predict recovery or deterioration after various brain disturbances of higher cerebral function? There are no clear answers to these questions, but, in principle, approximations of these function rules could be developed. The information could then be used to predict recovery and possible deterioration.

Many variables could influence the recovery of higher cerebral functions (Table 13-3), and various function rules could be affected differentially. Although others may exist, only seven variables are known to relate to recovery of higher cerebral functions after acquired brain injury: lesion location, size of lesion, type of neuropathology, initial severity of brain insult, patient's age at injury, time since lesion onset, and premorbid intelligence. A few findings highlight the role of some of the variables.

One to two years after lesion onset, auditory comprehension recovers better in global aphasic patients with subcortical lesions than in those with cortical lesions involving the temporal lobe (Naeser, et al., 1990). Speech fluency recovers more completely after left hemispheric ischemic infarction if the lesion does not extend into the rolandic cortical region (Knopman, et al., 1983). Both size and location of the lesion also relate to recovery of speech fluency. Lesion location, size, and type of brain insult influence the symptoms of a given aphasic condition, which change over time (Kertesz, 1993). Age and gender also may influence the recovery of aphasia, but these findings are more controversial (Kertesz, 1993).

Bisiach and Vallar (1988) summarized recovery phenomena associated with hemineglect following cerebrovascular lesions. They noted that during the first few weeks after onset, improvements could be seen in most patients. They noted that little is known regarding the neural mechanisms underlying such recovery but suggest that ipsilateral subcortical structures may play an important role. They noted that after frontal and parietal lesions, hypometabolism may occur in the subcortical regions. Return to normal metabolic activity at the subcortical level perhaps contributed to partial recovery of neglect phenomena. The dynamic interaction of cortical and subcortical structures is highlighted by their discussion.

Hier and colleagues (1983) studied a wide range of behavioral disorders associated with right cerebral hemisphere stroke. Different patterns of behavioral recovery were associated with different types of disturbances. For example, the estimated median duration of recovery from frank anosognosia was 9 weeks compared to 32 weeks for dressing apraxia. Hier and colleagues (1983) have also noted that the size of a lesion greatly influences the rate of recovery. Gender and age had little impact on recovery in an elderly group that they studied. Yet gender has been linked to rehabilitation outcomes (Prigatano, et al., 1997).

When differences in recovery of function between children and adults are considered, however, age clearly exerts an influence (Sabatini, et al., 1994). Motor recovery can be dramatic in children. In adulthood such patients provide intriguing insights about the possible neurophysiological mechanisms underlying the changes. Age relates to rehabilitation outcome, irrespective of how it influences specific higher cerebral functions (Ween, et al., 1996; Prigatano, et al., 1997).

The role of premorbid intelligence on recovery (and deterioration) phenomena at various stages after brain injury is another area of considerable interest. In a study of Vietnam veterans, Grafman and colleagues (1986) reported that preinjury scores on the Armed Forces Qualification Test (AFQT) predicted the veterans' cognitive performance after brain insult. The volumes of brain tissue lost (i.e., the amount of brain damage) also related to outcome but accounted for less variance than the preinjury AFQT scores. Premorbid intelligence, as measured by educational level, serves as a protective factor in neuropsychological disturbances seen in Alzheimer patients (Alexander, et al., 1997). Initial severity of TBI, as measured by the length of time before patients can follow commands, has been related to later level of neuropsychological impairments (Dikmen, et al., 1995). Furthermore, patterns of intelligence quotient (IQ) scores after TBI have been related to the duration of posttraumatic amnesia (Bond, 1975).

Other variables have been suspected to influence recovery of higher cerebral functions, but no clear data have convincingly demonstrated their role. These variables include gender, level of education, environmental reinforcers, and a variety of variables associated with rehabilitation therapies. The latter include the type of rehabilitation therapy, the amount of time spent in rehabilitation, and the frequency of rehabilitation therapies (Rattok, et al., 1992; Klonoff, et al., [1999]). The point at which rehabilitation is initiated may be an important variable for some

Table 13-3. Known and suspected factors influencing recovery of higher cerebral functions

Factors	Reference
Known	
Lesion location	Knopman, et al. (1983)
	Naeser, et al. (1990)
	Kertesz (1993)
Size of lesion (and degree other higher cerebral functions are affected)	Knopman, et al. (1983)
	Hier, et al. (1983)
Type of neuropathology	Kertesz (1993)
	Reitan and Wolfson (1994)
Severity of brain injury*	Bond (1975)
	Dikmen, et al. (1995)
Age of subject at injury	Rassmussen and Milner (1977)
Degree of atrophy present	Sabatini, et al. (1994)
Potential for plasticity of brain structure to perform different functions	
Time since lesion onset	Lezak (1979)
	Haaland, et al. (1994)
Premorbid intelligence (and hemispheric representation of functions before lesion onset in a given individual)	Grafman, et al. (1986)
Suspected	
Gender	Prigatano, et al. (1997)
Educational level of subject	Alexander, et al. (1997)
Actual time rehabilitation therapies began	

(continued)

patients. The environmental supports (i.e., reinforcers) used to initiate and maintain the desired functional outcome also appear crucial (Wolf, et al., 1989).

The patients' energy level for engaging rehabilitation and their motivation to learn from a given therapist are often important clinically (Prigatano, 1999). Therapists' level of motivation and skill in teaching or retraining a person are likewise important. Finally, the overall emotional and motivational characteristics of both therapists and patients and how they interact with one another would seem to contribute to the outcome picture (Prigatano and Wong, 1999).

Whatever factors are shown to contribute to recovery, strictly speaking, recovery is defined as the *reinstitution* of biological (and emergent psychological) "function rules" that would permit individuals to attain their previous level of adaptive problem-solving skills.

Table 13-3.—Continued

Factors	Reference
Time spent in rehabilitation therapies	
Frequency of rehabilitation therapies	
Type of rehabilitation therapies	Rattok, et al. (1992)
Environmental supports (reinforcers) to initiate and maintain the desired function	Wolf, et al. (1989)
Patient's motivation to learn from therapy	
Therapist's motivation to teach patient	
Presence of adverse moderating variables	
Biological examples	
Reduction of cerebral blood flow from carotid stenosis	
Hepatic encephalopathy	
Psychological examples	
Angry, distressed patient	
Anxious, depressed patient	
Presence of positive moderating variables	
Biological examples	
Adequate nutrition	
Return to normal sleep cycle	
Psychological examples	
Regained sense of "mental energy"	

*Severity is often measured by the Glasgow Coma Scale score or duration of posttraumatic amnesia after traumatic brain injury.

Models of Change or "Recovery"

The definition proposed here for recovery is innately mathematical. The correspondence or relationship that pairs each member of a given set with *exactly* one member of the other set must be reestablished for true recovery to occur. This process can occur completely for some functions but only partially for others over time.

What happens when recovery is complete? Typically, complete recovery has been described as *spontaneous* and, to some degree, effortless. For example, after a severe TBI that renders a patient unconscious, the patient is unable to produce a verbal or motor response to noxious stimuli [i.e., as defined by the Glasgow Coma Scale (GCS); Jennett and Teasdale, 1981]. As the patient emerges from coma, he or she often can verbalize and make motor responses to noxious stimuli. The underlying function rule that determines such recovery does not appear to be rewritten. Such recovery is thus termed spontaneous.

The simple mathematical model (Lynch and Olmstead, 1998) indicates that the input to the patient has not changed (i.e., the examiner asks the patient to open his or her eyes). Presumably, the function rules governing eye opening have not been altered. And, finally, the patient opens his or her eyes upon command (the output is the same). This model represents true restoration of function (Fig. 13-1A). Again, the recovery often appears "spontaneous" because the underlying function rule does not appear to have been permanently changed.

Spontaneous recovery, however, often takes time and should not be confused with instantaneous. Clinically, patients' behavior changes considerably, particularly during the first 3 months after brain injury. Although numerous biochemical explanations may underlie the observed changes in behavior and cognition, clinical neuropsychologists must recognize that spontaneous recovery is often gradual. If the mechanisms responsible for spontaneous recovery were understood, it might be possible to build upon them to facilitate rehabilitation outcomes.

A subtle form of compensatory behavior can create the impression of recovery (Fig. 13-1B). In this case, the input has been changed, but the function rules remain the same. Consequently, the output appears unchanged. For example, Bryan Kolb (1990), a noted neuroscientist, was unaware of a loss of vision in his right visual field after a left occipital infarction. Eventually, he found himself engaging in behaviors to compensate for the loss, such as tilting his head to change his point of central fixation. Apparently, the compensation appeared without his conscious intent and allowed him to navigate in space without bumping into objects or having difficulty reading. In his case, the underlying function rule remained the same but the input to the brain had to be changed for the behavior to appear normal. Such compensations are not examples of spontaneous recovery because the input must be changed for the function rule to operate properly. Many behaviors that give the impression of recovery are, in fact, compensatory behaviors (Gazzaniga, 1978).

True retraining or restitution of function typifies Luria's (1966) concept of what functional reorganization from neuropsychological rehabilitation might mean. In this model, the initial step is to conduct a careful neuropsychological examination to determine exactly the specific impairments of higher cerebral functions. In mathematical terms, this process is an attempt to determine which variables have been altered in a given function rule. If those variables can be identified, individuals might then be retrained so that the involved variable could be realigned. Theoretically, the function rule would only be slightly or minimally affected if direct retraining was to work (Fig. 13-1C).

Luria's (1966) clinical attempts at retraining were geared toward helping patients to make subtle adaptations so that they could overcome a disturbed functional rule. Some underlying change in the variables or

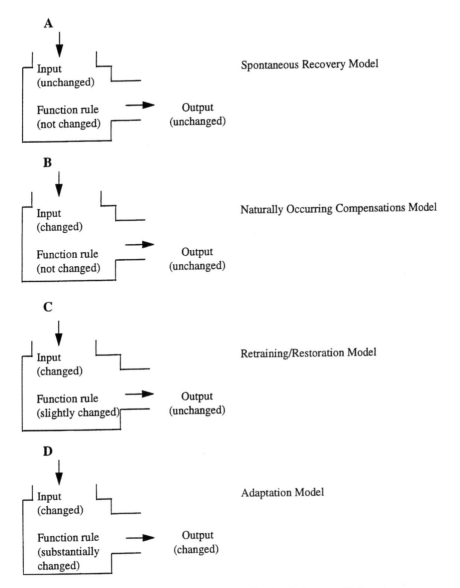

Figure 13-1. Models of change or recovery after brain injury. (A) Spontaneous recovery, (B) naturally occurring compensation, (C) retraining/restoration, and (D) adaptation.

their weighting becomes crucial. He emphasized that careful examination is needed to determine which variable is disturbed and then ongoing repetition and practice are needed to achieve retraining. If this process occurs, the model represents true restoration of function by retraining. Unfortunately, no data yet exist to support that such functional reorganization actually occurs as a result of retraining or rehabilitation. The theory, however, is logical, and this important and optimistic model should not yet be abandoned. Rather, continued work in this area is needed.

Perhaps most common after brain injury are patients who have suffered a significant brain injury and consequently their environment constantly changes how input is introduced to them (Fig. 13-1D). For example, others may speak slowly or repeat themselves to such patients. Functional augmented devices could also be used to facilitate communication. Patients could use checklists or some kind of schema to help them solve problems.

In such cases, input is clearly altered as others understand that these patients cannot handle information the way they once could. That is, the biological and psychological function rules that once governed the patients' higher cerebral functioning are permanently and severely altered. Therefore, their output will always be different, irrespective of how the input is presented.

This model (Fig. 13-1D) suggests a form of adaptation and adjustment to the permanent effects of brain damage as opposed to true retraining. Furthermore, patients' adaptation may deteriorate with time. Theoretically, the underlying reason is quite simple. Deterioration may occur because the altered function rules cannot handle the inputs provided by the environment. Another possibility is that the function rules may further deteriorate because cascading biological events associated with neuronal death may not stop at any given point (Geschwind, 1985).

What Is Deterioration of Function?

Strictly speaking, the deterioration of a function refers to a negative modification of a function rule that causes an adaptive problem-solving process to decline. When the underlying biological and psychological rules are changed, adaptation may decline because the direct activities of the brain can no longer sustain relationships that serve the process of adaptation. This situation would reflect a true decline as a direct consequence of brain damage. Function rules, however, could also be partially changed but not declining. Yet, the change renders the organism incapable of handling inputs from the environment. This case reflects deterioration of the indirect symptoms of brain damage. In clinical practice, many cases suggest that such mechanisms are operative.

The following case studies and group data highlight some of these points regarding recovery and deterioration of higher cerebral functions.

Various clinical observations and experimental findings relate to the models of change and recovery discussed above (Fig. 13-1). Understanding which of the four types of change may predominate in a given patient has the potential to help guide rehabilitation activities. It is important to determine whether direct or indirect symptoms have been affected, as described below.

Observations on "Spontaneous Recovery"

As noted, spontaneous recovery does not mean instantaneous recovery. Rather, it often refers to a return to a previous level of function that apparently requires no "relearning" and therefore appears "effortless." Spontaneous recovery phenomena can occur soon or several weeks (and perhaps months) after brain injury. Theoretically, spontaneous recovery is possible because the underlying function rule(s) have not been changed (Fig. 13-1A). Rather, some mechanism(s) seem to render the function rule(s) temporarily inoperable.

Laurence and Stein (1978) reviewed von Monakow's concept of diaschisis and considered it a possible mechanism underlying spontaneous restitution of function. In diaschisis, regions far removed from a relatively focal or regional brain insult might be rendered dysfunctional because of changes to the neural connections between the damaged and the nondamaged areas. When the changes diminish, nondamaged brain regions (mechanisms) return to "normal." How diaschisis might actually occur is unknown. Cerebral edema and changes in cerebral blood flow are often proposed as mechanisms underlying this phenomenon.

Two facts are important to the concept of diaschisis. First, spontaneous recovery may occur well past the time that cerebral edema is diminished and normal vascular blood flow is thought to be reinstituted. Second and perhaps more importantly, regions of the brain not thought to be directly damaged may never return to "normal."

Regarding this latter point, Perani and colleagues (1993) studied cerebral metabolism with positron emission tomography (PET) in two patients who suffered unilateral strokes. Both patients demonstrated hemi-inattention or "neglect" phenomena. During the acute phase (2 days after the stroke), the first patient showed "extensive reduction of metabolism in both cerebral hemispheres." Eight months later, "almost complete recovery of hypometabolism was demonstrated in the 'so-called' unaffected hemisphere." This recovery was paralleled by a substantial improvement in the patient's symptom of hemineglect. In the second patient, who had not recovered behaviorally at 4 months, "widespread metabolic reduction" was present in both cerebral hemispheres even though computed tomography (CT) confirmed that the lesion was unilateral.

This latter patient may represent a case in which spontaneous recovery is blocked because an underlying mechanism prevents intact functional rules to operate normally. Luria and colleagues (1969) suggested that such disturbed function could be reinstituted given the right "deinhibitory" therapies. If this theory is correct, the proper timing of "deinhibitory" rehabilitation therapies could result in substantial behavioral improvements in TBI patients. If nondamaged regions of the brain are rendered functionally useless, however, their failure to recover spontaneously may have long-term implications and ultimately result in further deterioration.

Many activities during the acute phase of neurological rehabilitation seem to focus on stimulating the disturbed function in hope that the activity will facilitate the natural course of recovery. In his review of the recovery of language disorders after brain insults, Kertesz (1988) notes that some type of reorganization may occur soon after injury. In some patients, for example, the right cerebral hemisphere appears to contribute to the partial return of language function (Basso, et al., 1989). Kertesz (1988) also observed that aphasic patients' symptoms may change considerably over time and that "aphasic syndromes" are anything but static.

Wilson and Baddeley (1993) reported a case that highlights that spontaneous recovery can occur well past a reduction in cerebral edema or the resumption of normal blood flow. A 55-year-old man showed a marked short-term memory deficit associated with a major disturbance in language comprehension. He was seen in a memory rehabilitation clinic 1 year after the onset of his brain dysfunction. He showed no substantial improvements after rehabilitation, which he completed about 2 years after onset. Six years after onset, he was reexamined as a part of a long-term follow-up study and his short-term memory and language comprehension had improved substantially. These improvements therefore occurred several years after rehabilitation had concluded and after no further recovery had been expected.

Serial follow-ups of severely impaired brain-injured children often produce equally dramatic findings. For example, a 13-year-old girl suffered a severe TBI that rendered her comatose for several days. When she emerged from her coma, she was globally aphasic and could not be given standardized neuropsychological tests until about 3 months after her injury (Table 13-4). Initially, she was so aphasic that she could only be given the performance section of the Wechsler Intelligence Scale for Children-Revised form (WISC-R).

Seven months after her injury, more extensive testing was possible as her aphasia resolved. She made numerous paraphasic errors but seemed to comprehend much of what was said. She could also be engaged in a variety of other psychometric tasks. At this time, her speed of finger tapping was extremely slow bilaterally, although it was better in the right hand than in the left. Fifteen months after her injury, her finger tapping improved significantly in both hands but especially in the right. She exhibited no parallel improvement in measures of intelligence. Speed of finger tapping, however, continued to improve and 2.5 years after injury was paralleled by an improvement in delayed verbal recall as measured by the Wechsler Memory Scale–Revised form. Five years after her TBI, the patient continued to show substantial improvements.

This case is complicated because the patient received ongoing speech and language therapy during this time. The point, however, is that despite a large area of encephalomacia (Fig. 13-2), her behavior recovered substantially. She not only graduated from high school but attended a college that specialized in helping children with learning disabilities. Clinically, she showed a slight hesitancy when speaking and signs of memory impairment on formal psychometric testing. Her language impairment, however, improved substantially.

An interesting question is whether her speed of finger tapping heralded her ultimate recovery—a question that must await further research before it can be answered. The pertinent point here is that with time and different therapies, higher cerebral functioning can sometimes improve substantially.

Naturally Occurring Compensations

If a functional rule is relatively intact but various brain disturbances preclude its natural operation, patients often attempt to change the sensory input. Assume that the function rules for "reading" were intact for Dr. Kolb after his left occipital stroke. Yet he was hampered by a visual field loss. Thus, he unconsciously tilted his head to change the point of central fixation so that he could continue to read relatively unhampered. Although he was still sometimes disturbed by the visual field loss, he nevertheless could read. Apparently, the functional rules for vision were partially but permanently damaged. In contrast, the functional rules for reading were not. In such cases, compensatory behaviors seem to emerge naturally. Dr. Kolb's compensatory behavior for reading was obviously adaptive. Numerous compensatory strategies, however, are nonadaptive and may lead to further disruptions.

For example, a middle-aged businessman suffered a mild head injury. His memory function was disturbed, but he did not acknowledge the disturbance and tolerated no feedback from others about it (possible evidence of denial of disability). His premorbid methods of coping with stressful issues ensued, and he became short with anyone he perceived as criticizing him. With time, the patient recognized that he had a partial memory impairment. He required others to speak to him slowly, which at times, embarrassed them (which he failed to recognize fully). When he responded to someone, he often did so quickly. In fact, when asked to recall a series of words during neuropsychological testing, he would

Table 13-4. Psychometric summary of a girl who sustained a severe TBI at 13 years

Psychometric Tests	Score at Age of Testing				
	13 yrs/ 6 mos*	13 yrs/ 10 mos†	14 yrs/ 6 mos‡	15 yrs/ 9 mos§	18 yrs/ 1 mo"
Trail Making Test					
Part A (sec)	56	16	41	60	31
Part B (sec)	70	29	75	81	90
WISC-R/WAIS-R					
Information	—	5	6	6	8
Similarities	—	5	5	10	12
Arithmetic	—	8	7	—	6
Vocabulary	—	6	n/a	9	10
Digit Span	1	6	8	8	5
Picture Completion	4	9	8	6	9
Picture Arrangement	9	13	12	11	12
Block Design	5	11	10	6	7
Coding	3	11	8	—	—
Digit Symbol	—	—	—	7	8
Wisconsin Card Sorting Categories					
Achieved	—	2 out of 6	—	—	—
Halstead Reitan Neuro-psychological Test Battery (Adult Form)					
Category Test (No. of errors)	—	—	28	31	25
Speech-Sounds Perception (No. of errors)	—	10	6	1	3
Seashore Rhythm Test (No. of errors)	—	8	4	6	7
Tactual Performance Test					
RH (min/sec)	—	7/5	6/20	7/25	10 (7 blocks)
LH (min/sec)	—	3/58	4/30	7/52	4/29

(continued)

say the words very quickly, presumably while they were still in his working memory. This impulsive behavior appeared to be an attempt to compensate for his memory deficit, but it was nonadaptive.

Naturally occurring compensations can therefore be both adaptive and nonadaptive. Other patients spontaneously reduce their workload or limit their contact with people. In some instances, this strategy will result in a positive adjustment. In others, it can lead to social withdrawal and isolation—a negative adjustment.

How patients adjust to their brain injury at every stage of the recovery process must be observed carefully. On acute brain injury rehabilitation

Table 13-4.—Continued

	Score at Age of Testing				
Psychometric Tests	13 yrs/ 6 mos*	13 yrs/ 10 mos†	14 yrs/ 6 mos‡	15 yrs/ 9 mos§	18 yrs/ 1 mo"
Both Hands (min/sec)	—	2/58	2/06	2/32	4/46
Memory Score	—	6	5	8	9
Localization Score	—	2	1	5	5
Manual Finger Tapping					
RH	—	22	41	41.2	44
LH	—	9.5	18	25.8	28.4
Wechsler Memory Scale-Revised					
Verbal Memory Index	—	—	61	66	88
Visual Memory Index	—	—	96	85	97
General Memory Index	—	—	64	65	90
Attention/Concentration Index	—	—	75	80	72
Delayed Recall Index	—	—	57	83	86
Rey Complex Figure					
Copy	—	—	—	—	34/36
Immediate	—	—	—	—	14.5/36
Delay	—	—	—	—	18.5/36
California Verbal Learning Test					
Trial 1	—	—	—	—	7/16
Trial 5	—	—	—	—	10/16
List B	—	—	—	—	2/16
Short-Term Free Recall	—	—	—	—	6/16
Short-Term Cued Recall	—	—	—	—	10/16
Long-Term Free Recall	—	—	—	—	9/16
Long-Term Cued Recall	—	—	—	—	V 10/16

Time since injury, *3 months; †7 months; ‡1 yr/3 mos; §2 yrs/6 mos; "4 yrs/10 mos; TBI = traumatic brain injury; RH = right hand; LH = left hand.

units, brain dysfunctional patients become agitated if overstimulated. If told to leave an area, they can respond belligerently and with hostility simply because they do not understand what is being asked of them. During the intermediate phase, patients may insist on returning to work as a normal method of compensating for anxiety. Blocking their wishes can create further anger and anxiety. During the postacute phase, patients may begin to carry memory notebooks or to avoid contact with certain individuals in attempts to compensate for their impaired ability to function. Careful analysis of patients' compensatory techniques can help determine if their strategies are adaptive or maladaptive. If the latter, the rehabilitation therapist needs to consider how to modify the strategy or to substitute more adaptive methods. Studies of brain dysfunc-

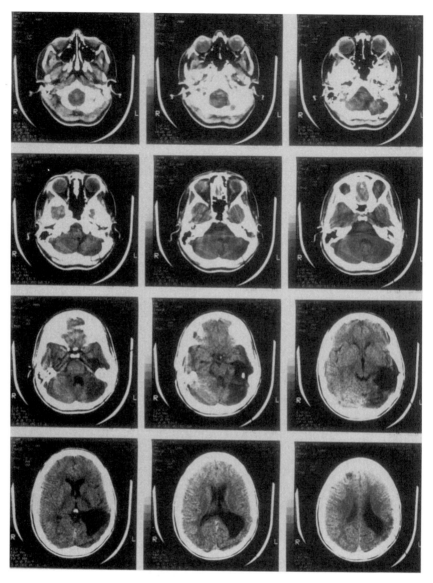

Figure 13-2. Magnetic resonance images of the brain of an adolescent girl who suffered a severe traumatic brain injury. Table 13-4 summarizes this girl's test scores.

tional patients' natural compensatory techniques and how to improve them are badly needed.

Observations on Retraining and Reorganization

The third model of change (Fig. 13-1C) suggests that altered functional rules can be reorganized under certain circumstances. What evidence supports this model? Recall that age and lesion location are important determinants of functional recovery (Table 13-3). More than 20 years ago, Rasmussen and Milner (1977) studied the effects of early brain injury on language representation in the brain and found that "childhood injuries to the left hemisphere occurring after the age of 5 years rarely changed the pattern of speech representation at maturity" (p. 367). Moreover, they attributed language recovery after age 5 to "intrahemispheric reorganization." For reorganization to occur, the frontal and parietal cortex needs to be relatively functional.

The frontal and parietal cortex has also been implicated in motor recovery after a capsular infarction in patients between the ages of 21 to 67 years (Weiller, et al., 1993). PET findings have suggested individual patterns of functional reorganization as soon as 7 weeks after injury and as late as 6 years after the ischemic infarction.

It is often difficult to demonstrate functional reorganization via training (i.e., rehabilitation) because the higher cerebral functions that are impaired appear to depend on complex laws of relationship among large neural networks (Luria, 1966; Mesulam, 1990). Cognitive tasks that might reveal an organizational effect produce complex findings on PET and functional magnetic resonance (MR) imaging. To demonstrate that reorganization occurs with or without specific training requires identifying a neuropsychological response that can easily be studied using modern, functional imaging techniques *and* that is clearly related to variables known to influence functional outcome (Table 13-3). Speed of finger tapping or oscillation may be one such measure.

The Halstead Finger Oscillation (or tapping) task is a part of the Halstead-Reitan Neuropsychological Test battery (Lezak, 1995). Numerous studies have shown that speed of finger movement is adversely affected by the type of brain damage (Reitan and Wolfson, 1994) and severity of TBI in both children (Bawden, et al., 1985) and adults (Dikmen, et al., 1995) and the time since injury (Haaland, et al., 1994). Speed of finger movement correlates with age in normal children (Seidman, et al., 1997) and adults (Vega and Parsons, 1967). Brain damage appears to attenuate that correlation (Vega and Parsons, 1967; Prigatano and Parsons, 1976).

Speed of finger movement also relates to the achievement of rehabilitation goals after a unilateral cerebrovascular accident (CVA) (Prigatano and Wong, 1997) and positively correlates with measures of quality of life 2 to 4 years after TBI (Klonoff, et al., 1986). As noted in Chapter 12, it also relates to measures of impaired self-awareness in TBI patients across cultures. Finally, the task is simple and can be measured quickly. Patients are rarely threatened by the task and often appear "motivated" to perform it. These results suggest that the speed and perhaps qualitative features of finger movement (see Prigatano and Hoffman, 1997) may have diagnostic and prognostic value.

Functional Organization and Reorganization After Brain Damage: Studies on Finger Movement

Cerebral blood flow studies of normal adults asked to oppose the thumb sequentially with the four fingers suggest that cerebral activation is not limited to the contralateral sensorimotor cortex (Roland, 1993; Roland and Seitz, 1991). Activation is seen in the ipsilateral sensorimotor cortex, the supplementary motor cortex, and the ipsilateral cerebellum, among other locations. Boecker and colleagues (1994) asked five healthy male volunteers (aged between 28 and 41) to do a self-paced tapping task with the middle finger. The contralateral primary sensorimotor cortex, the ipsilateral primary motor cortex, and the supplementary motor area were activated. The authors suggested that "the supplementary motor area is involved in self-paced finger tapping" (p. 1231).

These and other studies (e.g., Kawashima, et al., 1993) suggest that finger movements in normal individuals are associated with changes in blood flow (a measure of activation) in the primary sensorimotor, premotor, and supplementary motor regions. When the finger-tapping task is timed or paced, anterior cerebral activation increases, especially when training is required (Roland and Seitz, 1991). Cerebral blood flow has not yet been measured in normal persons performing the Halstead Finger Tapping Test. The present findings, however, suggest that the task most likely requires bilateral cerebral activation and may well involve supplementary motor regions. The converse of this proposition is that unilateral brain lesions may affect the speed of finger movement in the ipsilateral hand as well as in the contralateral hand, as recently reported by Prigatano and Wong (1997). Unilateral CVA patients showed bilateral impairments in speed of finger tapping at admission to an inpatient neurorehabilitation unit (typically 1 to 2 weeks after lesion onset). Patients who approached normal speeds of finger movement in the so-called unaffected hand had a higher incidence of achieving rehabilitation goals. This relationship was not true of measures of grip strength. Thus, some aspects of speed of finger movement seem to relate to recovery of function.

Two possible mechanisms could account for these findings. Either the so-called unaffected hemisphere (and hand) showed spontaneous recovery (via a resolving diaschisis), or alternative pathways could have assumed the processing for this task. Stein (1999), for example, suggests that one avenue to functional recovery may be the unmasking of latent neural pathways. This type of mechanism would favor a mechanism of true functional reorganization. Is there evidence for this model?

PET studies performed by Frackowiak and colleagues have provided evidence of functional reorganization after striatocapsular infarction (Weiller, et al., 1992; Chollet, et al., 1991). They reported the following:

When the normal fingers were moved, regional cerebral blood flow increased significantly in contralateral primary sensorimotor cortex and in the ipsilateral cerebellar hemisphere. When the fingers of the recovered hand were moved, significant regional cerebral blood flow increases were observed in both contralateral and ipsilateral primary sensorimotor cortex and in both cerebellar hemispheres. Other regions, namely, insula, inferior parietal, and premotor cortex, were also bilaterally activated with movement of the recovered hand. We have also demonstrated, by using a new technique of image analysis, different functional connections between the thalamic nuclei and specific cortical and cerebellar regions during these movements. Our results suggest that ipsilateral motor pathways may play a role in the recovery of motor function after ischemic stroke (Chollet, et al., 1991; p. 63).

These findings were followed by a second study in which patients who showed motor recovery after striatocapsular stroke were compared with normal subjects (Weiller, et al., 1992). In patients who showed recovery, activation was often increased in the frontal and parietal regions. The authors concluded as follows:

> We showed that bilateral activation of motor pathways and the recruitment of additional sensorimotor areas and of other specific cortical areas are associated with recovery from motor stroke due to striatocapsular infarction. Activation of anterior and posterior cingulate and prefrontal cortices suggests that selective attentional and intentional mechanisms may be important in the recovery process. Our findings suggest that there is considerable scope for functional plasticity in the adult human cortex (Weiller, et al., 1992; p. 463).

These conclusions are especially interesting given the previous discussion of impaired self-awareness that suggested that the integration of cognition and feelings permits self-awareness to emerge. In the present study, the activation of cingulate regions implies activation of both an affective component and a motor component during the recovery process. In the study by Weiller and colleagues (1992), the motor task consisted of sequential oppositional touching of the finger and thumb (i.e., a tapping task) performed to the rate of a metronome comparable to the speed of the task performed by normal persons. Subjects were between 28 and 69 years of age and were at least 3 months beyond the onset of their stroke. Evidence is therefore growing that recovery of finger movements to a normal speed may reflect a form of functional reorganization in some patients. Slow speeds may reflect a lack of recovery after diffuse TBI.

Haaland and colleagues (1994) studied the recovery of grip strength and the Halstead Speed of Finger Tapping in 40 TBI patients and 88 normal control subjects. Of the TBI patients, 75% had admitting GCS scores between 11 and 15 and 18% had scores between 8 and 10. Thus, most of these patients had mild to moderate brain injuries. Grip strength eventually returned to "normal" compared to control scores whereas finger tapping did not (Fig. 13-3).

Aizawa and colleagues (1991) found that the supplementary motor cortex is activated when monkeys tapped two small keys only *after* they had sustained a lesion in the precentral motor cortex. They argued that the supplementary motor area may initially be involved in performing

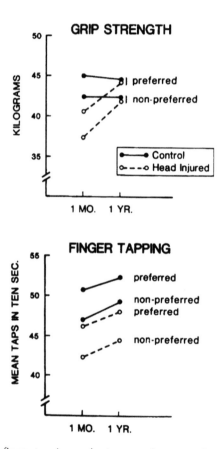

Figure 13-3. Mean finger tapping and grip strength scores obtained 1 month and 1 year after injury in a head-injured group without peripheral injuries (*n* = 40) and in a normal control group (*n* = 88). Standard errors for finger tapping ranged from 2.2 to 2.5 in the head-injured group and 2.2 to 2.4 in the control group. Standard errors for grip strength in both groups ranged from 3.3 to 3.5. From Haaland, K. Y., Temkin, N., Randahl, G., and Dikmen, S. (1994). Recovery of simple motor skills after head injury. *J. Clin. Exp. Neuropsychol.* 16(3), 448–456. © Swets & Zeitlinger Publishers. Used with permission

such motor tasks. Once the task has been learned, however, this region may not typically be activated. Therefore, this region may show activation again only after an injury.

This model suggests that pathways initially used to learn a task may become latent after several repetitions or after learning is well established. If the brain is damaged later in life, the latent pathways may have to be reactivated to perform the task. Thus, functional reorganization could mean reactivating previously used but latent pathways. The other possibility, of course, is that new pathways are recruited to perform the tasks. This option may be more likely to occur in younger rather than in more mature brains (Kolb, 1995).

Observations on the Adaptation Model

The three models of recovery described above suggest three corollaries. First, the concept of diaschisis may account for spontaneous recovery phenomena. Second, subtle behavioral compensation strategies may give a false impression of restoration of a function rule (i.e., the ability to read after a left cerebral hemisphere infarction). Third, brain reorganization, the reactivation of latent neural pathways, or both may explain the positive effects of retraining.

The fourth model that must be considered is based on adaptation. Here various compensations are used to aid survival and the quality of life after brain injury. In daily clinical practice, patients often use compensatory strategies and devices during the acute, subacute, intermediate, and long-term phases after significant brain damage.

In this fourth model (Fig. 13-1D), the functional rules are severely and permanently altered (i.e., damaged) and whatever partial recovery may occur is inadequate for an individual's survival and adjustment in life. Thus, some accommodations are necessary, and they often first appear in terms of changes in input. Because the functional rules have been damaged, even if input is changed, the final output will always remain altered compared to before the injury. Thus, individuals will not function "normally" even when a full range of compensations is provided.

The adaptation model applies to different brain dysfunctional patients to different degrees. The primary problem for some patients may be to find ways to preserve enough energy to meet the demands of the day's tasks (a common outcome after an unruptured cerebral artery aneurysm has been clipped). Others may need to compensate for subtle difficulties with memory and verbal fluency (very common after a mild or moderate TBI in young adults). Still others may need to adjust to permanent changes in their ability to function at work and in their interpersonal relationships (common with young adults who suffer severe TBIs and are in a coma for an extended period). The latter scenario, of course, is often associated with the significant personality and cognitive disturbances described in preceding chapters.

Perhaps the adaptation model is best recognized by the various mnemonic devices used to teach patients how to compensate for their permanently impaired memories and thereby reduce the impact of their disability. Kime and colleagues (1996), for example, reported a severely amnestic patient who was taught to use a systematic program of external cuing to increase her compliance within the day-treatment program. The procedure also helped the patient to maintain part-time voluntary work. Without such a compensatory strategy, she would have been unable to do so. Therefore, this approach can be extremely practical and associated with positive outcomes for both patients and those involved in their care.

As described here and elsewhere (Prigatano, et al., 1986), patients are not always willing to engage in such strategies. Many of the activities of postacute neuropsychological rehabilitation are aimed at helping them to recognize their need for such strategies and to find strategies that will work for them. Failure to do so leads to long-term psychosocial consequences such as depression, enhanced irritability, and the development of psychosomatic illness and, possibly, frank psychosis.

A key problem is associated with the adaptation model: Both the environment and the patient are constantly changing, albeit sometimes slowly. These changes must be monitored and adjusted to. If patients do not adjust, their condition may well deteriorate over time. Monitoring patients requires time and can be costly, but failure to do so can have devastating consequences.

Shortly, case examples will highlight some of the realities involved with partial recovery of both direct and indirect symptoms. Case examples of deterioration are also presented. Before these case examples are considered, however, the limited literature on deterioration after so-called "static" lesions of the brain is reviewed.

Deterioration of Function After So-Called "Static" Lesions of the Brain

There is a growing appreciation that no injury to the brain has a "static" effect because the brain, like other organs, is constantly changing. The aging process, for example, might interact differently with disordered higher cerebral functions than with "normal" ones. Injury could also increase the brain's susceptibility to various noxious agents. For example, many brain dysfunctional patients report a reduced tolerance for alcohol.

Deterioration of brain function after TBI has been recognized for several years. Its impact, however, is just beginning to be recognized. The most obvious example of deteriorating brain function is the late onset of epilepsy after TBI. Jennett and Teasdale (1981) noted that "in the study of 150 *severe* injuries followed for more than a year after injury, 15 percent had epilepsy; this would certainly have been higher had the follow-up been longer" (p. 281). These experienced authors acknowledge that epilepsy can appear for the first time several months or years after brain injury. Goetz and Pappert (1996) reviewed the literature on the development of movement disorders after TBI. Among other findings, they noted that the onset of dystonia after TBI can be delayed from 1 month to 9 years after injury.

Long-term psychiatric disturbances have also been reported. Thomsen (1984), for example, reported cases of posttraumatic psychosis that developed as long as 15 years after injury. The emergence of psychotic states may reflect not just years of frustration and confusion on the part of the patient but also continued structural and perhaps neurotransmitter disturbances.

Smith (1964) studied schizophrenic patients who underwent various forms of psychosurgery aimed at altering frontal lobe function 10 to 12 years after their surgery. Some patients' performance on psychometric tests declined. Lezak (1979) studied the recovery of memory and learning function in 24 male TBI patients up to 36 months after injury. Again, certain patients exhibited a decline in the more complex measures of immediate memory and retention.

Perhaps Corkin and colleagues (1989) reported the first convincing evidence that long-term deterioration can follow TBI. She and her colleagues followed World War II veterans for 40 years after their injury. Compared to their preinjury performance on the Army General Classification Test (AGCT, not the most sensitive neuropsychological measure), more than 50% of the patients with penetrating wounds to the head showed a decline in performance 40 years after injury (Fig. 13-4). The decline, however, was not obvious 10 years after injury. Citing the work of Walker and Erculei (1969), Corkin and colleagues (1989) noted that "... exacerbated cognitive decline following HI [head injury] becomes observable around or shortly after age 50."

Corkin and colleagues (1989) also cited Yakovlev's (1953) findings concerning patients who had undergone a frontal lobectomy but who had died at different intervals after surgery. Patients who lived the longest after their frontal lobectomy had more atrophic changes than could be explained on the basis of aging per se. The mechanism(s) underlying deterioration could include continued retrograde degeneration as well as a complex interaction between the presence of a lesion and a genetic predisposition for the development of Alzheimer's disease. In this latter regard, it has been suggested that recovery after various insults might be less in patients with a genetic predisposition for developing Alzheimer's disease (Roses and Saunders, 1997).

Normal aging may reduce the brain's reserve capacity (Corkin, et al., 1989; Chapter 3 on Satz). If the damage occurs early in life, it may deplete

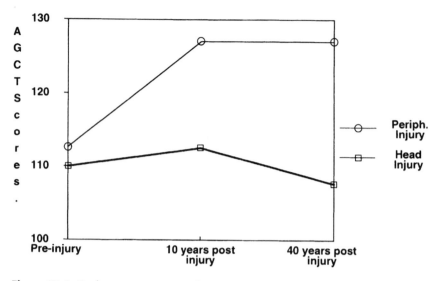

Figure 13-4. Performance scores on the Army General Classification Test before and 10 and 40 years after penetrating head injuries or peripheral injuries. Adapted from Corkin, et al. (1989).

these resources, which are then unavailable as a person ages. The findings of Corkin and colleagues (1989) and their interpretation are compatible with Goldman-Rakic's observations of the long-term effects of fetal frontal lesions. Discussing this work, Kolb (1990) observed the following:

> Further evidence for the emergence of deficits during development comes from the work of Patricia Goldman-Rakic and her colleagues. In her early studies she was impressed with apparent recovery of functions after frontal lobe injuries in infant monkeys (e.g., Goldman, 1974). As she continued her investigations it became clear that she and others had overestimated the extent of recovery because the animals were tested when still young. Thus, she found that as animals with dorsolateral prefrontal lesions developed they became progressively more impaired at cognitive tasks such as delayed alternation (Goldman-Rakic, Isseroff, Schwartz, and Bugbee, 1983; pp. 78–79)."

Kolb (1990) also noted that these types of experiments are important because they show ". . . that behavior may appear virtually normal early in life but become progressively less normal as animals develop" (p. 79).

Illustrative Cases

With these rather sobering observations in mind, let us consider clinical case examples of recovery and deterioration after brain injury and the lessons they offer regarding neuropsychological rehabilitation.

Partial Recovery of a Direct Symptom and Deterioration of an Indirect Symptom

A 22-year-old, right-handed, married man suffered a severe TBI from a motorcycle collision. He was immediately rendered unconscious, and no admitting GCS score could be recorded because he was intubated upon arrival to the emergency room. MR imaging of his brain 14 months after injury revealed multiple, bilateral intraparenchymal contusions in the frontal lobes (worse in the left than in the right). There were also areas of contusion within the splenium of the corpus callosum and evidence of multiple shear hemorrhages indicative of diffuse axonal injury. This pattern of lesions has been related to significant cognitive impairments (Johnson, et al., 1994).

Four months after injury, the patient was enrolled in a neuropsychological rehabilitation program (Chapter 8; Prigatano, et al., 1986). He was cooperative but showed a lack of spontaneous facial expression. When he smiled, his face had a childlike appearance. He also showed a classic pattern on IQ tests. Both his verbal and performance IQ were substantially affected, especially his performance IQ (Fig. 13-5). During the 9 months of rehabilitation, his performance IQ improved substantially while his verbal IQ improved mildly. At first glance, these improvements might suggest that rehabilitation had helped improve the cognitive functions responsible for the verbal and performance IQ measures. His performance on these tests 4.5 years after injury, however, suggests a different interpretation. His performance IQ continued to improve at the

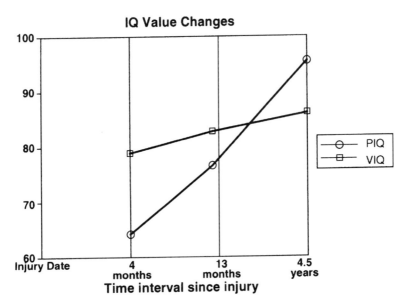

Figure 13-5. IQ scores of a man who sustained a severe traumatic brain injury at the age of 22 at various times after injury. PIQ = performance IQ; VIQ = verbal IQ.

same rate during the years following rehabilitation. Scores on the performance IQ are strongly dependent on speed of information processing. Reduced speed of information processing is often a direct effect of brain injury (Chapter 5). Thus, his increased performance IQ suggests that a direct symptom showed improvement with the passage of time.

At the end of the program, the patient was placed in a voluntary work setting. After spending several hundreds of hours devoted to helping him become realistically aware of his status, he commented: "Can I go back to work now as a mechanic?" The patient remained severely impaired with an almost complete frontal heteromodal syndrome of unawareness (see Chapter 12). The rehabilitation effort, at least as it related to helping him become realistic, appeared wasted.

He returned 4.5 years after his injury at the request of his wife. She noted that with time, he had become progressively more angry and had increased difficulties in controlling his temper (Fig. 13-6). When he had entered the rehabilitation program, he had no trouble controlling his temper because, in essence, he was adynamic. As he began to recover partially, his reactions became more affective. In fact, at discharge from the program 13 months after injury, his wife had begun to notice that his ability to control his temper had decreased. By 4.5 years after injury, this tendency had developed into a major problem. As noted in Chapter 6, the expression of anger is often an indirect consequence of brain injury. As the person becomes more frustrated and less able to cope, he or she is more likely to show intense anger reactions.

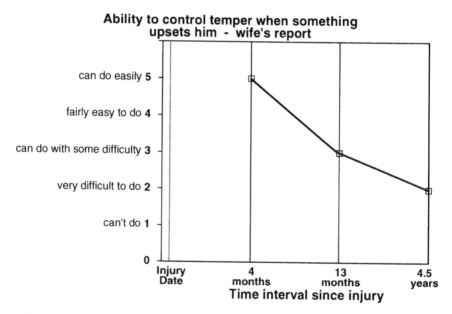

Figure 13-6. The ability of the patient described in Figure 13-5 to control his temper as reported by his wife on the Patient Competency Rating Scale.

This case is typical of many patients who are enrolled in neuropsychological rehabilitation programs too early. They may recover considerable cognitive function during the first 12 months after their TBI, but many remain severely impaired, particularly in terms of their awareness of their disabilities. During this early phase of recovery, group experiences and individual therapeutic work may have little impact on helping them become aware of the level of their abilities. In fact, this patient, as well as others that I have followed over the years, noted that he had no appreciation of his true cognitive difficulties during this early period. Group or individual feedback simply frustrates such patients. Only as this patient accumulated more life experiences did he begin to appreciate the nature of his difficulties.

This case represents partial recovery of a direct symptom of brain injury (easily measured by speed of information processing) several years after injury. It also reflects deterioration of an indirect symptom (i.e., temper control) as the patient endured several years with little insight into the nature of his impairments.

Partial Recovery of a Direct Symptom Followed by Deterioration and Remediation of an Indirect Symptom

A left-handed, single college student suffered severe anoxia at the age of 21. He was seen within 3 weeks of the anoxic episode and at that time was densely amnestic. Xenon CT (1 month after the insult) revealed diminished perfusion in the left frontal and occipital lobes. Two months after the injury, he was still clearly amnestic. His general memory index score as measured by the Wechsler Memory Scale-Revised form was less than 50. The patient began rehabilitation about 4 months after the insult. By that time, his WMS-R General Index score was 71 and his Delayed Memory Index score was 61.

Several months of intensive neuropsychological rehabilitation ensued. The patient progressed in terms of his physical functioning and on various measures of speed of information processing, but he continued to show severe memory impairment. He also appeared to lack insight about his impairments. He resisted the suggestions of others that he not return to his old college. After several months of neuropsychological rehabilitation, he returned to his old university with an altered course load. At this time, however, he would not identify himself as a student with a disability.

As he attempted to resume his old lifestyle, he began to develop intense headaches followed by panic attacks. After several months of unsuccessful psychological and medical treatment, he returned to his hometown. Again, a regimen of medical therapies was instituted to reduce his headaches but none worked. The patient and family then turned to holistic remedies, which also failed to produce any substantial changes. During this time, the patient saw no connections among his somatic symptoms, his panic attacks, and his inability to function in his daily environment. Because a good working relationship had been established with this patient, however, he agreed to work within the context of psychotherapy.

After several months of psychotherapy, he agreed to attend another, much less demanding college. An experienced vocational rehabilitation counselor helped smooth the transition by going to the university with the patient and explaining his medical history to university officials. He now was able to identify himself as a student with a disability and received appropriate help (see Chapter 9). As he succeeded in his new environment, his headaches decreased substantially (but were not completely eliminated). His panic attacks, however, stopped.

After enjoying considerable success in school with fewer headaches and no panic attacks, he was asked whether his inability to function and his somatic symptoms were connected. He stated "I have no headaches or panic attacks—I guess you're right." Note his choice of words. Despite the significant change, he still did not fully recognize the connection between being overwhelmed by his environment and his symptoms.

This patient has been followed for 7 years and periodically is seen in supportive psychotherapy. Against the background of this lengthy working relationship, he can now say that he had little insight into his disabilities and only gained understanding with time (and perhaps the therapeutic relationship). This case represents partial recovery of a memory disturbance (a direct symptom of a brain dysfunction) and also the initial deterioration of indirect symptoms of brain injury (e.g., headache and anxiety) followed by remediation of those problems. Management of this case can be considered successful.

Delayed Deterioration of Direct Symptoms

A 32-year-old woman suffered a severe TBI from a motor vehicle accident. She was first seen within 10 days of her injury and has now been followed for almost 10 years. Her admitting GCS score was 6. CT revealed hemorrhagic contusions in the left frontal and temporal lobes as well as in the basal ganglia. The patient was given neuropsychological tests throughout this period and followed closely. The results of her neuropsychological test findings highlight how both recovery and deterioration can occur (Table 13-5).

At 3.5 months after TBI, this woman's speed of information processing was severely restricted, as reflected by her digit symbol subtest score of 6. Her scores on the vocabulary and block design subtests were in the low average range (9 and 7, age-corrected scale scores, respectively). This woman was accomplished and had successfully graduated from a major university. Her scores reflected brain dysfunction and a reduction of her overall abilities.

Three and a half *months* after injury, her finger tapping was extremely slow bilaterally. Gradually, her speed of finger tapping and

Table 13-5. Psychometric summary of a woman who sustained a severe TBI at the age of 32

Psychometric Tests	Score at Testing Time After Injury				
	3.5 mos	1 yr/2 mos	2 yrs/2 mos	3 yrs/6 mos	8 yrs
WAIS-R (age-corrected score)					
Digit symbol	6	5	7	7	7
Vocabulary	9	8	9	13	8
Block design	7	8	9	10	10
Halstead Finger Tapping*					
Raw scores					
RH	28.8	33.4	35.4	34.2	27.2
LH	30.6	39.4	42.6	39	43.4
T scores					
RH	26	30	34	34	27
LH	30	46	50	46	51

TBI = traumatic brain injury; RH = right hand; LH = left hand.

cognitive functions improved. For example, 3.5 *years* after injury, her block design subtest score improved one standard deviation and her vocabulary score improved at about the same level. Speed of finger tapping also improved.

Just before her evaluation 8 years after injury, however, she developed unexplained choreiform movements of the right hand. It was thought that this disturbance essentially affected motor functions: Her right hand finger-tapping score decreased to a level that was comparable to her performance at 3.5 *months* after injury. There was a possible decrease in her vocabulary score. Her left hemisphere appears to have been affected by the onset of the disturbance, of which the motor disturbance was only one manifestation. This patient continues to be followed. Her course, unfortunately, demonstrates delayed deterioration of direct symptoms of brain injury, in her case, 8 years after TBI.

Delayed Deterioration of Direct and Indirect Symptoms

A 20-year-old, left-handed man suffered a TBI in a small airplane crash. He was unconscious for a lengthy but undocumented period. He was referred for a neuropsychological rehabilitation program 4 years after his injury. At that time, his Wechsler Adult Intelligence Scale-Revised verbal IQ score was 89 and his Wechsler Memory Quotient was 69. He has been followed for 18.5 years.

This patient's story is complex but highlights some features of late-

onset psychosis. Four years after injury, the patient complained of headaches that were not relieved by medication. Unlike the earlier patient,
however, he could not be helped to recognize the connection between
his somatic difficulties and his cognitive impairments. During the course
of cognitive retraining, for example, he would comment: "Dr. Prigatano,
I could do this (cognitive) task if only I didn't have this headache." I
would respond: "If you could do the cognitive tasks, perhaps you would
not develop a headache."

During the course of rehabilitation, the patient was cooperative, but
his lack of insight into his disabilities persisted. He was placed in voluntary work settings, which were of some help. He insisted on working
in paid positions and finally got a sales job in a department store, saying
he was "a people person." Throughout the neuropsychological rehabilitation program, this man had insisted that the marks of success were a
college degree and a fair income.

His family lived some miles from the rehabilitation program. During
the early stages of this work, we did not fully recognize the importance
of having a close working relationship with his family. So although the
working relationship with his family was cordial, they never developed
a really good understanding of this young man's deficits. Despite our
recommendations to the contrary, the patient finally returned home and
began to work in the family business. This venture was unsuccessful,
and he eventually moved to a resort community in hope of a better
lifestyle. With time, however, his condition began to deteriorate.

When he developed psychotic delusions about 18 years after injury,
he insisted that an attorney who had handled his case (and whom he
had incorrectly identified as a Rhodes scholar) was out to get him. During this time, he also had many incorrect memories of how I had spoken
to him or treated him 14 years earlier.

His psychotic state also precluded neuropsychological testing. He did,
however, complete the Patient's Competency Rating Scale with a total
score of 137 out of 150 points. As noted earlier, a total score of 150 points
means that persons can perform everyday activities *absolutely perfectly.*
Eighteen and a half years after injury, he still insisted that he had, in
essence, no cognitive deficits. In contrast, his parents rated him as 77 out
of the 150 points, indicating that his daily functioning was significantly
limited.

Eighteen and a half years after injury, an MR image of his brain demonstrated moderate encephalomalacia in the left anterior frontal lobe. A
small deposit of hemosiderin suggested an old contusion. There was evidence of subcortical white matter lesions in both frontal lobes and mild
atrophy of the midbrain and pons.

The actual mechanism underlying this man's psychosis is unknown.
Clinically, however, it appears that his persistent frontal heteromodal
cortical unawareness syndrome did not resolve with time. After years of

failure and persistent anosognosia, he began to develop delusions. Interestingly, the delusions centered around very personal concerns (i.e., his intellectual level as reflected by his inability to obtain a college degree and his desire to make a lot of money). In this case, postacute and late-onset psychosis appears to reflect a complex interaction between direct and indirect symptoms of brain injury. The case clearly demonstrates neuropsychological deterioration several years after trauma.

Summary, Conclusions, and Geschwind's Observations

This chapter discussed recovery and deterioration after so-called static brain lesions. The cases presented indicate the importance of conceptualizing whether a direct or indirect symptom is changing with time and/or rehabilitation. Cognitive rehabilitation, as well as other neuropsychological rehabilitation activities, should be planned according to the patients' readiness to engage in specific rehabilitation tasks. All patients should be worked with soon after injury, but the amount of time spent on various rehabilitation tasks depends on a thorough understanding of which functions appear to be recovering spontaneously and which are not.

When possible, rehabilitation activities should try to deinhibit functions that appear to be functional but that have not returned to their normal level of activity for unknown reasons. Therapy that attempts to reactivate latent pathways should also be attempted to foster the reorganization of new neural networks. Therapists should be clear about whether they are attempting to facilitate recovery or the process of adaptation. Obviously, interventions need to be timed appropriately, particularly when few financial resources are available for intensive neuropsychological rehabilitation.

This chapter also attempts to highlight the importance of Geschwind's (1985) observations about "mechanisms of change after brain lesions." He made three key points. The first point introduced this chapter. Namely, "... one can probably never speak of a fixed neurological lesion" (p. 2). The intent of this chapter was to demonstrate the truth of this statement. Some changes are positive and some are negative. Many changes occur soon after injury, but some may occur as late as 40 years after lesion onset. The nature of the changes is dynamic and obviously interacts with variables such as lesion location, size, the nature of the neuropathology, and the individual's age at the time of observation.

Geschwind also noted that "... there must be many other cases in which the capacity for recovery is latent, but revealed by some future manipulation ..." (p. 1). This point is extremely important and dovetails with the discussion of spontaneous recovery and reorganization of higher cerebral functions using the ideas of Luria and others. The future awaits further investigations to highlight this principle.

Finally, Geschwind (1985) noted that the "study of ... unfavorable

mechanisms may be even more important than investigation of spontaneous recovery in leading to improved methods of therapy" (p. 2). Apparently, Geschwind intended this comment for those studying the unfavorable biological changes associated with brain injury. Clinical
neuropsychologists involved in rehabilitation, however, can also identify
with this point. It was precisely the failure of existing rehabilitation programs that led to the postacute milieu-oriented day-treatment programs
developed by Ben-Yishay and colleagues (1985) and Prigatano and colleagues (1986).

These programs were developed in response to the unfavorable psychosocial changes associated with untreated higher cerebral deficits, primarily in young TBI patients. The patients provided ample evidence that
indirect symptoms associated with brain injury could deteriorate. With
time, methods were developed to help manage these indirect symptoms
in a more substantial way, as some of the case studies have highlighted.
Long-term follow-up of many patients in these programs, however, reveals that negative changes can also include direct symptoms of brain
injury. This sobering observation should lead us to develop more innovative ways of understanding the underlying mechanisms. Undoubtedly,
technology such as PET and functional MR imaging will facilitate these
efforts. However, these methods do not replace the need for careful clinical observations of the changes that TBI patients exhibit.

The observations described in this chapter support the earlier points
made by Jackson, Shephard Ivory Franz, and Lashley. Recall that John
Hughlings Jackson (Chapter 1) suggested that patients who recover from
hemiplegia do so by compensation. He suggested that "nervous arrangements near to those destroyed, having closely similar duties, come to
serve, not as well, but, according to the degree of gravity of the lesion, next
and next as well as those destroyed" (Jackson, 1888; p. 114). This observation can now be expanded based on the recent PET studies of recovery
of motor deficits. Frackowiak and colleagues (Weiller, et al., 1992; Chollet,
et al., 1991) have shown that not only areas near the lesion may take over
functional activities but regions far removed may do so as well.

Shephard Ivory Franz emphasized that neuropsychological phenomena cannot be understood until they are followed from onset to termination. He emphasized that the study of the phenomena associated with
recovery was just as important as understanding the primary phenomenon underlying the defect (i.e., the specific neuropsychological syndrome). We can now add to his observation. Long-term study of recovery may well define periods of deterioration in some patients.
Understanding the pattern of recovery and decline after various types of
brain injury may substantially increase our understanding of brain–
behavior relations. Shephard Ivory Franz, however, led the way in emphasizing this point.

Finally, Lashley emphasized that several mechanisms were potentially responsible for recovery and that all involved mechanisms that had to be understood to maximize a given patient's recovery. Geschwind's (1985) comments further support this notion. The hope is that continued clinical insights paired with sophisticated investigations of brain activity will lead to further scientific insights that could help patients recover their higher cerebral functions after TBI and avoid deterioration of those functions later in life.

References

Aizawa, H., Inase, M., Mushiake, H., Shima, K., and Tanji, J. (1991). Reorganization of activity in the supplementary motor area associated with motor learning and functional recovery. *Exp. Brain Res.* 84: 668–671.

Alexander, G. E., Furey, M. L., Grady, C. L., Pietrini, P., Brady, D. R., Mentis, M. J., and Schapiro, M. B. (1997). Association of premorbid intellectual function with cerebral metabolism in Alzheimer's disease: implications for the cognitive reserve hypothesis. *Am. J. Psychiatry* 154: 165–172.

Basso, A., Gardelli, M., Grassi, M. P., and Mariotti, M. (1989). The role of the right hemisphere in recovery from aphasia: two case studies. *Cortex* 25: 555–566.

Bawden, H. N., Knights, R. M., and Winogron, H. W. (1985). Speeded performance following head injury in children. *J. Clin. Exp. Neuropsychol.* 7(1): 39–54.

Ben-Yishay, Y., Rattok, J., Lakin, P., Piasetsky, E. D., Ross, B., Silver, S., Zide, E., and Ezrachi, O. (1985). Neuropsychological rehabilitation: quest for a holistic approach. *Semin. Neurol.* 5: 252–258.

Bisiach, E., and Vallar, G. (1988). Hemineglect in humans. In F. Boller and J. Grafman (eds), *Handbook of Neuropsychology* (Vol. 1, pp. 195–222). Elsevier, Amsterdam.

Boecker, H., Kleinschmidt, A., Requardt, M., Hänicke, W., Merboldt, K. D., and Frahm, J. (1994). Functional cooperativity of human cortical motor areas during self-paced simple finger movements: a high-resolution MRI study. *Brain* 117: 1231–1239.

Bond, M. R. (1975). Assessment of psychosocial outcome after severe head injury. Ciba Foundation Symposium 34 (new series). *Outcome of Severe Damage to the Central Nervous System* (pp. 141–158). Elsevier, Amsterdam.

Chollet, F., DiPiero, V., Wise, R. J. S., Brooks, D. J., Dolan, R. J., and Frackowiak, R. S. J (1991). The functional anatomy of motor recovery after stroke in humans: a study with positron emission tomography. *Ann. Neurol.* 29: 63–71.

Corkin, S., Rosen, T. J., Sullivan, E. V., and Clegg, R. A. (1989). Penetrating head injury in young adulthood exacerbates cognitive decline in later years. *J. Neurosci.* 9(11): 3876–3883.

Dikmen, S. S., Machamer, J. E., Winn, H. R., and Temkin, N. R. (1995). Neuropsychological outcome at 1-year post head injury. *Neuropsychology* 9(1): 80–90.

Forrester, G., and Geffen, G. (1991). Performance measures of 7- to 15-year-old children on the Auditory Verbal Learning Test. *Clinical Neuropsychologist* 5(4): 345–359.

Gazzaniga, M. S. (1978). Is seeing believing: notes on clinical recovery. In S. Finger (ed), *Recovery from Brain Damage. Research and Theory* (pp. 410–414). Plenum, New York.

Geffen, G., Moar, K. J., O'Hanlon, A. P., Clark, C. R., and Geffen, L. B. (1990). Performance measures of 16-to 86-year-old males and females on the Auditory Verbal Learning Test. *Clinical Psychologist* 4(1): 45–63.

Geschwind, N. (1985). Mechanisms of change after brain lesions. In F. Nottebohm (ed), *Hope for a New Neurology* (pp. 4–11). New York Academy of Sciences, New York.

Goetz, C. G., and Pappert, E. J. (1996). Movement disorders: post-traumatic syndromes. In R. W. Evans (ed), *Neurology and Trauma* (pp. 569–580). W. B. Saunders, Philadelphia.

Goldman, P. S. (1974). An alternative to developmental plasticity: heterology of CNS structures in infants and adults. In D. G. Stein, J. J. Rosen, and N. Butters (eds), *Plasticity and Recovery of Function in the Central Nervous System* (pp. 149–174). Academic Press, New York.

Goldman-Rakic, P. S., Isseroff, A., Schwartz, M. L., and Bugbee, N. M. (1983). The neurobiology of cognitive development. In P. H. Mussen (ed), *Handbook of Child Psychology: Biology and Infancy Development* (pp. 311–344). Wiley, New York.

Grafman, J., Salazar, A., Weingartner, H., Vance, S., and Amin, D. (1986). The relationship of brain-tissue loss volume and lesion location to cognitive deficit. *J. Neurosci.* 6(2): 301–307.

Haaland, K. Y., Temkin, N., Randahl, G., and Dikmen, S. (1994). Recovery of simple motor skills after head injury. *J. Clin. Exp. Neuropsychol.* 16(3): 448–456.

Hier, D. B., Mondlock, J., and Caplan, L. R. (1983). Recovery of behavioral abnormalities after right hemisphere stroke. *Neurology* 33: 345–350.

Jackson, J. H. (1888). Remarks on the diagnosis and treatment of diseases of the brain. *British Medical Journal* July 21: 111–117.

Jennett, B., and Teasdale, G. (1981). *Management of Head Injuries.* F. A. Davis, Philadelphia.

Johnson, S. C., Bigler, E. D., Burr, R. B., and Blatter, D. D. (1994). White matter atrophy, ventricular dilation, and intellectual functioning following traumatic brain injury. *Neuropsychology* 8(3): 307–315.

Kawashima, R., Yamada, K., Kinomura, S., Yamaguchi, T., Matsui, H., Yoshioka, S., and Fukuda, H. (1993). Regional cerebral blood flow changes of cortical motor areas and prefrontal areas in humans related to ipsilateral and contralateral hand movement. *Brain Res.* 623: 33–40.

Kertesz, A. (1988). Recovery of language disorders: homologous contralateral or connected ipsilateral compensation? In S. Finger, T. E. Levere, C. R. Almi, and D. G. Stein (eds), *Brain Injury and Recovery. Theoretical and Controversial Issues* (pp. 307–322). Plenum, New York.

Kertesz, A. (1993). Recovery and treatment. In K. M. Heilman and E. Valenstein (eds), *Clinical Neuropsychology* (3rd ed, pp. 647–674). Oxford University Press, New York.

Kime, S. K., Lamb, D. G., and Wilson, B. A. (1996). Use of a comprehensive program of external cuing to enhance procedural memory in a patient with dense amnesia. *Brain Inj.* 10(1): 17–25.

Klonoff, P. S., Costa, L. D., and Snow, W. G. (1986). Predictors and indicators of quality of life in patients with closed-head injury. *J. Clin. Exp. Neuropsychol.* 8(5): 469–485.

Klonoff, P. S., Lamb, D. G., Henderson, S. W., and Shepherd, J. (1999). New considerations for assessing outcome after milieu-oriented rehabilitation. *Arch. Phys. Med. Rehabil.* (in press).

Knopman, D. S., Selnes, O. A., Niccum, N., Rubens, A. B., Yock, D., and Larson, D. (1983). A longitudinal study of speech fluency in aphasia: CT correlates of recovery and persistent nonfluency. *Neurology* 33: 1170–1178.

Kolb, B. (1990). Recovery from occipital stroke: a self-report and an inquiry into visual processes. *Canadian Journal of Psychology* 44: 130–147.

Kolb, B. (1995). *Brain Plasticity and Behavior*. Lawrence Erlbaum, Mahwah, NJ.

Laurence, S., and Stein, D. G. (1978). Recovery after brain damage and the concept of localization of function. In S. Finger, T. E. Levere, C. R. Almi, and D. G. Stein (eds), *Recovery from Brain Damage. Research and Theory* (pp. 369–407). Plenum, New York.

Lezak, M. D. (1979). Recovery of memory and learning functions following traumatic brain injury. *Cortex* 15: 63–72.

Lezak, M. D. (1995). *Neuropsychological Assessment* (3rd ed). Oxford University Press, New York.

Luria, A. R. (1966). *Higher Cerebral Functions in Man*. Basic Books, New York.

Luria, A. R., Naydin, V. L., Tsvetkova, L. S., and Vinarskaya, E. N. (1969). Restoration of higher cortical function following local brain damage. In P. J. Vinken and G. W. Bruyn (eds), *Handbook of Clinical Neurology* (Vol. 3, pp. 368–433). North-Holland, Amsterdam.

Lynch, C., and Olmstead, E. (1998). *South-Western Mathmatters. An Integrated Approach*. South-Western Educational, Cincinnati.

Mesulam, M-M. (1990). Large-scale neurocognitive networks and distributed processing of attention, language, and memory. *Ann. Neurol.* 28(5): 597–613.

Naeser, M. A., Gaddie, A., Palumbo, C. L., and Stiassny-Eder, D. (1990). Late recovery of auditory comprehension in global aphasia. Improved recovery observed with subcortical temporal isthmus lesion vs Wernicke's cortical area lesion. *Arch. Neurol.* 47: 425–432.

Perani, D., Vallar, G., Paulesu, E., Alberoni, M., and Fazio, F. (1993). Left and right hemisphere contribution to recovery from neglect after right hemisphere damage—an [18F] FDG PET study of two cases. *Neuropsychologia* 31(2): 115–125.

Prigatano, G. P. (1999). Motivation and awareness in cognitive rehabilitation. In D. Stuss and I. H. R. Robertson (eds). *Cognitive Rehabilitation*. Cambridge University Press, Cambridge.

Prigatano, G. P., and Hoffmann, B. (1997). Finger tapping and brain dysfunction: a qualitative and quantitative study. *BNI Quarterly* 13(4): 14–18.

Prigatano, G. P., Fordyce, D. J., Zeiner, H. K., Roueche, J. R., Pepping, M., and Wood, B. C. (1986). *Neuropsychological Rehabilitation After Brain Injury: Theoretical and Clinical Issues.* Johns Hopkins University, Baltimore.

Prigatano, G. P., and Parsons, O. A. (1976). Relationship of age and education to Halstead test performance in different patient populations. *J. Consult. Clin. Psychol.* 44: 527–533.

Prigatano, G. P., and Wong, J. L. (1997). Speed of finger tapping and goal attainment after unilateral cerebral vascular accident. *Arch. Phys. Med. Rehabil.* 78:847–852.

Prigatano, G. P., and Wong, J. L. (1999). Cognitive and affective improvement in brain dysfunctional patients who achieve inpatient rehabilitation goals. *Arch. Phys. Med. Rehabil.* (in press).

Prigatano, G. P., Wong, J. L., Williams, C., and Plenge, K. L. (1997). Prescribed versus actual length of stay and inpatient neurorehabilitation outcome for brain dysfunctional patients. *Arch. Phys. Med. Rehabil.* 78: 621–629.

Rasmussen, P., and Milner, B. (1977). The role of early left-brain injury in determining lateralization of cerebral speech functions. In S. J. Dimond and D. A. Blizard (eds), *Conference on Evolution and Lateralization of the Brain.* New York Academy of Sciences, New York.

Rattok, J., Ben-Yishay, Y., Ezrachi, O., Lakin, P., Piasetsky, E., Ross, B., Silver, S., Vakil, E., Zide, E., and Diller L. (1992). Outcome of different treatment mixes in a multidimensional neuropsychological rehabilitation program. *Neuropsychology* 6(4): 395–415.

Reitan, R. M., and Wolfson, D. (1994). Dissociation of motor impairment and higher-level brain deficits in strokes and cerebral neoplasms. *Clinical Neuropsychologist* 8(2): 193–208.

Roland, P. E. (1993). *Brain Activation.* Wiley-Liss, New York.

Roland, P. E., and Seitz, R. J. (1991). Positron emission tomography studies of the somatosensory system in man. Ciba Foundation Symposium 163. *Exploring Brain Functional Anatomy with Positron Tomography* (pp. 113–124). John Wiley & Sons, Chichester, England.

Roses, A. D., and Saunders, A. M. (1997). ApoE, Alzheimer's disease, and recovery from brain stress. *Ann. N. Y. Acad. Sci.* 826: 200–212.

Sabatini, U., Toni, D., Pantano, P., Brughitta, G., Padovani, A., Bozzao, L., and Lenzi, G. L. (1994). Motor recovery after early brain damage: a case of brain spasticity. *Stroke* 25: 514–517.

Seidman, L. J., Biederman, J., Faraone, S. V., Weber, W., and Ouellette, C. (1997). Toward defining a neuropsychology of attention deficit–hyperactivity disorder: performance of children and adolescents from a large clinically referred sample. *J. Consult. Clin. Psychol.* 65(1), 150–160.

Shimoyama, I., Ninchoji, T., and Uemura, K. (1990). The finger-tapping test: a quantitative analysis. *Arch. Neurol.* 47(6): 681–684.

Smith, A. (1964). Changing effects of frontal lesions in man. *J. Neurol. Neurosurg. Psychiatry* 27, 511–515.

Stein, D. G. (1999). Brain injury and theories of recovery. In Goldstein, L. (ed). *Advances in Pharmacotherapy in Recovery after Stroke*. Futura, Armonk, NY (in press).

Stein, D. G. (1996). Recovery of function. In J. G. Beaumont, P. M. Kenealy, and M. J. C. Rogers (eds), *The Blackwell Dictionary of Neuropsychology* (pp. 608–613). Blackwell, Cambridge, Mass.

Thomsen, I. V. (1984). Late outcome of very severe blunt head trauma: a 10-15 year second follow-up. *J. Neurol. Neurosurg. Psychiatry* 47: 260–268.

Vega, A., Jr., and Parsons, O. A. (1967). Cross-validation of the Halstead-Reitan tests for brain damage. *Journal of Consulting Psychology* 31: 619–623.

Walker, A. E. and Erculei, F. (1969). *Head Injured Man: Fifteen Years Later*. Charles C. Thomas, Springfield, IL.

Ween, J. E., Alexander, M. P., D'Esposito, M., and Roberts, M. (1996). Factors predictive of stroke outcome in a rehabilitation setting. *Neurology* 47:388–392.

Weiller, C., Chollet, F., Friston, K. J., Wise, R.J.S., and Frackowiak, R.S.J. (1992). Functional reorganization of the brain in recovery from striato-capsular infarction in man. *Ann. Neurol.* 31:463–472.

Weiller, C., Ramsay, S. C., Wise, R.J.S., Friston, K. J., and Frackowiak, R.S.J. (1993). Individual patterns of functional reorganization in the human cerebral cortex after capsular infarction. *Ann. Neurol.* 33: 181–189.

Wilson, B. A., and Baddeley, A. (1993). Spontaneous recovery of impaired memory span: does comprehension recover? *Cortex* 29: 153–159.

Wolf, S. L., Lecraw, D. E., Barton, L. A., and Jann, B. B. (1989). Forced use of hemiplegic upper extremities to reverse the effect of learned nonuse among chronic stroke and head-injured patients. *Exp. Neurol.* 104:125–132.

Yakovlev, P. I. (1953). Fronto-pontine bundle and associated projection fibers of the frontal lobe following frontal leucotomy. *Transactions of the American Neurological Association* 78:286–291.

14

Science and Symbolism in Neuropsychological Rehabilitation

> A simple rule that every great man knows by heart, it's smarter
> to be lucky than lucky to be smart!
>> From the musical *Pippen*, song: "War is a Science"

> ... scientific psychology, as far as it has gone today, leaves much
> to be desired in the understanding of man and has little to tell us
> about how to live wisely and well.
>> D. O. Hebb, "What psychology is about," 1974, p. 74

This text has attempted to demonstrate the need for continued scientific study of brain–behavior relationships (i.e., neuropsychology) and the importance of applying that information to rehabilitation. It has also attempted to illustrate the importance of understanding patients' experiences (Principle 1) during a neuropsychological examination or rehabilitation program.

The cognitive and personality problems of brain dysfunctional patients can be formidable, and understanding how the problems interrelate is badly needed (Principle 5). A sophisticated understanding of the direct and indirect effects of brain injury improves understanding of how to approach patients and, thereby, how to educate them and their family members about the effects of brain damage (Principle 4). Such an analysis also improves understanding of the complicated disturbances in higher cerebral functioning labeled as disorders of impaired self-awareness (Principle 11). Finally, understanding the complex changes associated with brain damage that occur over time is relevant to planning neuropsychological rehabilitation and to treating patients

---

The impetus for this last chapter, as well as the plan for this text, was based in part on the Tenth Annual James C. Hemphill Lecture: "Science and symbolism in neuropsychological rehabilitation after brain injury," presented by George P. Prigatano, Ph.D., at the Rehabilitation Institute of Chicago on November 7, 1991.

from a prospective rather than a retrospective manner (Principle 12). These scientific efforts are crucial to working with brain dysfunctional individuals.

This book has concluded that to be effective, practitioners of neuropsychological rehabilitation must also attempt to understand their patients' personal struggles. Achieving this goal often requires supplementing the scientific approach with a phenomenological approach. This approach is not antiscience or subjective science (as Hebb labeled them, 1974). Instead, it is a serious attempt to understand patients' personal experience, particularly the nature of their personal struggles, their need for personal meaning in life despite the inevitable losses associated with brain injury, and their need to use personally relevant symbols to guide them during troublesome times.

By its nature, neuropsychological rehabilitation requires both a scientific and a phenomenological approach. They do not weaken each other. Instead, they maximize our capacity to help patients realistically and to facilitate their adjustment to the permanent effects of brain injury. This strategy may also prove useful in the overall recovery process (Principle 13). This final chapter attempts to highlight this principle and to suggest that symbols may be especially important not only in understanding patients' phenomenological experiences but also in helping them adjust to their permanent losses. This point was also discussed in the chapter on psychotherapy.

Toward Resolving Paradox

Chapter 1 noted Karl Pribram's comment that in science we often just collect facts, but true knowledge emerges when we resolve paradox. The scientific portion of this text focuses on three paradoxical areas that are slowly being resolved.

The first is the paradox noted by Brodal (1973) and quoted in Chapter 11. An accomplished neuroscientist, Brodal observed "two aspects" of the central nervous system that are "apparently contradictory." "There is an extremely high degree of specificity and at the same time, a far going diffuseness in the patterns of organization" (p. 687).

The modest modification of Luria's (1966) definition of higher cerebral functions partially addresses this paradox. Higher cerebral functions are integrative precisely because a high degree of specificity exists. From this integration, however, other properties emerge that seem to affect the entire nervous system simultaneously. These emergent properties are difficult to define, but they are the psychological (or neuropsychological) laws that govern brain–mind relationships. Understanding that higher cerebral functions are, by nature, integrated and emergent may help us appreciate the paradoxes involved in the organization of the nervous system.

I personally believe that human consciousness is the best example of these integrative and emergent properties. These properties are reflected in the natural integration of thoughts and feelings and how this integration leads to ideas unbounded by the space-time continuum. Given how the brain is organized, individuals can imagine events that have not yet occurred and that may never occur but that are possibilities.

The second paradox concerns disorders of self-awareness. If these disorders are the result of brain dysfunction, why do cultural factors influence their expression? The Japanese study discussed earlier (Prigatano et al., 1997) suggests how we might begin to answer this question. Damage to the anterior regions of the brain (frontal lobes systems) may affect the ability to perceive the context of a behavior or cognition. Culture, however, determines the context. Thus, the interaction of culture and brain dysfunction may determine what experience is altered and how that experience is reported and expressed. Thus, disorders of self-awareness inherently reflect this dynamic interaction between the brain and its environment.

The third paradox is that so-called unilateral lesions often result in bilateral cerebral dysfunction. Given von Monokaw's theory of diaschisis, this tendency, by itself, is not paradoxical. The so-called unaffected brain regions of some persons with unilateral lesions, however, eventually recover but others do not. For example, two patients with right-hemisphere lesions showed hemi-inattention or unilateral neglect (Perani, et al., 1993). One patient recovered and one did not. In the patient who recovered, the metabolic activity in the left hemisphere returned to normal. In the patient who did not recover, the metabolic activity in the left hemisphere never returned to normal. What mechanism underlies these phenomena?

Is it possible that temporarily disturbed functions that do not "spontaneously" regain normal metabolic activity initiate a cascade of events that cause further deterioration or permanent dysfunction? If diaschisis fails to resolve spontaneously or via deinhibitory training (i.e., Luria, et al., 1969), will a permanent higher cerebral dysfunction develop that could have been remediated with appropriate treatment?

The work of Corkin and colleagues (1989) shows that brain dysfunctional individuals in the fifth decade of life may exhibit a precipitous decline in function not characteristic of their earlier years after brain injury. Thus, a dynamic interaction among age, lesion location and type, and the possible role of temporarily inhibited functions appears not only possible but probable at the ultimate level of neuropsychological recovery.

The paradoxes surrounding recovery and deterioration await further investigation and are clearly the future of neuropsychology. Clinical neuropsychologists will do well if they study these phenomena carefully and apply their insights to patient care. These and many other interesting paradoxes await resolution via the application of the scientific method. Clinical neuropsychologists need to participate in this venture to improve the profession and the quality of life of the patients whom they serve.

Against this background, it is crucial to consider the role of phenomenology in patient care. The importance of the role of symbols in human existence cannot be minimized, particularly after brain injury.

The Symbols of Intelligence and Brain Damage

Unequivocally, brain damage adversely affects various cognitive functions (see Chapter 5). With time, patients may sense that they are no longer as intelligent or smart as they once were. In our culture, such a loss is tremendous and can threaten people's sense of personal value and security (see Prigatano, 1991). Fear of being ridiculed, sensing a diminished intellectual capacity to handle arguments or to fight for one's position, feeling confusion and associated frustrations (see Chapter 2) about one's life increase feelings of despair and frustration. Some patients simply cannot overcome this experience and find it extremely difficult to articulate. Consequently, they often use symbols from music or other arts to convey their experience.

Even articulate patients often find it extremely difficult to describe their sense of loss about their declining intelligence. An accomplished professor, for example, played John Lennon's song "Yesterday" to describe his feelings of being "half the man that he was yesterday." This patient, who had a right hemisphere lesion, often appeared euphoric and sometimes socially inappropriate. His choice of music reflected his existential despair that could not be detected from formal neuropsychological examinations or interviews.

How do clinical neuropsychologists deal with this issue in the context of their clinical practice? Parents who have a child with subnormal intelligence worry about their child's present and future functioning. Many of these parents, however, report that their child's lower intelligence in no way diminishes their love for that child. The child's value is reflected in so many other capacities than his or her IQ. It is reflected in the child's honesty, the child's caring and loving attitude, the child's capacity for humor, and the child's capacity to work hard in the face of adversity. These are the virtues that often enable the human spirit to overcome subnormal intelligence or any other hardship. In some form, this spirit must be recaptured when a young adult, a middle-aged adult, or senior citizen suffers a brain injury associated with cognitive losses.

Anyone who has ever been frightened or intimidated by his or her inability to solve a problem or to use logic defensively knows that nothing short of courage is needed to maintain one's position and sense of hope during such time. Courage is an extremely important quality that helps many people to cope with adversity. This is also true after brain damage.

In our society, the symbol of intelligence is a symbol of survivability and power. It is perhaps best personified by our culture's preoccupation with science. In many ways, quality of life has improved because the scientific method has been applied to a variety of problems. Yet many people who are totally engrossed in intellectual pursuits and who have not been in touch with the affective side of life find themselves in a state of despair. As Marie Louise von Franz has commented: "Science is a wasteland for the human soul."

Franz, a Jungian analyst, understood that a purely rational approach to the world misses some of the essential ingredients in what it means to be human. Humans function both cognitively and affectively. They are both rational and irrational (see the description of the higher cerebral functions in Chapter 2). They are driven by their animal heritage as much as by their capacity to reason, speak, or make tools (see Chapter 6). Once this dual aspect of humanity is understood, clinical neuropsychologists are in a much better position to help patients with the consequences of brain damage. The symbol of intelligence can be placed into perspective. It is no longer the golden idol that all must worship. It is an important aspect of human behavior, but it need not be the only symbol that offers a sense of personal strength and security (Prigatano, 1991).

Patients who can put the symbol of intelligence into a meaningful perspective are in a much better position to cope with the effects of their brain injury. Neuropsychological rehabilitation, which often incorporates psychotherapy, can help with this process (see Chapters 8 and 9). If patients are not helped to place the symbol of intelligence into perspective, their loss of cognitive functioning can ultimately lead to severe depression. For many the consequence is social isolation; for a few it is suicide. Thus, more than the symbol of intelligence is needed as a guiding symbol in life.

Chapter 9 attempted to show that the symbols of work, love, and play can help patients establish meaning in life. Adapting these symbols to an individual's condition after brain injury can aid the process of rehabilitation. These symbols often help persons learn how to live well and wisely, aspects of living for which scientific psychology has offered little.

One might argue that luck is needed to live well and wisely. Thomas Jefferson reportedly responded to comments that he was lucky by saying "The harder I work, the luckier I get." Jefferson's observations reflect American culture and its belief system. Hard work often overcomes many forms of adversity. Therefore, hard-working people appear to be more fortunate than others. Although hard work and motivation can help patients to cope with a number of aspects of brain injury, motivation by itself is an insufficient condition for recovery (Prigatano, 1999). No matter how hard one tries, the effects of brain injury sometimes cannot be reversed. People can, however, learn to adapt to the effects of brain injury. Yet, this goal requires more than a knowledge of scientific psychology or neuropsychology.

Psychologists can be too intimidated to approach knowledge bases beyond their scientific training. They may fear being ridiculed as non-scientific, unethical, or inept by their colleagues. At some point, however, clinical neuropsychologists must find the courage to do what other disciplines have done—namely, to describe what they see and to try to deal with it using *all* the information available to them. One such avenue is to combine the strength and insight of science with the wisdom of the humanities.

A Return to Hebb's Observation

In 1973 Donald Hebb gave an invited address to the American Psychological Association entitled "What Is Psychology About?" His address was later published (Hebb, 1974) and represents an important article for psychologists. In it Hebb clarified that psychology is a biological science devoted to difficult questions (e.g., how does the brain produce mind?). He delineated the strengths and limitations of scientific psychology but noted that scientific psychology has a poor track record for teaching people to live well or wisely. When brain dysfunctional patients attend rehabilitation, they typically want more than a scientific analysis of their problems. They want help in dealing with the effects of these problems on their life. It is the responsibility of the psychologist to assist in this process. Avoiding this responsibility decreases the credibility of the field in the perceptions of both the public and the medical community.

In my experience, the scientific training of neuropsychologists often neglects this important component of therapy. Hebb points out that the humanities (the study of philosophy, art, history, and literature) offer valuable clues about how to live well and wisely. He also warns that combining the two (into what he refers to as a humanistic psychology) often ruins both.

His statement, however, must be interpreted cautiously. It applies to attempts to study the humanities scientifically. The converse also applies—decreasing the rigor of science through introspective methods. The scientific method is thereby damaged and no objective information can be obtained. His statement, however, does not preclude scientifically trained psychologists from using knowledge of the humanities in their clinical practice.

Remember what the terms clinical practice mean. Practice means exerting continual effort to do something better. Clinical means, or at least implies, that the effort being practiced is related to improving another person's health. Consequently, I argue that more than a scientific approach is needed when working with brain dysfunctional patients.

The recent Houston Conference on Specialty Education and Training in Clinical Neuropsychology, for example, made no reference to the importance of psychotherapy as a skill that clinical neuropsychologists should develop. Any experienced psychotherapist, however, recognizes that one is essentially impotent as a psychotherapist without a firm grasp of what the humanities have to teach. Although useful at times, behavioral therapy falls exceedingly short because it fails to deal with patients' subjective experiences (Prigatano, 1997) or to help them with broader philosophical or existential questions. What, then, should be involved in the training of clinical neuropsychologists involved in neuropsychological rehabilitation?

The Training of Clinical Neuropsychologists and Neuropsychological Rehabilitation

If neuropsychologists limit their work to research or neuropsychological assessment, current standards of training are probably adequate. If, however, psychologists trained in neuropsychology will apply their clinical skills to the rehabilitation of people with brain injuries, considerably more training is needed. In this case, individuals should first be trained as clinical psychologists and then pursue postdoctoral training in clinical neuropsychology. The reason is simple. Besides understanding brain–behavior relationships and the relevant history, therapists also need to understand psychiatric disturbances and their history. Such studies include a variety of theorists who have deeply considered the nature of human beings: Freud, Jung, Harry Stack Sullivan, Maslow, Carl Rogers, and B. F. Skinner.

The training of clinical psychologists includes considerable supervision of clinical work. The goal is to determine how well students will interact with patients during psychological assessments and interventions aimed at helping patients to cope with life's problems. Clinical psychologists also receive specific training in psychotherapy. Clinical neuropsychologists from a background of physiological psychology or human neuropsychology often miss this type of training.

Training a psychotherapist is complicated. It involves not only formal course work but often years of personal supervision and personal psychotherapy. Most experienced psychotherapists confess that they did not develop their psychotherapeutic skills in graduate school or even during the first 5 years thereafter. Rather, their skills developed over many years of clinical practice and cannot be separated from their own personal life experiences. By midlife, people have typically experienced enough changes or losses in life to have gained a sense of maturity. In contrast, the typical 27-year-old graduating with a Ph.D. has undergone formal academic training but little else.

Formal training is crucial, but learning to become a clinical neuropsychologist never ends. The process of evolution as it influences the biological and psychological activities of organisms must be studied. Animal behavior and its great parallels to human behavior are also important, as described in Chapter 6. All too often these relevant connections are missed unless persons have a specific interest to understand their own behavior or they are fortunate enough to have professors who mentor them.

The essence of the training of clinical neuropsychologists involved in neuropsychological rehabilitation allows them to apply multiple sources of information to understand a given patient's suffering. A broad knowledge of science as well as an understanding of the humanities can combine to optimize clinical care. I am not advocating a humanistic form of science. Rather, both sources of knowledge complement each other and should be integrated to train clinicians to help patients during the rehabilitation process after significant brain damage.

Illustrative Cases

Three cases highlight Principle 13.

". . . you don't know the meaning of a brain injury until later in your life."

A middle-aged man suffered a moderate TBI when he fell down a flight of stairs. He was involved in a neuropsychological rehabilitation program, and his approach to rehabilitation was exceptionally practical. He had cognitive deficits but seemed able to cope with them. He did not appear to be overwhelmed by his memory difficulties or by his reduced speed of information processing. He worked diligently at all cognitive retraining activities and engaged a work trial with an uncommon level of maturity. During the relatives' group, his wife described her husband and how he had changed—his memory problems, for example. At times, she was moved to tears while describing her husband's condition. Her husband, however, did not seem to be overwhelmed by his situation and yet had good insight about his condition. Why?

During the time of his neuropsychological rehabilitation program, I discussed the potential use of fairy tales in psychotherapy. We invited group psychotherapy patients to either read their favorite fairy tales or to relate stories that they felt had influenced their life. This patient, who was from Vietnam, was not raised with fairy tales but did relate a story that he had learned as a child.

There was an old man named Thong who lived in Vietnam. Thong was a farmer and had one horse to plow his field in order to raise his crops to care for his family. One day, Thong went out to the barn to fetch his horse and discovered that the horse had run away. Other villagers came to console him, stating that it was certainly bad luck he lost his horse. The old man looked at his friends and said, "Maybe it is and maybe it isn't, only time will tell."

A few weeks later the horse returned, not only by himself but brought along a female companion. The female companion was expecting. The villagers once again gathered around Thong proclaiming his great luck. Now he was the envy of the whole village! They stated that he was indeed fortunate to have his horse back with an expecting companion. Again the old man looked and shrugged his shoulders and said, "Maybe it is and maybe it isn't, only time will tell."

Then, as the story goes, Thong's son went out one day to ride the horse. The horse bucked him off, and the young man suffered a brain injury. The villagers once again gathered around Thong stating what a tragedy this was for him. Again, the old man looked at the villagers and shrugged his shoulders and said, "Maybe it is and maybe it isn't, only time will tell" (Prigatano, 1991; p. 7).

This patient, who had lived through the horrors of the Vietnam War, finished the story by saying that when war had come to this small village, only the young healthy men were taken to serve in combat and most were eventually killed. The boy who had suffered the brain injury was not recruited into the army and thus survived. The power of this story was that the meaning of events cannot be known immediately. What had first appeared to be a tragedy (i.e., a brain injury) turned out to be good fortune (i.e., the boy survived as opposed to being killed in war).

This patient had maintained the philosophy of life reflected in this story from his childhood. This patient did not need psychotherapy; in fact, he taught the psychotherapist much about the meaning of life and the importance of a personal philosophy. The patient's phenomenological experience not only helped him to adjust to his brain injury but helped others recognize that their adjustment could also improve if they internalized the wisdom of such a story.

Childhood stories can have a tremendous impact as reflected by this particular vignette. These stories symbolize important human experiences that have been reported over the ages. Maintaining contact with these symbols helps us cope with adversity with considerably less anxiety and perhaps more foresight than we might otherwise.

"The Man in the Mirror"

A second patient with a more severe brain injury has been described elsewhere (Prigatano, 1991; p. 7). An athlete headed toward a promising academic and athletic career, she suffered a severe brain injury in an automobile accident. When she was first seen (about a year after injury), she was angry and frequently had violent outbursts. Despite hemiplegia, she would strike out and hit others, often with minimum provocation.

Several times a day she yelled that she did not wish to live. At various times during her psychotherapy, she voiced confusion about her sexual orientation and identity. She had many of the cognitive and affective disturbances associated with severe TBI (see Chapters 5, 6, and 7).

Working with her in the context of group psychotherapy seemed futile. But after months of working with her and of her observing other patients, her mood and behavior slowly changed. She progressively recognized the true impact of her brain injury on herself as well as on others. During group psychotherapy, she played Michael Jackson's song: "Man in the Mirror." (The reader might wish to listen to this song.) The lyrics emphasize that individuals should take a good look at themselves and recognize that they are not the only ones suffering in life. The song helped the patient make the next step in her commitment to life. Her violent outbursts, her negative attitude, and her severe depression slowly receded. She was able to accept (as were her parents) her need to work as a volunteer and to abandon hopes of functioning at a higher level. The song was an extremely important turning point in this patient's life. She had severe cognitive deficits, but with the right therapeutic relationship and the right use of symbols she was able to find a renewed sense of direction in her life. These two cases highlight that the symbols and the values that they point to can be extremely important in brain injury rehabilitation.

". . . I guess you're right."

Not all patients, however, improve so dramatically. In fact, the previous two cases highlight the underlying principle but are rare in clinical practice. A third patient represents a more common presentation, but his case still highlights the importance of symbols. The patient, discussed throughout this text, suffered cardiac arrest and clear cerebral anoxia in his early twenties. Recall that initially he was grossly amnestic. His memory improved but he lacked insight as to the extent of his memory problems or the problems he would face returning to an academic life.

With his lack of insight, he attempted to resume his previous lifestyle only later to develop panic attacks and severe headaches. He had little insight that his cognitive disturbances made it impossible to function in his previous environment. He saw absolutely no connection between his cognitive failures and the emergence of his anxiety and the development of severe headaches.

After repeated failures, he finally agreed to be reevaluated and to resume work with the psychotherapist who had worked with him in neuropsychological rehabilitation. Numerous discussions ensued aimed at showing the patient the connection among his cognitive deficits, his academic and job failures, and the development of his psychiatric and somatic symptoms. Despite these discussions, he still failed to perceive the connection.

This patient, however, trusted in caregivers, which was an important symbol in his life. His father was a physician and he trusted his father. Consequently, he trusted the health care system and the psychotherapist who was a part of it. Thus, with no insights about the connection between his neuropsychological disturbances and his psychiatric and somatic complaints, the patient agreed to follow the advice of his psychotherapist, who recommended that he change universities and embark on a less demanding career.

At the new university, an experienced vocational rehabilitation counselor helped the patient to identify himself as a student with a disability. This step was major because the young man did not want to acknowledge his disability. The concept of disability is a powerful symbol that means one does not function normally. The problem of lost normality after brain injury is discussed elsewhere (Prigatano, 1994). This particular patient, however, had a difficult time accepting this symbol (i.e., the symbol of a disabled individual) in relation to himself.

As he followed the advice of his psychotherapist and made a variety of changes in his daily life, his ability to cope improved. Life became more secure and predictable, his panic attacks disappeared, and his headaches diminished markedly.

As his functioning improved, the psychotherapist again asked the patient if he perceived a connection between his neuropsychological difficulties and his somatic and psychiatric problems. The patient looked at the therapist quizzically. He still could see no connection, but because his ability to function had improved noticeably, he said "I guess you're right."

This case highlights the importance of two symbols in guiding the patient's behavior. The first symbol was trust in a caregiver. Relating to that symbol, the patient could follow the guidance of the psychotherapist. The second symbol, that of disability, was extremely difficult for this patient to relate to. However, once he did and recognized that his disability did not mean that he lacked value, he was able to adjust to life much better. By identifying with or, at least, relating to these symbols, the patient could confront his life realistically.

Concluding Comments and Observations

I wrote this text to help clarify a number of issues concerning the nature of higher cerebral deficits, how they emerge after brain injury, and how neuropsychological rehabilitation attempts to help brain dysfunctional patients.

The field has made slow but steady progress toward understanding the nature of higher cerebral functions and how they are affected by various forms of brain damage. The course of recovery is also better appreciated, and the myth of a static brain injury has been dispelled. Confronting these realities allows more innovative rehabilitation programs to be developed.

What do studies of brain-injured people reveal about the nature of human beings, and, conversely, what does our philosophy of human nature reveal about brain damage? During a seminar in Zurich, Tony Frey, a Jungian analyst, once remarked that he believed that human beings have exactly the same amount of "good" and "evil" in them. He stated that if this were not the case, humanity would surely have either eliminated wars or destroyed itself by this time. Any practicing psychotherapist (or astute observer in human behavior) can attest that both positive and negative forces reside within every human being.

Although people often say that they want to be happy, considerable evidence suggests that they often behave in a manner that perpetuates their unhappiness. Paul Watzlawick (1983) captured this reality in the title of his book: *The Situation is Hopeless, but not Serious: The Pursuit of Unhappiness*.

Given their eternal struggle with the forces of life (i.e., libido) and those of death or destruction (i.e., Thanatos; Freud 1924; Kaplan, et al., 1994), human beings continue to ask important questions about the nature of their existence and their struggles to survive. Eventually, these questions lead to the ultimate question: What is the meaning of one's existence? Freud (1930/1961) recognized the importance of this question to people in his monograph *Civilization and its Discontents*: "It is impossible to escape the impression that people commonly use false standards of measurement—that they seek power, success, and wealth for themselves and admire them in others, and that they underestimate what is of true value in life" (p. 11).

Later, considering the purpose of life, he noted that various philosophical answers have been unsatisfactory and suggested that direct observation of behavior is needed to answer the question (p. 23). He stated that "as we see, what decides the purpose of life is simply the program of the pleasure" (p. 23). He then noted how the capacities to work and love derive from this basic principle. Yet, toward the end of his life, Freud recognized that he had suffered a great deal to express his own individuality by insisting on the verity of his psychoanalytic insights despite their unpopular reception. The meaning Freud derived from his own life appeared to be enhanced by his desire to assert his own individuality.

Jung emphasized the importance of seeking one's individuality as an extremely important component of a meaningful life. Consequently, I prefer a Jungian perspective on the purpose or meaning of life. In the introduction to her work, *The Myth of Meaning and the Work of C. G. Jung*, Aniela Jaffé (1984) begins with the following quote from Camus: "I have seen many people die because life for them was not worth living. From this I conclude that the question of life's meaning is the most urgent question of all" (p. 3).

The question of meaning in life, as well as the reality of death, haunts every human existence. When tragedy befalls individuals, these question momentarily attain a clear focus. Goldstein (1951/1971) provided an especially constructive critique of Freudian psychology when he noted that both unconscious (he prefers the term nonconscious, as does Kihlstrom, 1987) and conscious aspects of human behavior are important in defining human beings.

The "creative power" of human nature, which ultimately separates man from animals, is but a matter of degree. Language and toolmaking are not necessarily unique to humanity. They are elevated to a higher form, presumably because of the development of the cerebral cortex and its associated structures. The human brain, however, not only develops language but constructs symbols.

Symbols can be distinguished from signs. A sign means the same thing irrespective of its context (e.g., no smoking sign). In contrast, symbols can only be interpreted within a specific context. Thus, symbols, by their nature, require frontal-limbic connections (Pribram, 1971, 1991; Prigatano, 1989). Jung (1964) suggested that symbols not only reflect what one is experiencing but help define (but not necessarily explain) aspects of reality not easily grasped by consciousness. Thus, individuals are often drawn to symbols as a means of expressing the complexity of their existence as well as their hopes and fears for the future.

Symbols emerge from the arts. They can be found in poetry. They are reflected in drawings and in paintings. They are represented in music. Many symbols recur across cultures and times. Such symbols therefore continue to reveal an important aspect of human nature. C. G. Jung was perhaps the most outspoken psychological theorist who recognized the universal aspect of some symbols. Jung has been criticized for many things, but those who know his work can appreciate not only his courage but his creativity in helping individuals grapple with the problems associated with the second half of life.

In various places I have argued that brain injury, regardless of chronological age, catapults individuals into the second half of life. That is, life is no longer the same after brain injury—individuals function with less intelligence, less capacity for memory, less physical strength, and fewer opportunities for the future. Jung recognized that during middle age, people without brain injuries struggle with similar kinds of problems, albeit at a less severe level. He reviewed the use of symbols and how they have guided human beings at various stages in their life. It was his insight and inspiration that led to the recognition of the importance of symbols in working with brain dysfunctional individuals.

At times I am asked whether patients with severe cognitive deficits can actually benefit from psychotherapy. The answer is yes. Much depends, however, on the psychotherapist's capacity to understand patients' neuropsychological problems and to identify symbols that the patients can relate to. This process is the true spirit of the phenomenological approach and its reliance on the humanities.

Are the 13 principles listed in this text useful? Will they survive the ravages of managed care? Are they oversimplifications of complex realities that neuropsychologists must face in their clinical work and research? Do they provide guidance for research or for how to approach brain dysfunctional patients clinically? As my Vietnamese patient emphasized in his story about his own brain injury, "Maybe it will and maybe it won't; only time will tell."

In the spirit of that patient, who taught me so much about the use of psychotherapy and the strengths and limitations of neuropsychological rehabilitation, I conclude this text with a quote from my favorite fairy tale, *Jack and the Beanstalk*. The tale conveys many important aspects of life: courage, taking chances, confronting fears, and, if we are a little "lucky," finding the "goose that lays the golden egg." But not everybody finds the prize. The willingness to take a chance and to pursue one's individuality, however, can become the cornerstone for a meaningful life—with or without brain damage. Thus a phrase from *Jack and the Beanstalk* may serve to guide not only our clinical work with patients but our ability to report empirical observations regardless of their popularity or unpopularity with colleagues:

"So we have learned he who takes a chance, has a chance."

References

Brodal, A. (1973). Self-observations and neuro-anatomical considerations after a stroke. *Brain* 96: 675–694.

Corkin, S., Rosen, T. J., Sullivan, E. V., and Clegg, R. A. (1989). Penetrating head injury in young adulthood exacerbates cognitive decline in later years. *J. Neurosci.* 9(11): 3876–3883.

Freud, S. (1924). *A General Introduction to Psychoanalysis* (24th ed). Simon and Schuster, New York.

Freud, S. (1930/1961). *Civilization and its Discontents*, J. Strachey (ed). W. W. Norton, New York.

Goldstein, K. (1951/1971). On emotions: Considerations from the organismic point of view. *J. Psychology* 31: 37–49). Reprinted in A. Gurwitsch, E. M. Goldstein Haudek, and W. E. Haudek (eds), *Kurt Goldstein Selected Papers*. Martinus Nijhoff, The Hague.

Hebb, D. O. (1974). What psychology is about. *Am. Psychol.* 29(2), 71–79.

Jaffé, A. (1984). *The Myth of Meaning in the Work of C. G. Jung.* Daimon, Zurich, Switzerland.

Jung, C. G. (1964). *Man and His Symbols.* Doubleday Windfall, Garden City, NY.

Kaplan, H. I., Sadock, B. J., and Grebb, J. A., (1994). *Kaplan and Sadock's Synopsis of Psychiatry. Behavioral Sciences. Clinical Psychiatry* (7th ed). Williams & Wilkins, Baltimore.

Kihlstrom, J. F. (1987). The cognitive unconscious. *Science* 237: 1445–1452.

Luria, A. R. (1966). *Higher Cerebral Functions in Man.* Basic Books, New York.

Luria, A. R., Naydin, V. L., Tsvetkova, L. S., and Vinarskaya, E. N. (1969). Restoration of higher cortical function following local brain damage. In P. J. Vinken and G. W. Bruyn (eds), *Handbook of Clinical Neurology* (Vol. 3, pp. 368–433). North-Holland, Amsterdam.

Perani, D., Vallar, G., Paulesu, E., Alberoni, M., and Fazio, F. (1993). Left and right hemisphere contribution to recovery from neglect after right hemisphere damage—an [^{18}F] FDG PET study of two cases. *Neuropsychologia* 31: 115–125.

Pribram, K. H. (1971). *Languages of the Brain: Experimental Paradoxes and Principles in Neuropsychology.* Prentice-Hall, Englewood Cliffs, NJ.

Pribram, K. H. (1991). *Brain and Perception: Holonomy and Structure in Figural Processing.* Lawrence Erlbaum, Hillsdale, NJ.

Prigatano, G. P. (1989). Work, love, and play after brain injury. *Bull. Menninger Clin.* 53(5): 414–431.

Prigatano, G. P. (1991). Science and symbolism in neuropsychological rehabilitation after brain injury. The Tenth Annual James C. Hemphill Lecture, November 7, 1991, Rehabilitation Institute of Chicago.

Prigatano, G. P. (1994). Disordered mind, wounded soul: the emerging role of psychotherapy in rehabilitation after brain injury. *Journal of Head Trauma Rehabilitation* 6(4): 1–10.

Prigatano, G. P. (1995). 1994 Sheldon Berrol, MD, Senior Lectureship: The problem of lost normality after brain injury. *Journal of Head Trauma Rehabilitation* 10(3): 87–95.

Prigatano, G. P. (1997). Learning from our successes and failures: Reflections and comments on "Cognitive rehabilitation: How it is and how it might be." *Journal of International Neuropsychological Society* 3:497–499.

Prigatano, G. P. (1999). Motivation and awareness in cognitive rehabilitation. In D. Stuss and I. H. R. Robertson (eds), *Cognitive Neurorehabilitation.* Cambridge University Press, Cambridge.

Prigatano, G. P., Ogano, M., and Amakusa, B. (1997). A cross-cultural study on impaired self-awareness in Japanese patients with brain dysfunction. *Neuropsychiatry, Neuropsychology, and Behavioral Neurology* 10(1): 135–143.

Watzlawick, P. (1983). *The Situation is Hopeless, But Not Serious: The Pursuit of Unhappiness.* W. W. Norton, New York.

Index

Page references followed by the letter *f* are for figures
Page references followed by the letter *t* are for tables

Attention disorders after traumatic brain
injury, 98*t*, 100–102
Attitude of brain-injured patient, 217
AVM. *See* Arteriovenous malformation

Behavior
caused by brain dysfunction, 50–51
compensatory, in recovery, 302, 303*f*
driving forces of, 204
focal brain lesions and, 75
problems, sensitivity to distress, 78
self-destructive, 206
Ben-Yishay, Yehuda, 17–19
BNI Screen for Higher Cerebral Functions, 58,
151, 278
Boredom, 101, 104
Brain
damage. *See* Brain injury
dysfunction. *See also specific types of dysfunction*
behaviors caused by, 50–51
dementia in, 52
memory impairment in, 51–52
mental fatigue and, 37–38
evolution, 7–8
animal behavior and, 118–123, 119*f*,
120*f*
cognition and, 123–125, 125*f*
personality and, 123–125, 125*f*
higher functions. *See* Higher cerebral
functions
organization/function, 7–8
Brain injury
clinical evidence, 30–32
disability
extent of, inability to recognize, 218
influence on self-reports,
278
experience of, 29–30
human nature and, 343
lesions
localization of, 5
size of, recovery level and, 12
"static," deterioration of function
and, 316–318, 318*f*
tissue mass loss and, 91, 91*f*
meaning, childhood stories and, 339–
340
rehabilitation. *See* Rehabilitation, neuropsychological
symptoms. *See* Symptoms; *specific symp-
toms/impairments*
traumatic. *See* Traumatic brain injury
Brief Psychiatric Rating Scale, 135, 136*f*
Broca's area, speech/speech planning and,
109

California Verbal Learning Test (CVLT),
59, 102
Catastrophic reaction, 13
Cerebral artery aneurysm
clinical evidence, 30–31
cognitive/behavioral/emotional
changes, 75
Cerebral blood flow, regional
changes, speech/speech planning and,
109
in finger movement studies, 312–313
Cerebral edema reduction, spontaneous recovery after, 306
Cerebral functions, higher. *See* Higher cerebral functions
Cerebral hemisphere
dysfunction, unilateral *vs.* bilateral, 283
lesions
anosognosia for hemiplegia and, 272–
274, 273*t*
emotional responses of "affected"
side, 267–268
size of, recovery rate and, 299
unilateral, bilateral dysfunction and,
334
neglect, 305
organization of, 282–283
unaffected regions, 334
finger movement studies and, 312
hypometabolism in, 305
Cerebral metabolism, positron emission
imaging of, 305
Cerebrovascular accident (CVA)
anosognosia for hemiplegia and, 272–
274, 273*t*
cognitive rehabilitation for, 250–251
finger tapping speed, 311
Change mechanisms, after brain injury,
325–326
Characterological problems, 133
Children, impact of brain injury on, 81, 83*f*
Cingulate gyrus, emotion/motivation and,
132
Clinical sensibility in psychotherapy after
brain injury, 202–203
Clinician, understanding of patient and, 28–
29
Cognition
brain evolution and, 123–125, 125*f*
feelings and, 125
flexibility, 107
focal brain lesions and, 75
interaction with social demands, 94
motivation and, 124
Cognitive disorders after brain injury
arousal and, 100–102, 98*t*

Hypersexuality, Klüver-Bucy syndrome of, 123, 129, 132*t*
Hysterical paralyses, 267

Identity, fidelity and, 214–215
Indirect symptoms. *See* Symptoms, indirect or positive
Individual cognitive retraining (IZED), 183
Individuality, importance of, 343–344
Individuation, 214
Inertia, energy and, 126
Information
  domains, in assessing personality, 149
  processing speed after traumatic brain injury, 97, 100, 98*t*
Initiation disorders after traumatic brain injury, 98*t*–99*t*, 103–105, 104*f*, 105*f*
Insurance companies, documentation of rehabilitation progress, 235
Integrative functions, higher. *See* Higher cerebral functions
Intellectual level, symptoms and, 58–60
Intelligence quotient (IQ)
  partial recovery, with anger/frustration, 318–321, 319*f*, 320*f*
  premorbid, 59
Intelligence symbols, brain injury rehabilitation and, 335–337
Interdisciplinary rehabilitation team
  advantages of, 236–237, 237*t*
  candidate selection, 239
  change in, 240–241
  disadvantages of, 237–238, 237*t*
  division of labor and, 230
  efficacy of interventions and, 236
  flexibility of, 237
  group dynamics and, 229–233, 241
  leadership, 233
  management, methods of, 236–240, 240*t*
  members/staff, 241
    conflict with patient, 237–238
    interstaff relations, review of, 239
    personality of, 238–239, 239*t*
    relations with patient, review of, 239
    respites for, 240
    selection of, 239
  need for, 229
  orchestration, difficulties with, 229
  scapegoat for, 233
  vocational rehabilitation and, 74
  "we" versus "us" focus, 230–232
Interpersonal relationships, objective, 214
Intimacy, 210–211
IQ. *See* Intelligence quotient

Irritability, frustration of brain dysfunctional patients and, 34
IZED (individual cognitive retraining), 183

Jackson, John Hughlings, 5–6
Judgment disorders after traumatic brain injury, 99*t*, 105–107
Jung, Carl Gustav, 21–22, 127, 205

Klüver-Bucy syndrome of hypersexuality, 123, 129

Language
  brain regions in, 42
  development, emotional content and, 95–96
  disorders
    after traumatic brain injury, 99*t*, 107–109
    nonaphasic or subclinical, 108
  skills, in early brain damage, 157
Lashley, Karl S., 9–12
Learning
  disorders, after traumatic brain injury, 98*t*
  emotional content and, 95–96
  retardation, brain injury and, 9–10
Libido, 127
Life, meaning of, 343
Life failures after brain injury, 73
Limbic system
  disruptions, 132
  frontal lesions, 121
  regions of, 282
  sensory input
    first, 119–120
    second, 121
  subdivisions, functions of, 120–121, 120*f*
  thalamic-cingulate area, damage to, 122–123
  visual information from, 122
Love
  symbols of
    adaptation to brain injury and, 336
    after brain injury, 210–211, 211*f*
  triangular theory of, 211, 211*f*
Luria, Alexander Romanovich., 14–17

MacLean, Paul, 118–123
Memory impairments
  compensation for, 252
  depression and, 94
  negative symptoms, 98*t*, 102
  persistence of, 78, 79*t*
  positive symptoms, 98*t*, 102–103
  types of, 51–52

Personality *(continued)*
  neuropsychiatric/neuropsychologically
    based, 132–133
  organismic theory of, 33–34
  premorbid
    of brain dysfunction patients, 54
    definition of, 61
    patient's description of impairments
      and, 171–172
Phenomenological field of patient
  artistic expression and, 40–41
  barriers to entering, 38–40
Planning disorders after traumatic brain in-
    jury, 98t–99t, 103–105, 104f, 105f
Plasticity, 94–95
Play, symbol of
  adaptation and, 336
  description of, 211–213, 212f
Positive symptoms. *See* Symptoms, indirect
    or positive
Postmorbidity in personality assessment,
    150
Posttraumatic amnesia, 29
Premorbid conditions
  intelligence, recovery and, 299
  personality
    clinical manifestations, 61–62
    research, related, 62–64, 64t
    symptoms and, 61–64, 64t
    in personality assessment, 149–150
  symptom picture and, 53–61
  symptoms and
    cultural milieu, 61
    psychosocial setting, 60–61
Pribram, Karl, 20–21
"Primary process thinking," 126
Problem solving, 44
Productivity
  status, outcome and, 246–247, 247t
  symbol of work and, 208
Protected work trial, 187–189
Psychiatric disturbances
  etiological factors in, 64
  faulty learning patterns and, 132
Psychological development, biological
    brain changes and, 126
Psychology
  humanistic, 336
  scientific, strengths/weaknesses of, 336
Psychometric tests, 249
Psychosis, posttraumatic, 78
Psychosocial development stage, symp-
    toms and, 54–57
Psychotherapy, postinjury, 201–202
  adjustment to permanent impairments
    and, 254–256

analogies, 224–225
benefits of, 345
case examples, 215–216
clinical sensibility in, 202–203
cost-benefit ratio, 255
definition of, 204–205
efficacy, indirect measurement of, 254–
    255
emerging role of, 202–203
fairy tales in, 339–340, 345
family members
  practical considerations for, 223–224
  recurring issues for, 219–223
focus of, 218
function of, 205–206
goal of, 219
"hero's journey," 213–214, 258
limitations of, 216–219
practical considerations for, 218–219
in rehabilitation, 183, 185–186
strengths of, 215–216
supportive, 206
therapeutic alliance in. *See* Therapeutic
    alliance

RAVLT (Rey Auditory Verbal Learning
    Test), 295–297, 297t
Reactionary problems, 133
Recovery
  adaptation model
    description of, 304, 303f
    observations on, 315–316
  cognitive disorders and, 96–97
    partial, of direct symptom with de-
      terioration/remediation of indi-
      rect symptom, 321–322
    rate/completion of, 16
    retraining/reorganization, observa-
      tions on, 310–311
    spontaneous, 301–302, 305–307, 308–
      309t, 303f, 310f
  compensations, naturally occurring, 6–
    7, 302, 303f, 307–310
  of function
    age and, 296–297, 299
    definition of, 294–300, 298t, 300t–
      301t
    higher cerebral, 298
  of higher cerebral functions, influenc-
    ing factors, 300t–301t
  historical aspects, 8
  mechanisms of change and, 325–327
  models, 301–302, 304, 303f
  partial, 318–321, 319f, 320f
Reeducation after brain injury, 8
Referrals, 74

Symptoms *(continued)*
  direct or negative
    definition of, 52–53
    delayed deterioration of, 322–323,
      323*t*
    and indirect, delayed deterioration
      of, 323–325
    partial recovery with deterioration
      of indirect symptom, 318–321,
      319*f*, 320*f*
  indirect or positive
    definition of, 53
    delayed deterioration, with delayed
      direct of, 323–325
  lesion location and, 13
  location of brain injury and, 56
  neurobiological approach, 49
  premorbid condition and, 64–65
    age, 54–55
    cultural milieu, 61
    education, 57–58, 57*f*
    intellectual level and, 58–60
    psychosocial development stage
      and, 54–57
    psychosocial setting, 60–61
  psychosocial approach, 49
  severity, brain injury severity and,
    63
  size of brain injury and, 56
  type of brain injury and, 56

Tactual Performance Test, 59
TBI. *See* Traumatic brain injury
Teaching process, 89
Temper, control of, 320, 320*f*
Temporal lobe, heteromodal disorders,
  283, 285*t*
Temporal-occipital cortex infarction, MRI
  of, 35–36, 36*f*
Tension release in brain-injured patients,
  34, 170
Thalamic-cingulate connections, disruption
  of, 140
Therapeutic alliance
  establishing, 204
  guidance and, 209, 217
  outcome and, 246
Therapeutic milieu, 180–181, 194–195
Therapeutic relationship, information re-
  vealed in, 139–140

Therapist
  barriers to entering patient's phenome-
    nological field, 38–40
  dealing with frustration/confusion of
    patient, 32–37, 36*f*
  outcomes and, 241
  psychological resources, drain on, 39
  time constraints of, 39
Tower of London Test, 54
Training, of clinical neuropsychologists,
  338–339
Traumatic brain injury (TBI)
  depression after, symptoms of, 135–137
  experience of, 29–30
  indirect effect, of depression, 135, 136*f*,
    137*t*
  premorbid personality and, 61–64, 64*t*
  speed of information processing after,
    97, 100, 98*t*–99*t*
Treatment outcome. *See* Outcome, treatment

Unilateral lesions, bilateral cerebral dysfunction and, 334
Unimodal cortex, 282–283

Verbal control, 217
Vocational rehabilitation, rehabilitation
  team and, 74

"Wake-up call," brain injury as, 218
Wall chart, 192–193
Wechsler Adult Intelligence Scale Perfor-
  mance-R, Performance IQ, 97
Weinstein, Edwin A., 19–20, 171–172
Well-being, sense of, daily stressors and,
  235
Well chart for Cognitive Group Therapy,
  183, 184*f*
Word choice in personality assessment, 150
Work
  inability, 247, 248*t*
  return to after TBI, 79–80
  symbols of
    adapting to brain injury condition,
      336
    description of, 208–210, 208*f*
Work trial, protected, 187–189, 195

Young brain-injured adult, rehabilitation
  of, Holistic rehabilitation, for
  young brain–injured adult